Clinical Gynecologic Oncology Review

Clinical Gynecologic Oncology Review

Third Edition

TUNG VAN DINH, M.D.
William Osler Scholar in the J. P. McGovern Academy of Oslerian Medicine
Professor of Obstetrics and Gynecology
Professor of Pathology
Division of Gynecologic Oncology
Department of Obstetrics and Gynecology
The University of Texas Medical Branch at Galveston
Galveston, Texas

EDWARD V. HANNIGAN, M.D.
Frances Eastland Connally Professor in Gynecologic Oncology
Director of the Division of Gynecologic Oncology
Associate Vice-Chairman of the Department of Obstetrics and Gynecology
Professor of Radiation Therapy
Chief of Staff, UTMB Hospitals
The University of Texas Medical Branch at Galveston
Galveston, Texas

MARK G. DOHERTY, M.D.
Texas Oncology, P.A.
Sammons Cancer Center
Baylor University Medical Center
Methodist Medical Center
Dallas, Texas

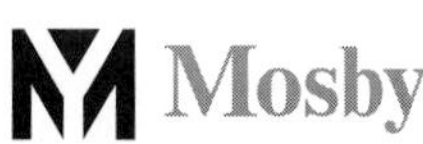

An Affiliate of Elsevier Science
St. Louis Philadelphia London Toronto Sydney

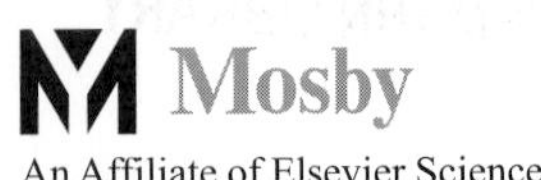

An Affiliate of Elsevier Science

11830 Westline Drive
St. Louis, Missouri 63146

CLINICAL GYNECOLOGIC ONCOLOGY REVIEW ISBN 0–323–01621–9

Notice

Obstetrics and Gynecology is an ever-changing field. Standard safety precautions must be followed, but as new research and clinical experience broaden our knowledge, changes in treatment and drug therapy may become necessary or appropriate. Readers are advised to check the most current product information provided by the manufacturer of each drug to be administered to verify the recommended dose, the method and duration of administration, and contraindications. It is the responsibility of the treating physician, relying on experience and knowledge of the patient, to determine dosages and the best treatment for each individual patient. Neither the Publisher nor the editor assumes any liability for any injury and/or damage to persons or property arising from this publication.

The Publisher

First Edition 1993. Second Edition 1998.

Library of Congress Cataloging-in-Publication Data
Dinh, Tung Van
Clinical gynecologic oncology review / Tung Van Dinh, Edward V. Hannigan, Mark G. Doherty—3rd ed.
p. ;cm.
Complements: Clinical gynecologic oncology / Philip J. DiSaia, William T. Creasman. 6th ed. c2002.
ISBN 0–323–01621–9
1. Generative organs, Female—Cancer—Examinations, questions, etc. I. Hannigan, Edward V. II. Doherty, Mark G. III. DiSaia, Philip J. Clinical gynecologic oncology. IV. Title.
[DNLM: 1. Genital Neoplasms, Female—Examination Questions. WP 145 D611c 2002 Suppl. 2003]
RC280.G5 D46 2002 Suppl.
616.99′465′0076—dc21 2002071927

Acquisitions Editor: Judy Fletcher
Developmental Editor: Heather Krehling
Project Manager: Lee Ann Draud
Designer: Steven Stave

KI/MVY

Printed in the United States of America.

Last digit is the print number: 9 8 7 6 5 4 3 2 1

This book is dedicated to our wives and children

Tonia and Tuan, Tue, Tri, and Tho
Mary and Casey, Patrick, and Brendan
Blanca and Robert, little Blanca, Colin, and Morgan
for their love and support

FOREWORD

In *Clinical Gynecologic Oncology Review*, 3rd edition, Drs. Dinh, Hannigan, and Doherty provide a wonderful tool that reinforces many of the basic principles of gynecologic oncology discussed in our textbook, *Clinical Gynecologic Oncology*, sixth edition. Their orderly presentation follows formats that are popular on many standardized examinations, affording a "practice" facet to the use of the review book. Some questions elicit recall primarily, whereas many others require interpretation and/or problem solving. Recall items typically test the examinee's knowledge of definitions or isolated facts (e.g., details of human anatomy). Interpretation items require the student to review some information, in tabular or graphic form, and reach a conclusion (e.g., a diagnosis). Problem-solving items present a situation and require the examinee to take some action (e.g., the next step in patient management). All of these are important to solidify or refresh one's knowledge.

In the spirit of our textbook, the *Review* focuses almost exclusively on clinically relevant situations. We congratulate the authors and are pleased to have their assistance in the mission of teaching, which we hold dear to our hearts.

Philip J. DiSaia, M.D.
William T. Creasman, M.D.

PREFACE

The third edition of *Clinical Gynecologic Oncology Review* has been written to complement the sixth edition of *Clinical Gynecologic Oncology*, by Philip J. DiSaia and William T. Creasman. The purpose of the review book is to emphasize the main ideas without altering the philosophy of the text's original authors. Its intended audience is practicing physicians, residents, and students interested in gynecologic oncology. It can be used to identify areas of weakness, to reinforce new information, or to reassure oneself that the subject matter is understood.

In this third edition, the section "Key Points to Remember" has been revised and expanded. All questions have been reviewed, and questions have been written to cover the new material. The questions are written in simple format—best answer and matching questions. An Answer section refers the reader to specific pages in *Clinical Gynecologic Oncology*, 6th edition, with a rationale for each answer. We recommend that the reader read a chapter of the textbook, then read the Key Points in this book, and answer all questions from the chapter before verifying the answers. To reinforce the material, read all comments and refer to the textbook.

We wish to thank Drs. Philip J. DiSaia and William T. Creasman for giving us again the honor of writing this third edition, Mrs. Judith Fletcher from Elsevier Science for her patience and invaluable editorial assistance, and Ms. Lee Ann Draud for her help in producing this book.

Thanks are also due to our secretary, Mrs. Marsha Corona, for her hard work on the manuscript.

Tung Van Dinh
Edward V. Hannigan
Mark G. Doherty

CONTENTS

chapter 1

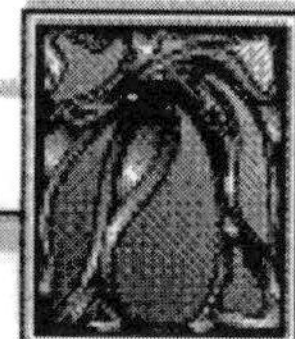

PREINVASIVE DISEASE of the CERVIX

Key Points to Remember

- The mean age of patients with carcinoma in situ is 15.6 years younger than that of patients with invasive squamous cell carcinoma of cervix.
- All women who are or have been sexually active, or who have reached age 18, should undergo an annual Pap and pelvic examination. After three negative findings, the Pap smear may be performed less frequently.
- In the United States, death rates from cervical cancer have dropped from number 1 to number 12 among all cancers in women. In 2000, 12,800 new cervical and 4600 deaths will occur. Approximately 600,000 women are identified with cervical intraepithelial neoplasia (CIN) per year.
- Worldwide, it is estimated that 500,000 cervical cancers will be diagnosed, and half of these patients will die.
- A large number of older women (average age 65) are not being screened with cervical cytology. Screening of the patient older than 65 years of age results in a 63% improvement of 5-year mortality. Pap smear screening should continue for a lifetime. There is a high false-negative Pap smear rate in the United States.
- Ostor noted that in CIN I, 60% will regress and only 10% will progress to carcinoma in situ. One third of CIN III will regress to normal. Melnikow found that progression to cancer was 0.25% with ASCUS (atypical squamous cells of undetermined significance), 0.15% with LSIL (low-grade squamous intraepithelial lesion), and 1.44% with HSIL (high-grade intraepithelial lesion). Regression to normal occurred in 68% of ASCUS, 47% LSIL, and 35% HSIL.
- Annual Pap smear testing reduces a woman's chance of dying of cervical cancer from 4/1000 to about 5/10,000, a difference of almost 90%.
- Factors associated with the development of cervical cancer are low socioeconomic status, early first coitus, multiple sexual partners, high-risk sexual partners, and smoking.
- Human papilloma virus (HPV) has been found to be associated with cervical neoplasia. Eighty-five percent of all cervical cancers contain high-risk HPV sequences (16, 18, 31, 33, 35, etc.). Integration of HPV DNA into the human genome occurs in the E_1–E_2 region. E_6 and E_7 genes are expressed in HPV-positive cervical cancer. E_6 causes rapid degradation of *P53*; E_7 inactivates *PRB*.
- Transmittal of HPV DNA appears to be sexual, but nonsexual transfer is not rare. The prevalence and incidence of HPV DNA appear to vary greatly, depending on age, sexual activity, the number of times tested, and the laboratory technique used.
- The use of routine screening using HPV DNA probes and of HPV DNA typing in patients with ASCUS or LSIL does not appear to be clinically indicated and is not cost-effective at the present time. The virus cannot be eliminated with any known therapy.
- Case definition of AIDS includes HIV-positive women with invasive cervical cancer. HIV-positive women have a higher incidence of CIN, the treatment of which has a high failure rate. All HIV-positive women should have a Pap smear every 6 months. Recurrences of CIN are associated with CD4 and T-lymphocyte counts, but not with a grade of CIN. HIV-positive women have more advanced cervical cancer with a poor prognosis.
- CIN I progresses to cancer only 1% of the time; CIN III progresses to cancer 15% of the time. The mean age for CIN III is 28 years old. The mean transition time from normal to CIN III is 4.5 years. No method is available to predict which CIN will progress to invasive cancer.
- ACOG Committee opinion noted that the new diagnostic technology (Thin Prep, Papnet) increases the cost and the number of patients with LSIL and is not currently the standard of care.
- ASCUS and SIL on Pap smears should have histologic confirmation of CIN before treatment. A diagnosis of ASCUS should be no more than 5% of Pap findings.
- ECC should be performed on all patients undergoing colposcopy, unless they are pregnant.
- Colposcopy only suggests an abnormality; final diagnosis should be based on histologic diagnosis.
- Management of ASCUS Pap smears: repeat Pap smear every 4–6 months. If second ASCUS: colposcopy. ASCUS favoring a neoplastic process requires colposcopy. HPV typing may be helpful.
- Management of LSIL Pap smears: either repeat Pap smear or colposcopy.
- Management of HSIL Pap smears: colposcopy.
- AGUS is a misnomer. It detects more squamous lesions (36% CIN) than glandular lesion (6%). Management of AGUS Pap smears consists of colposcopy on all patients plus endometrial biopsy on those older than 35 years old.
- Fifty percent or more of adenocarcinoma in situ of cervix (ACIS) are seen with squamous CIN. Ninety-five percent occur at the squamocolumnar junction. Cold knife conization with free margins may be adequate therapy

for ACIS. Hysterectomy is suggested for patients not interested in fertility.

- Diagnostic conization must be performed when the ECC findings are positive or when the upper limits of the lesion cannot be visualized. Cone biopsy is rarely indicated in pregnancy. Pregnant patients with preinvasive or microinvasive disease of cervix should be allowed to deliver vaginally.
- Cryotherapy has a total failure rate of 8%. Compared with cryotherapy, laser treatment for CIN is more painful and expensive for the patient and more time-consuming for the physician and patient. Therapeutic results are equivalent.
- LEEP should not be performed on patients with ASCUS or LSIL cytology without colposcopy. Complications of LEEP are cervical stenosis (1%) and bleeding (5%).
- Post-cone patients should be followed up with cytology only, irrespective of surgical margins. Patients treated with hysterectomy for CIN should be followed indefinitely.

QUESTIONS

Directions for Questions 1–40: Select the one best answer.

1. Patients with carcinoma in situ of the cervix are younger than patients with invasive squamous cell carcinoma by an average of:
   A. 5 years
   B. 10 years
   C. 15 years
   D. 20 years
2. Recommendations for optimal screening interval to reduce the mortality of cancer of cervix are the following *except:*
   A. all women who are, or who have been, sexually active should have a yearly Pap smear
   B. all women who have reached age 18 should undergo an annual Pap test
   C. after two negative Pap smears, the high-risk woman should be screened every 2 years
   D. after three negative Pap smears, cervical screening may be performed less frequently at the discretion of the physician
3. Reasons found at the Connecticut study (1985–1990) that cervical cancer was not detected before it became invasive are the following *except:*
   A. one fourth of patients never had a Pap smear and one fourth had a Pap smear only 5 years before the diagnosis of cancer
   B. a large number of older women were not screened
   C. all patients had complete evaluation of abnormal Pap smears
   D. one fifth of normal Pap smears re-read after cancer diagnosis were abnormal
4. The following are true concerning cervical cancer in older patients *except:*
   A. the older patient is at increased risk for cervical cancer
   B. increasing age is associated with more advanced disease
   C. age has an effect on disease-free survival
   D. Pap smear screening should continue for a lifetime
5. The minimum transit time from carcinoma in situ to invasive cancer of the cervix is said to be:
   A. 2 years
   B. 4 years
   C. 8 years
   D. 10 years
6. Annual Pap smear testing reduces a woman's chance of dying of cervical cancer by:
   A. 30%
   B. 50%
   C. 75%
   D. 90%
7. Factors associated with an increased occurrence of carcinoma of cervix are the following *except:*
   A. first coitus at an early age and multiple sexual partners
   B. smoking
   C. husband with more than 20 sexual partners
   D. alcohol and drug abuse
8. Mature HPV (human papilloma virus) particles are found in nuclei of koilocytotic cells that are located:
   A. in the stroma of the cervix
   B. in the endocervix
   C. in the basal layers of the squamous epithelium
   D. in the superficial layers of the squamous epithelium
9. Types of HPV most commonly associated with genital condylomata:
   A. 6/11
   B. 16/18
   C. 31/33
   D. 39/45
10. HPV viral factors necessary for immortalization of human genital epithelial cells are:
   A. E_1 and E_2
   B. E_2 and E_4
   C. E_5 and E_6
   D. E_6 and E_7
11. Types of HPV most commonly affected with carcinoma of cervix:
   A. 6/11
   B. 16/18
   C. 31/33
   D. 45/51
12. The following are true concerning HPV and neoplasia of the cervix *except:*
   A. there is no epidemiologic study that demonstrates HPV causes cancer
   B. routine screening for HPV does not appear to be appropriate at the present time
   C. HPV can be eliminated with laser therapy
   D. treatment of the male partner does not significantly improve treatment outcome
13. The mean transition time from normal to carcinoma in situ of the cervix is:
   A. 2 years
   B. 3 years
   C. 4.5 years
   D. 6.5 years

14. Recommendations of the Bethesda System in 1988 for cervicovaginal cytology consist of the following *except:*
    A. a statement on adequacy of the specimen
    B. report of infections and cell atypias
    C. report of low-grade squamous intraepithelial lesions (SIL) comprising HPV changes and CIN I, and high-grade SIL comprising CIN II and CIN III
    D. report of Papanicolaou classes
15. Concerns expressed by DiSaia and Creasman on the Bethesda System include:
    A. koilocytosis is a descriptive term and not diagnostic. Colposcopy of all Pap smears with koilocytosis results in overtreatment and increased costs.
    B. separation of LSIL and HSIL represents a splitting of cells
    C. increased confusion with the designation of ASCUS and LSIL
    D. all of the above
16. The following are *not* true concerning Pap smears *except:*
    A. it is a diagnostic tool
    B. one can treat a patient for CIN based solely on the Pap smear result
    C. Pap smears can always be used to identify malignancies of uterus, tubes, and ovaries
    D. it is valid for screening only
17. CDC recommendations for HIV-positive women are to have a Pap smear every:
    A. 3 months
    B. 6 months
    C. 9 months
    D. year after two negative Pap smears
18. Indication for follow-up of a Pap smear with atypical glandular cells of undetermined significance (AGUS) suspicious of adenocarcinoma in situ consists of:
    A. repeating Pap smear
    B. colposcopy, biopsy, and endocervical curettage
    C. B plus conization
    D. hysterectomy
19. Abnormal patterns recognized with colposcopy are the following *except:*
    A. leukoplakia
    B. acetowhite epithelium
    C. punctation and mosaicism
    D. atypical vessels
20. The normal physiologic transformation zone is most active during which period(s) of a woman's life?
    A. fetal development
    B. adolescence
    C. first pregnancy
    D. all of the above
21. Indications for conization of cervix include:
    A. inadequate colposcopy or positive endocervical curettage results
    B. microinvasive disease or adenocarcinoma in situ on biopsy
    C. great discrepancy between cytologic and histologic findings
    D. all of the above
22. A specimen from colposcopically directed biopsy of the cervix shows early invasive carcinoma. What is the next step of management?
    A. repeat biopsy
    B. conization of cervix
    C. endocervical curettage
    D. total abdominal hysterectomy
23. A colposcopy is unsatisfactory because the entire transformation zone cannot be visualized. The endocervical curettage result is negative for dysplasia and the biopsy sample reveals CIN III. One should:
    A. repeat endocervical curettage
    B. repeat colposcopy and biopsy
    C. perform conization of cervix
    D. perform total abdominal hysterectomy
24. Pap smear results suggest invasive disease. The colposcopy is adequate. Biopsy specimen shows CIN III. Endocervical curettage is negative for dysplasia. Recommended therapy for this patient is:
    A. repeat ECC
    B. repeat biopsy
    C. conization of cervix
    D. total abdominal hysterectomy
25. A 34-week pregnant patient has a Pap smear result suggestive of CIN III. Colposcopy is adequate and shows a small area of coarse punctation on the anterior cervix. Appropriate therapy may include:
    A. small biopsy
    B. biopsy and endocervical curettage
    C. conization of cervix
    D. cesarean section followed with simple hysterectomy
26. Decisions about the choice of therapy for cervical intraepithelial neoplasia (CIN) depend on the following factors *except:*
    A. age of patient and desire for fertility
    B. experiences of the physician
    C. reliability for follow-up
    D. histologic grade of the lesion
27. Management of cervical intraepithelial neoplasia includes:
    A. loop electrosurgical excision, cryosurgery
    B. laser vaporization
    C. conization
    D. all of the above
28. Based on a single treatment, the lowest rate of failure occurs in which method of treatment of CIN?
    A. electrocoagulation
    B. cryosurgery
    C. laser
    D. loop electrosurgical procedure
29. The following are true concerning laser vaporization of the cervix *except:*
    A. successful treatment is not related to the severity of the histologic grade
    B. an intermittent beam gives better results than a continuous beam
    C. destruction should attain a depth of 5 to 7 mm
    D. pain and bleeding can be a problem
30. Major complications of conization of the cervix include the following *except:*
    A. hemorrhage

B. cervical stenosis
C. infertility
D. increased risk of adenocarcinoma of cervix

31. Hysterectomy is a common treatment for CIN. The following are true *except:*
A. the recurrence rate after hysterectomy is less than the recurrence rate after conization
B. removing a vaginal "cuff" of upper vagina at the time of hysterectomy does not decrease the recurrence rate
C. the abdominal approach is preferable to a vaginal hysterectomy
D. the ovaries need not be removed to treat CIN

32. Metaplastic transformation of the cervical transformation zone from columnar to squamous epithelium:
A. probably occurs throughout a woman's life
B. is probably unrelated to estrogen or progesterone levels
C. is hastened by an alkaline vaginal pH
D. is probably quiescent during fetal life and pregnancy

33. Advantages of loop electrosurgical excision procedure (LEEP) include the following *except:*
A. the procedure can be done on an outpatient basis
B. tissue is available for study
C. diagnosis and therapy are all done at one time and at the same visit
D. there is no hemorrhage

34. Percentage of LEEP specimens showing no abnormalities is:
A. 10%–15%
B. 15%–29%
C. 15%–25%
D. 25%–50%

35. How many patients are identified with CIN per year in the United States?
A. 100,000
B. 300,000
C. 500,000
D. 600,000

36. It is estimated that in 2000 there were how many new cases of cancer of the cervix and how many deaths?
A. 10,000 cases and 5,000 deaths
B. 12,800 cases and 4,600 deaths
C. 18,000 cases and 6,000 deaths
D. 25,000 cases and 10,000 deaths

37. The most likely reason to account for the fact that CIN is being detected in females of younger and younger age groups is:
A. sexual activity at much earlier ages
B. improved screening for CIN in younger age groups
C. increased prevalence of tobacco use in younger age groups
D. increased prevalence of HPV in younger age groups

38. The definition of the cervical transformation zone is:
A. the squamocolumnar junction
B. the endocervix
C. the portio vaginalis
D. parts of the cervical epithelium undergoing or having undergone squamous metaplasia

39. According to Ostor, the percentage of regression of CIN I and CIN III to normal is:
A. 50% and 50%
B. 60% and 33%
C. 10% and 30%
D. 25% and 25%

40. The ACOG Committee opinion suggested that the new techniques (Thin Prep and Papnet) are:
A. important because they can lower the incidence of invasive cancer and increase survival
B. not expensive compared to the value of increased life expectancy
C. better in detecting CIN and carcinoma
D. problematic with the higher cost and the increased number of LSIL

Directions for Questions 41–57: For each numbered item, select the letter of the most appropriate answer. Each letter may be used once, more than once, or not at all.

41–45. Treatment modalities for cervical intraepithelial neoplasia:
A. cryosurgery
B. laser vaporization
C. both
D. neither

41. Less expensive
42. Outpatient treatment
43. Bleeding
44. Vaginal discharge after treatment
45. Specimen for histologic evaluation

46–52. Concerning cervical intraepithelial neoplasia (CIN):
A. CIN I
B. CIN III
C. both
D. neither

46. Undifferentiated cells cover the entire epithelial thickness
47. More frequently harbors HPV 6/11
48. Cryotherapy
49. Hysterectomy
50. Radiation
51. Radical hysterectomy
52. Undifferentiated cells cover the lower third of the epithelium

53–57. In Figure 1–1*A* and *B*, match the lesions (letters) with the appropriate management (numbers):
A. a lesion seen at colposcopy
B. histology of a cervical lesion
C. both
D. neither

53. Radical hysterectomy
54. Simple hysterectomy
55. Biopsy for diagnosis
56. Subtotal hysterectomy
57. Conization for treatment

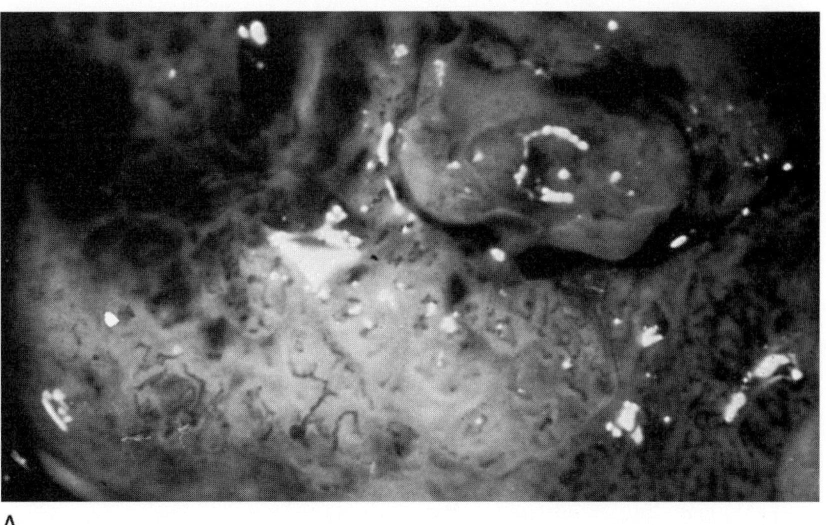

A

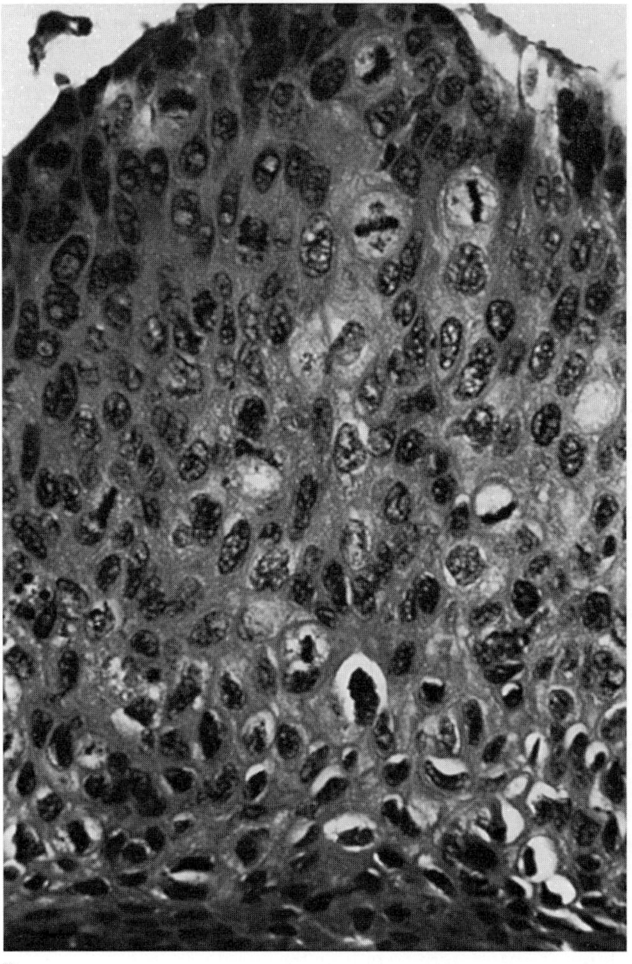

B

FIGURE 1–1. (Courtesy Dr. Kenneth Hatch, Birmingham, Alabama.)

ANSWERS

1. **C** page 1
   According to data from the Third National Cancer Survey, the mean age of patients with carcinoma in situ was 15.6 years younger than that of patients with invasive squamous cell carcinoma of the cervix. This difference is greater than previously observed (10 years).
2. **C** page 2
   A high-risk patient (early intercourse, multiple sexual partners) should be screened every year. The above

recommendations formulated by the American College of Obstetricians and Gynecologists and the American Cancer Society are reasonable for decreasing the incidence and death rate from cervical cancer and for detecting a larger number of women with preinvasive neoplasia. Note also that there is a high false-negative Pap smear rate (10% to 20%).

3. **C** page 2
About 10% of women in the Connecticut study had incomplete evaluation of abnormal Pap smears. Many physicians do not comply with existing cancer screening guidelines. It is estimated that about 11 million white women aged 65 or older in the United States did not have a Pap smear in the past year. Adenocarcinomas were seen about twice as often in women who developed cancer within 3 years of a negative Pap smear.
4. **C** page 2
When stratified by stage of disease, there is no effect of age on disease-free interval. Screening of patients older than 65 years of age would benefit most with a 63% improvement of 5-year mortality. Data from the 1992 National Health Interview Survey indicated that one half of women older than 60 years of age did not have a Pap smear during the last 3 years.
5. **C** page 3
Although transit time from carcinoma in situ to invasive cancer is said to require 8, 10, or possibly 20 years, some patients make this transition in a short time. Remember that cervical intraepithelial neoplasia (CIN) does not necessarily progress in an orderly fashion to invasive cancer; an earlier CIN lesion can progress directly to invasive cancer. Masterson found that 28% of 25 untreated patients demonstrated invasive carcinoma at the end of 5 years.
6. **D** page 4
Annual testing reduces a woman's chance of dying of cervical cancer from 4/1000 to 5/10,000, a 90% difference. It also reduces the cost of treatment because treating a preinvasive or early invasive disease is considerably less expensive than treating a late invasive disease.
7. **D** page 4
Alcohol and drug abuse have no relationship to the occurrence of carcinoma of the cervix. However, it is noted that women who are HIV positive may be at high risk for CIN.
8. **D** page 5
A koilocyte is a superficial squamous cell with cytoplasmic perinuclear cavitation and a degenerated irregular, hyperchromatic nucleus. HPV antigen has been demonstrated in the nucleus by immunoperoxidase technique. HPV DNA also has been elucidated using molecular hybridization. The koilocyte is the histologic hallmark of HPV infection.
9. **A** page 5
Nearly 70 types of HPV have been identified. Types 6/11 are associated with genital condylomata and the minor CIN groups. When HPV 6/11 are found with CIN, the regression rate is high.
10. **D** page 6
E_6 binds with *P53* to prevent *P53* normal function of responding to DNA damage induced by radiation or chemical mutagen. E_7 binds to *PRB* (retinoblastoma susceptibility gene) to inactivate *PRB* and push the cell cycle into S-phase and induce DNA synthesis.
11. **B** page 6
Although types 6/11, 31/33/35, 39/45/51, and 52/56/58 of HPV have been identified in carcinoma of the cervix, HPV 16/18 are most often found. More than 85% of all cervical cancers contain high-risk HPV sequences.
12. **C** page 9
At present, there is no known therapy that can totally eliminate HPV. As a result, there is probably no benefit to know HPV subtypes for clinical management. Neither treatment of sexual male consorts nor sexual abstinence significantly improves treatment outcome of the female patient, according to studies by Campion and Riva. Also, according to some investigators, HPV DNA is ubiquitous and endemic.
13. **C** page 12, Table 1–3
The transition time from normal to carcinoma in situ of the cervix is 4.51 years; the transition time from normal to CIN I–II is 1.62 years. Carcinoma in situ of the cervix is usually asymptomatic. The lesion is frequently not observed grossly. Recognition of the lesion is assisted by cytology and colposcopy. The diagnosis must be confirmed by histology.
14. **D** page 11
The Papanicolaou classification has been changed so many times that the numbers have no constant meaning. The Bethesda system in 1988 is an attempt to clarify the varied terminology.
15. **D** page 13
DiSaia and Creasman think that CIN is a neoplastic continuum and there should not be a two-tier designation of SIL. The cervical epithelium is only 0.25 mm thick; separation of LSIL and HSIL represents a splitting of cells. Managing koilocytosis in the same way as CIN I results in overtreatment and increased cost.
16. **D** page 14
The Pap smear is not a diagnostic tool; it is only a screening mechanism. Diagnosis rests with a tissue biopsy. The Pap test must be performed with care by sampling the transformation zone to yield optimal accuracy. Evaluation of an abnormal Pap smear includes colposcopy, biopsy, and endocervical curettage (ECC). The false-negative rate is thought to be 10% to 20% for CIN, up to 40% for invasive cervical cancer, and less sensitive for upper genital neoplasms.
17. **D** page 10
CDC recommends that all HIV-positive women have a Pap smear. If normal, repeat in 6 months, then yearly if the Pap is normal. Pap smear with severe inflammation should be repeated in 3 months, and Pap smear with ASCUS or SIL should be further evaluated with colposcopy. False-negative Pap smear rate is 10% to 19%. Treatment of CIN in HIV-positive patients has a high failure rate.

18. **C** page 18
Colposcopy, biopsy, and ECC should be done to detect invasive disease. If histology shows only adenocarcinoma in situ, conization is the diagnostic technique of choice. Conization of the cervix may be adequate therapy for adenocarcinoma in situ if surgical margins are free. For patients more than 35 years old, an endometrial biopsy is suggested.
19. **A** page 21
Leukoplakia is a heavy, thick, white lesion seen with the naked eye. A biopsy should be performed to identify the tissue lesion under the hyperkeratotic layer. Acetowhite epithelium, punctation, and mosaicism denote CIN; a biopsy should also be performed on these. Atypical vessels are often associated with invasive cancer. Abnormal colposcopic patterns are not specific enough for final diagnosis; biopsy is necessary for histologic diagnosis.
20. **D** page 20
The normal physiologic transformation zone is most active during fetal development, adolescence, and first pregnancy. The process is enhanced by an acid pH and influenced by estrogen and progesterone levels.
21. **D** page 22
The goal of evaluating a patient with abnormal Pap smear is to rule out invasive cancer. All the above findings are incomplete for confidently eliminating invasive disease. A conization should be performed to enable the pathologist to look at the entire transformation zone.
22. **B** page 22
Conization of the cervix should be performed to evaluate the extent of the invasion. Further treatment varies depending on the depth of invasion, i.e., microinvasive or frankly invasive cancer.
23. **C** page 22
Conization of the cervix should be performed because the transformation zone or the lesion cannot be visualized entirely (unsatisfactory colposcopy). The procedure is done to rule out occult invasive disease.
24. **C** page 22
Biopsy and endocervical curettage results do not explain the Pap smear that shows invasive disease. Conization is indicated to rule out invasive carcinoma.
25. **A** page 23
A small biopsy of the most abnormal area could be performed for diagnosis. Endocervical curettage should not be done during pregnancy. If there is no invasion, the patient is allowed to deliver vaginally. Some experienced colposcopists prefer to defer all biopsies to the postpartum period because the cervix is very vascular during pregnancy. Regression of 68% to 78% was noted postpartum in pregnant women with CIN II and CIN III, respectively. Regression rates did not depend on the type of delivery.
26. **D** page 23
Except for microinvasive and invasive cancers, which are treated differently, CIN is considered a continuum of the disease and treated with different modalities irrespective of the histologic grade. The other cited factors should be included in the choice of therapy.
27. **D** page 24
Besides the above modalities, local excision, electrocoagulation, and hysterectomy can be used effectively for the treatment of CIN.
28. **A** page 24, Table 1–9
Based on a single treatment, electrocoagulation, reported by Chanen and Rome, has the lowest failure rate (2.7%). However, this treatment modality requires hospitalization and general anesthesia.
29. **B** page 26
A continuous laser beam gives better results than an intermittent beam. It is also necessary to avoid the use of flammable agents and to use nonreflective surfaces.
30. **D** page 29, Table 1–13
There is no increase in adenocarcinoma of cervix in patients with conization. Other major complications include uterine perforation, incompetent cervix, rupture of membranes, and increased preterm delivery.
31. **C** page 29, Table 1–15
Vaginal hysterectomy is a common and effective treatment for CIN in a patient who desires permanent sterilization. The removal of additional vaginal tissue is unnecessary unless vaginal extension of intraepithelial neoplasia has been identified colposcopically. After conization, Kolstad and Klem noted a 2.9% recurrence rate of CIS and a 0.9% incidence of subsequent invasive cancer. Corresponding figures for patients after hysterectomy were 1.2% and 2.1%. Boyes et al. noted a 6.3% of persistence CIS and 0.6% recurrence of cancer in patients treated with conization vs. 0.9% and 0.3% in patients treated with hysterectomy. Although the chance of subsequent recurrence of invasive disease is small, it can occur. Patients treated with hysterectomy must be observed indefinitely.
32. **A** page 20
The process of transition from columnar to squamous epithelium probably occurs throughout a woman's lifetime. However, it has been demonstrated that this process is most active during three periods of a woman's life: fetal development, adolescence, and first pregnancy. It is known that the process is enhanced by an acid pH environment and is considerably influenced by estrogen and progesterone levels.
33. **D** page 28
Secondary hemorrhage occurs in 1% to 10% of patients according to the experience of the surgeon.
34. **C** page 28
Fifteen percent to 25% of LEEP specimens have negative histology. The indiscriminate use of LEEP before colposcopy, or for evaluating ASCUS or LSIL Pap smears, should be avoided.
35. **D** page 2
It is estimated that as many as 600,000 women per year are identified with CIN in the United States, among whom 55,000 have CIN III. Screening has decreased the incidence and death rate from cervical cancer and also has identified a large number of women with preinvasive neoplasia.

36. **B** page 2
In 2000, the American Cancer Society estimated 12,800 new cervical cancer cases and 4600 deaths from cancer.
37. **B** page 11
Recent studies show that CIN is being diagnosed at a much younger age. In DiSaia and Creasman's material, the median age for CIS of the cervix has decreased approximately from 40 to 28 years of age. This may reflect that screening of high-risk patients is done at an earlier time, resulting in diagnosis at a younger age. Analysis of 800 CIN patients at Duke University Medical Center showed that 30% were 20 years of age or younger at the time the diagnosis was established.
38. **D** page 19
The transformation zone is that area of the cervix and vagina that was initially covered by columnar epithelium and through a process referred to as metaplasia has undergone replacement by squamous epithelium. Colposcopy is based on study of the transformation zone.
39. **B** page 3
Ostor noted that 60% of CIN I will regress and only 10% will progress to CIS. In patients with CIS, one third will regress to normal. Melnikow found that regression to normal occurred in 68% of ASCUS, 47% of LSIL and 35% of HSIL.
40. **D** pages 13–15
In most studies comparing Thin prep technique (TP) and conventional Pap (CP), there is only increase in the LSIL category, and no increase in HSIL category Pap smears. The reduction of benign biopsies and the increase in confirmed CIN I–III was not statistically significant, comparing TP to CP. The new technologies increase life expectancy by 5 hours to 1.6 days with an increased cost of $30 to $257. An ACOG Committee opinion noted that they currently are not standard of care.
41. **A** pages 24–26
42. **C** pages 24–26
43. **B** pages 24–26
44. **C** pages 24–26
45. **D** pages 24–26
Laser ablation and cryotherapy may be done as outpatient procedures. Cryotherapy is less expensive than laser ablation because of the cost of instruments. Patients will have vaginal discharge after either modality of treatment. After cryotherapy there may be discharge for as long as 6 weeks. The discharge after laser ablation is usually of shorter duration. Although patients may rarely bleed after cryosurgery, cervical bleeding is not uncommon during and after ablation with laser therapy because the destruction is deep. Neither method will provide tissue for histologic study.
46. **B** page 15
47. **A** page 15
48. **C** page 15
49. **B** page 15
50. **D** page 15
51. **D** page 15
52. **A** page 15
Depending on the presence of undifferentiated cells in the lower, middle, and upper third of the epithelium, the CIN is graded I, II, or III. Most CIN I lesions contain low-risk HPV viruses (6/11), whereas CIN III harbors high-risk HPV viruses (16/18). Both CIN I and CIN III can be treated with cryosurgery. A hysterectomy can be performed in a patient who has CIN III and has completed her family. Radiation is primarily used for invasive cancer. Radical hysterectomy is performed only in invasive cancer.
53. **D** Figure 1–9, page 22
54. **B** Figure 1–2, page 15
55. **A**
56. **D**
57. **B**
Figure 1–1*A* shows a colposcopic view of atypical vessels, which is indicative of invasive cancer. Figure 1–1*B* shows histology of CIN III. Lesion A requires histologic confirmation by biopsy. Radical hysterectomy is the treatment for invasive carcinoma of cervix. Total hysterectomy is a treatment of CIN III in patients who have completed their families. CIN III can be treated also with electrocautery, cryosurgery, laser vaporization, cold knife conization, or LEEP. Subtotal hysterectomy, which does not remove the cervix, is not an appropriate therapy for either lesion. Conization is a modality of treatment for CIN III but not for invasive cancer.

chapter 2 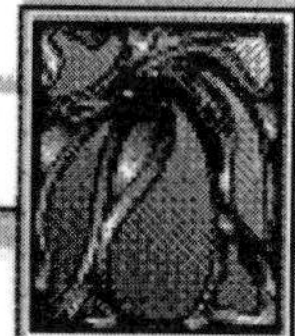

PREINVASIVE DISEASE of the VAGINA and VULVA and RELATED DISORDERS

Key Points to Remember

- For the year 2000, an estimated 2100 cases of cancer of vagina will be diagnosed.
- Patients with abnormal cytologic findings in the absence of cervix should be subjected to a thorough examination of the vaginal and vulvar epithelium.
- The upper third of the vagina is the portion most frequently involved by preinvasive disease.
- One to two percent of patients have vaginal recurrences after hysterectomy for a similar lesion in the cervix.
- Twenty-five percent of cases of post-irradiation dysplasia of vagina can progress to invasive disease if left untreated. VAIN tends to be multifocal; examination of the entire vagina should be done.
- Management of VAIN consists of local excision, topical 5-FU, and laser. Laser destruction of 1.0 to 1.5 mm of epithelium is safe. 5-FU or laser is used for multifocal lesions.
- Adenosis is more common in patients whose mothers took DES before the 18th week of gestation (60% have vaginal adenosis). Acquired vaginal adenosis can occur in patients after treatment of VAIN with laser or 5-FU. Vaginal adenosis has been observed in patients without a history of exposure to DES.
- Twenty percent of women exposed to DES show an anatomic deformity of the upper vagina and cervix: transverse vaginal and cervical ridge, cervical collar, vaginal hood, and cockscomb cervix.
- Follow-up of DES-exposed women consists of yearly examinations at age 14 or at menarche with examinations of vagina and cervix, careful digital palpation of vagina, and colposcopy, with biopsies if necessary.
- There is an increased incidence (15%) of CIN in women with in utero exposure to DES.
- There is no recommended treatment for vaginal adenosis at the present time if cytology results and examination are normal. Routine cytology should be continued for life.
- New classification of non-neoplastic intraepithelial disorders of vulva includes lichen sclerosus, squamous cell hyperplasia, and other dermatoses.
- Microscopic features of lichen sclerosus and squamous hyperplasia are characteristic.
- Treatment of lichen sclerosus consists of clobetasol or testosterone ointments. Treatment of squamous cell hyperplasia is steroid ointment.
- Squamous hyperplasia is associated with 27% to 35% of women with lichen sclerosus (LS). VIN was associated with 5% of LS. Only 4% of women with LS developed vulvar cancer.
- The average age of the patient with VIN is 50 years.
- The incidence of VIN has almost doubled to 2.1 per 100,000 women years in the last two decades.
- In the year 2000, 3400 women would be diagnosed with vulvar cancer and 800 women would die from it.
- VIN III is asymptomatic in 50% of cases; the predominant symptom is pruritus.
- HPV DNA type 16/18, 31, 33, 35 has been found in 80% to 90% of VIN but the incidence of HPV DNA in vulvar cancer decreases with age.
- Vulvar biopsy should be performed for diagnosis before treatment of VIN.
- Untreated VIN progresses rapidly to carcinoma in older or immunocompromised patients.
- Treatment of VIN includes local excision, skinning vulvectomy with skin graft procedure, or laser, which is usually reserved for multifocal extensive disease.
- Pain, bleeding, and infection are the complications of laser treatment of VIN, but cosmetic results appear excellent.
- Excision can rule out microinvasive disease. Recurrences are threefold higher when margins are positive for VIN II–III. Laser treatment has a high rate of success (94%) but requires multiple treatments.

Questions

Directions for Questions 1–22: Select the one best answer.

1. Characteristics of carcinoma in situ (CIS) of the vagina are the following *except*:
   A. it may develop as a primary lesion
   B. it may appear after irradiation therapy for carcinoma of the cervix
   C. it tends to be unifocal
   D. patients tend to have an antecedent or coexistent neoplasia of the lower genital tract
2. Frequent localization of CIS of the vagina is:
   A. upper third
   B. middle third
   C. lower third
   D. all of the above

3. The mainstay of therapy for CIS of the vagina is:
   A. laser vaporization
   B. large excision
   C. cryotherapy
   D. 5-FU topical application
4. Acquired vaginal adenosis
   A. should be considered premalignant
   B. is related to DES use after menarche
   C. is columnar epithelial metaplasia often seen after vaginal 5-FU therapy and laser therapy
   D. is not seen after laser therapy of vagina
5. In reference to laser therapy for VAIN,
   A. destruction to a 1- to 1.5-mm depth should not damage underlying structures
   B. this modality is most appropriate for multifocal lesions
   C. success rate is superior to that of 5-FU
   D. success rate is superior to that of local excision
6. Disruption of the transformation of columnar epithelium of müllerian origin to stratified squamous epithelium by administration of DES results in adenosis. This is present in the vagina in the following forms *except:*
   A. glandular cells lining the vagina
   B. glandular cells beneath the squamous lining
   C. glandular cells mixed with squamous metaplasia
   D. squamous and transitional epithelia
7. The administration of DES will not increase the incidence of adenosis after which week of pregnancy:
   A. 12th
   B. 14th
   C. 16th
   D. 18th
8. Anatomic deformities of the upper vagina and cervix observed in 20% of women exposed to DES include:
   A. transverse vaginal and cervical ridges
   B. cervical collar, vaginal hood
   C. cockscomb cervix, cervical pseudopolyp
   D. all of the above
9. True statements regarding the relationship of in utero DES exposure to later squamous disease include all *except:*
   A. no increased risk of squamous cell carcinoma has been noted
   B. no increased risk of squamous CIN has been noted
   C. more than one half of women exposed to DES will have vaginal adenosis
   D. no therapy is necessary for most patients exposed to DES
10. Observations and recommendations concerning the use of colposcopy in women exposed to DES include all *except:*
    A. physical examinations, cytologic monitoring, and colposcopic examinations should continue for life
    B. vascular mosaic and punctate patterns are commonly seen but are not usually associated with preinvasive or invasive potential
    C. careful digital palpation of the entire vagina combined with thorough cytologic and colposcopic examination are necessary parts of the initial evaluation of the woman exposed to DES
    D. the initial colposcopic evaluation should occur at 14 years of age
11. The following statements regarding the therapy of vaginal adenosis are false *except*:
    A. judicious use of cryotherapy should be considered for areas of the genital tract that have abnormal colposcopic appearance (e.g., punctation, mosaicism)
    B. acidifying jellies are recommended to speed the process of metaplasia and enhance squamous maturation
    C. in general, therapy of adenosis is not recommended
    D. laser therapy of areas of adenosis is an effective substitute for cryotherapy
12. True statements relative to VIN include all *except:*
    A. the frequency of VIN is increasing in younger women
    B. the risk of later invasive cancer is less than 20% and the disease is usually asymptomatic
    C. human papilloma viruses have been associated with development of VIN
    D. HPV subtyping is a recommended investigation to determine degree of risk
13. The following statements in regard to VIN are true *except:*
    A. the physical appearance of VIN is highly varied and depends on location and severity of disease
    B. VIN is graded based on degree of thickness of the epithelial abnormality (e.g., VIN I, VIN II, and VIN III)
    C. the behavior of VIN in regard to progression to more serious disorders is similar to that of CIN
    D. the term *Bowen's disease*, a synonym for VIN III, should no longer be used
14. The revised classification of non-neoplastic epithelial disorders of the vulva is composed of:
    A. hyperplastic dystrophy, lichen sclerosus, mixed dystrophies
    B. leukoplakia, hyperplastic dystrophy, and vulvar atypias
    C. squamous hyperplasia, lichen sclerosus, and other dermatoses
    D. squamous cell carcinoma in situ and Paget's disease of vulva
15. The following statements concerning vulvar squamous cell hyperplasia are false *except:*
    A. excision is treatment of choice
    B. usually involves only the labia majora
    C. microscopically appears as thinned epithelium
    D. if associated with VIN, it should be reported as VIN
16. The following statements in regard to lichen sclerosus are true *except:*
    A. clobetasol propionate is the new treatment of choice
    B. usually progresses to invasive malignancy if untreated
    C. the process often extends around the anal region
    D. a zone of subepithelial cellular collagen with underlying chronic inflammatory cells is seen microscopically

17. The predominant symptom of vulvar intraepithelial neoplasia (VIN) is:
    A. bleeding
    B. discharge
    C. pain
    D. pruritus
18. Types of HPV associated with squamous intraepithelial lesions of the vulva are:
    A. type 16/18
    B. type 31, 33, 35
    C. type 51
    D. all of the above
19. Intraepithelial neoplasia of the vulva is best called:
    A. bowenoid papulosis
    B. Bowen's disease
    C. erythroplasia of Queyrat
    D. VIN III
20. Accepted treatments for VIN III include:
    A. large excision
    B. laser surgery
    C. skinning vulvectomy and skin graft procedure
    D. all of the above
21. The main complication of vulvar laser surgery is:
    A. pain
    B. hemorrhage
    C. infection
    D. all of the above
22. The most likely location of this lesion (Fig. 2–1) of the vulva is:
    A. clitoris
    B. labium majus and labium minus
    C. perineum
    D. mons pubis

Directions for Questions 23–31: For each numbered item, select the letter of the most appropriate answer. Each letter may be used once, more than once, or not at all.

23–26. Match the different modalities of treatment of VAIN, their advantages, and inconveniences:
    A. surgical excision
    B. laser vaporization
    C. cryotherapy
    D. 5-FU topical applications
23. Tremendous local reaction with prolonged use
24. Rarely used, not very successful
25. Treatment of choice at the present time
26. Pain and bleeding, excellent healing, can destroy minute multifocal lesions

27–31. Match clinical presentation and treatment of non-neoplastic disorders of the vulva:
    A. lichen sclerosus
    B. squamous hyperplasia
    C. both
    D. neither

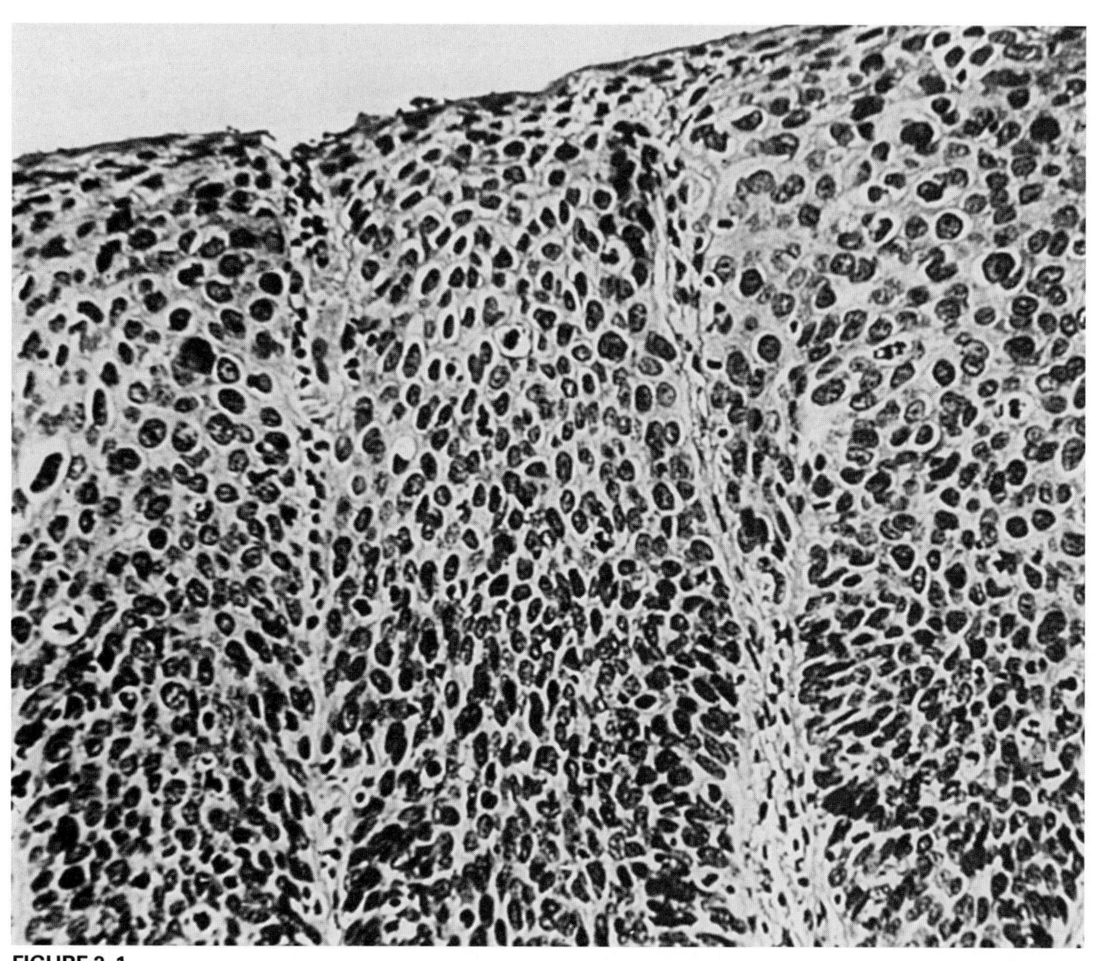

FIGURE 2–1.

27. Erythematous, macular
28. Topical steroids
29. Biopsy should precede therapy
30. Testosterone ointment
31. 5-FU ointment

Answers

1. **C** page 36
Contrary to cervical intraepithelial neoplasia, vaginal intraepithelial neoplasia (VAIN) is often multifocal. The necessity to perform an adequate colposcopy on the entire vaginal tube is obvious.
2. **A** page 36
In most series, the upper third of the vagina is most frequently involved by VAIN, as is invasive carcinoma of the vagina.
3. **B** page 36
Local large excision is the treatment of choice for CIS of the vagina at the present time. 5-FU topical ointment requires a long treatment and is irritative; laser vaporization gives excellent results but requires special skills to avoid injuries to bladder and rectum; cryocautery is not as successful as in the treatment of cervical intraepithelial neoplasia (CIN).
4. **C** page 37
Columnar epithelium and chronic inflammation are often seen in the reddened areas of vaginas treated with 5-FU or with laser therapy. It is not associated with DES use and is thought to be a reparative rather than a premalignant condition.
5. **A** page 37
Benedet demonstrated that involved epithelium had a mean thickness of 0.46 mm and proposed that a 1- to 1.5-mm laser depth would satisfactorily vaporize VAIN while sparing underlying structures. 5-FU is more appropriate for multifocal lesions. Krebs demonstrated efficiency of laser equal to that of 5-FU. Laser therapy has not been shown to be superior to other modalities.
6. **D** page 37
Adenosis may be found in the first three forms in the vagina. Squamous epithelium is normal in the vagina; transitional epithelium belongs to the urinary tract.
7. **D** page 39
Adenosis is more common in patients whose mothers began DES treatment early in pregnancy. Its frequency is not increased if administration of DES began after the 18th week of gestation.
8. **D** page 39
All described anatomic deformities can be observed in 20% of women exposed to DES.
9. **B** page 40
An increase in squamous CIN has been described in individuals exposed to DES. The DESAD project demonstrated a twofold incidence over the control group not exposed to DES.
10. **A** page 40
Physical examinations and cytologic monitoring should continue for the life of the patient. Clinicians treating women exposed to DES disagree about whether routine colposcopy is warranted beyond the initial examination (in the patient with no cytologic abnormality). Most agree that it is unnecessary beyond the time of complete resolution of adenosis, if examination and cytology results remain normal.
11. **C** page 40
Adenosis is a self-limiting process. Almost all areas of adenosis will undergo metaplasia to squamous epithelium. The vigorous metaplastic changes of adenosis commonly have a colposcopic appearance usually associated with CIN, but biopsy results are negative. Specific treatments should not be undertaken unless there is histologic documentation of premalignant change.
12. **D** page 45
Although high-risk HPV subtypes such as 16 and 18 are isolated in a substantial number of cases of VIN, the clinical usefulness of HPV subtyping has not been established.
13. **C** page 47
The comparative behavior of VIN to CIN is not known.
14. **C** page 42
The nomenclature of non-neoplastic epithelial disorders of the vulva was changed in 1987 by the International Society for the Study of Vulvar Disease (ISSVD). It includes squamous cell hyperplasia (formerly hyperplastic dystrophy), lichen sclerosus, and other dermatoses.
15. **D** page 43
Topical corticosteroids are the treatment of choice. Excision often results in recurrence. Squamous cell hyperplasia may involve any of the areas of the vulva. Microscopically, hyperkeratosis, parakeratosis, and acanthosis thicken the epithelium.
16. **B** page 44
Only 4% of patients with lichen sclerosus are later found to have vulvar malignancy. Clobetasol provided relief of symptoms in 75% of patients vs. 20% for testosterone in double-blinded study.
17. **D** page 44
The predominant symptom of VIN is pruritus. The disease is asymptomatic in more than 50% of cases.
18. **D** page 45
VINs are associated with HPV, particularly types 16/18, 31, 33, 35, and 51. HPV DNA has been found in 80% to 90% of VIN, but the incidence decreases with age. At present, subtyping of HPV in patients with VIN has no clinical application.
19. **D** pages 39 and 42
The new term used by ISSVD is VIN III. Other terms should be discarded.
20. **D** page 47
All of the above modalities are acceptable treatments for VIN III. Excision of the lesion has the advantage of obtaining the specimen for pathologic examination. Laser should be used only after multiple biopsy results rule out invasive disease.
21. **A** page 47
Pain, which is severe in some patients, is the main complication of the laser. Bleeding and infection have been reported also. General anesthesia should be used if one elects to treat a large area of the vulva. Cosmetic results appear to be excellent. Greater

expertise with the laser is required for this therapy than for cervical vaporization.

22. **C** Figure 2–6, page 45
VIN III is usually multifocal. The perineum is involved in 92% of patients, and the clitoris is involved in 70% of patients.
23. **D** page 37
24. **C** page 37
25. **A** page 37
26. **B** page 37
Local excision has been the mainstay of therapy for VAIN. Weekly insertions of 5-FU cream (1.5 g) deeply into the vagina once a week at bedtime for 10 consecutive weeks is also efficacious. Cryosurgery was found not to be successful because of the flaccidity of the vaginal wall and the lack of good freezing contact. Laser therapy gave good results in experienced hands, but it required thorough diagnostic investigation to rule out invasive disease. Pain and bleeding are the main complications, but these appear to be minimal. Healing is excellent.
27. **D** page 44
28. **C** page 44
29. **C** page 44
30. **A** page 44
31. **D** page 44
It is necessary to perform a biopsy on any vulvar lesion before treatment. Lichen sclerosus appears as a pale skin, sometimes shiny or wrinkled. Squamous cell hyperplasia has a thickened, hyperplastic, white keratinized surface that can simulate VIN. Lichen sclerosus is treated with clobetasol ointment, which is a high-potency steroid. Squamous cell hyperplasia is treated with mid-potency or low-potency steroids (triamcinolone, hydrocortisone). 5-FU ointment is used for treatment of vaginal intraepithelial neoplasia, not for non-neoplastic intraepithelial disorders of the vulva.

chapter 3

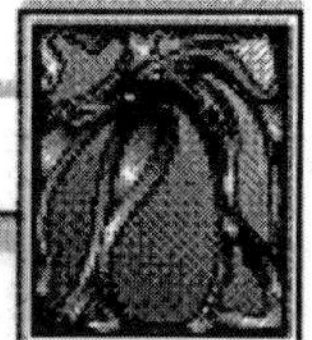

INVASIVE CERVICAL CANCER

KEY POINTS TO REMEMBER

- Cancer of the cervix is more prevalent in women of lower socioeconomic status and in those who have first coitus at an early age, multiple sexual partners, and husbands who had sexually transmitted diseases and many sexual partners. Squamous cell carcinoma of cervix is almost nonexistent in a celibate population.
- Human papilloma virus (HPV) is strongly associated with the etiology of cancer of the cervix.
- FIGO stage Ia squamous cancer of the cervix defines a microscopic lesion.
- Ia_1 has a lesion with stromal invasion up to 3 mm in depth and no greater than 7 mm in width.
- Ia_2 has stromal invasion present at 3 to 5 mm in depth and no greater than 7 mm in width. Lymphatic/vascular space involvement is not included in the definition. Survival of patients with stages Ia_1 and Ia_2 approaches 99% to 98%, respectively. Recurrence rate of patients in these two substages is no more than 1% to 2%.
- Management of patients with FIGO stage Ia_1 (3 mm depth and 7 mm width) and SGO criteria (no lymph vascular involvement) is conservative: conization with free margins or total hysterectomy. The recurrence rate is 0.7%, the death rate is 0.2%, and the percentage of positive nodes is 1.2%. Although still in dispute, a growing number of investigators do not use capillary-like space involvement as an exclusion criterion for this stage.
- Patients with stage Ia_2 (3 to 5 mm invasion, 7 mm width) have a low incidence of lymph node metastasis (6.3%). The recurrence rate is 4%, and the death rate is 2%. They can be evaluated with laparoscopy or retroperitoneal lymphadenectomy, and if results are negative simple hysterectomy or even conization may be reasonable. GOG reported 50 patients with 3- to 5-mm invasion undergoing radical hysterectomy and pelvic lymphadenectomy. There were 23% with lymph space involvement (LSI), no node involvement, and no recurrence. Data are accumulating for the adequate evaluation of and appropriate therapy for patients with stage Ia_2.
- Clinically evident lesions, even with superficial invasion, are considered stage Ib.
- Cytology and colposcopy are valuable tools for eradication of cervical cancer, the incidence of which is around 8 to 10/100,000/year in the United States.
- The most common routes of spread of carcinoma of the cervix are (1) direct extension to vaginal mucosa, myometrium, parametria, and pelvic sidewalls; and (2) lymphatics: paracervical lymphatic, then to obturator, hypogastric, and external iliac nodes.
- Lymph node involvement in stage I: 15% to 20%; stage II: 25% to 40%; stage III: 50% or higher.
- Six percent of patients with stage I disease have positive periaortic nodes, 16% with stage II, and 8% with stage III.
- According to GOG experience with staging laparotomy, mis-staging occurs in the magnitude of 23% in stage IIb and 64% in stage IIIb.
- Twenty percent of stage IIb–IVa patients have metastatic disease to periaortic nodes. Twenty-five percent of these patients demonstrated a 3-year, disease-free survival with extended postoperative field irradiation.
- Eighty-five to ninety percent of cervical cancers are squamous cell; 10% to 15% are adenocarcinomas.
- Adenocarcinomas are often bulky neoplasms and create "barrel-shaped" lesions of cervix.
- The spread pattern of adenocarcinoma of cervix is similar to that of squamous carcinoma. It more readily spreads hematogenously. Local recurrence is more common.
- Microinvasive adenocarcinoma of cervix, using the 1994 FIGO definition of stage Ia: stage Ia_1 (3-mm depth and 7-mm width) adenocarcinoma of cervix can be treated with conservative surgery (hysterectomy). There were recurrences with stage Ia_2.
- Combined treatment with intracavitary radium followed by hysterectomy gives an improved 5-year survival for adenocarcinoma of the cervix. Survival was correlated with tumor size and grade. Lesions greater than 3 cm have 90% 5-year survival.
- Most studies suggest no difference in survival when adenocarcinomas are compared with squamous carcinomas after correction for stage.
- A study from GOG on stages Ia_2 and Ib concludes that survival is worse with adenosquamous cancer than with squamous cancer and adenocarcinoma (72%, 82%, 88%, respectively).
- Neuroendocrine small cell carcinoma has a very poor prognosis (14% 5-year survival) despite aggressive therapy including surgery, radiation, and chemotherapy.
- Glassy cell carcinoma, a poorly differentiated adenosquamous carcinoma, is associated with a poor outcome, regardless of the modality of therapy (5-year survival, 45% for Ib lesions).
- Staging of cancer of the cervix is a clinical appraisal; it cannot be changed later. It should remain constant and does not limit the treatment plan. Stages 0: in situ; I: cervix; Ia_1: microscopic lesion with invasion of 3-mm depth and 7-mm width; Ia_2: microscopic lesion with invasion 3- to 5-mm depth and 7-mm width; Ib: clinical

lesion or microscopic lesion greater than that in Ia_2; Ib_1: lesion smaller than 4 cm; Ib_2: lesion larger than 4 cm; II: vagina and parametrium; IIa: involvement of two thirds of vagina; IIb: infiltration of parametria; III: vagina, pelvic side walls; IIIa: involvement of lower one third of vagina; IIIb: extension to pelvic side wall or hydronephrosis; IV: bladder, rectum, distant metastases; IVa: involvement of mucosa bladder or of the rectum; IVb: distant metastasis.

- In early stages (Ib and IIa) comparable survival rates result from both treatment techniques: radical surgery or radiotherapy. The advantage of radiotherapy is that it is applicable to virtually all patients, whereas radical surgery excludes certain medically inoperable patients. Above stages I and IIa, all patients should be treated primarily with radiotherapy. In many institutions, surgery for stages I–IIa is reserved for young patients (ovarian function and vaginal preservation).
- Five-year survival of cervical cancer (FIGO data 1998) treated with

Stage	Surgery (%)	Radiation Only (%)*	Surgery + Radiation (%)
Ib	90	72	80
IIa	66	65	68
IIb	80	64	64
IIIa		45	
IIIb		36	
IV		14	

*Data from MD Anderson Hospital.

- A GOG study based on 277 patients with stage Ib2 cancers and negative lymph nodes showed no improvement in overall survival if radiation is added to surgery.
- Postoperative radiotherapy is recommended in patients with positive lymph nodes after surgery. VSI (vascular space invasion) is also a factor for irradiation.
- Major complications after radical surgery are postoperative bladder dysfunction, lymphocyst formation, pulmonary embolism, ureteral fistulae, pelvic infection, and hemorrhage.
- Recurrence can occur in 10% to 20% of patients treated with radical hysterectomy and bilateral lymphadenectomy. Fifty-eight percent of the recurrences occur within the first 12 months and 83% occur within the first 2 years after surgery. Radiation therapy is the treatment of choice for patients with pelvic recurrences with a survival rate of 25%. Recurrences outside the pelvis carry a poor prognosis.
- Early recognition of a centrally located, recurrent lesion appears to give the best prognosis for salvage.
- The maximal effect of ionizing radiation on cancer is obtained in the presence of a good and intact circulation and adequate cellular oxygenation.
- Radiation dose tolerances for the following are: vaginal mucosa, 20,000 cGy; rectovaginal septum, 6000 cGy; bladder mucosa, 7000 cGy; colon and rectum, 5000 cGy; small bowel in the pelvis, 4000 cGy; and small bowel in the abdomen, 2500 cGy.
- Cesium (half-life 30 years) provides a very adequate substitute for radium (half-life 1620 years).
- Radiation therapy consists of local application of radium/cesium (intracavitary techniques, interstitial therapy) and whole pelvic irradiation. Total dose approximates 7000 cGy delivered to paracervical tissues.
- Techniques for the application of radium consist of three intracavitary (Stockholm, Paris, and Manchester) and one interstitial directly into the tumor. In the United States, oncologists use fixed radium applicators with the intrauterine tandem and vaginal colpostats with flexible afterloading system (Fletcher-Suit).
- Whole pelvic irradiation is usually administered with brachytherapy (e.g., intracavitary cesium) in a dose range of 4000 to 5000 cGy. High-energy megavoltage equipment has definite advantages over orthovoltage, because the hard, short rays of megavoltage pass through the skin without much absorption and cause little injury to it. Extended field irradiation to treat periaortic metastases delivered at a dose of 4000 to 5000 cGy in 4 to 6 weeks. Complication rate is 5%.
- Late complications of radiation therapy include small bowel obstruction (20% with extended fields), sigmoiditis (3%), rectovaginal fistula, rectal stricture, vesicovaginal fistula, ureteral structure (1% each).
- Stage for stage, the outcome for the pregnant patient with cervical cancer (incidence 0.01% of pregnancies) is the same as that for the nonpregnant patient.
- Concomitant cisplatin with radiation therapy emerges as the treatment of choice when radiation is used in cervical cancer. A GOG study shows that both progression-free survival and overall survival were significantly higher in the radiation-cisplatin group, compared with that in the radiation-only group, for patients with stage Ib followed for 4 years (83% vs. 74%; $P = 0.008$).
- Radical hysterectomy is acceptable during any trimester for stage I and early stage II lesions, and radiation can be used before 24 weeks' gestation. Therapy may be delayed for a few weeks until fetal viability is reached for patients at 24 weeks' gestation or more.
- Cancer in a cervical stump should be treated by radical cervicectomy if stage and medical conditions allow.
- After suboptimal surgery in patients with stage I or II disease, radiation therapy *or* radical parametrectomy and lymphadenectomy give good survival rates (80% to 90%).
- The incidence of pelvic recurrence after irradiation alone for stages Ib, IIa, and IIb carcinomas of the cervix increases with increasing tumor diameter. Data from MD Anderson Hospital show an improved pelvic control rate and small increase in survival when patients with barrel-shaped lesions were treated with preoperative irradiation followed by extrafascial hysterectomy. A large prospective, randomized study is lacking.
- Factors influencing survival include lymphatic and blood vessel invasion; size of carcinoma, which correlates with the frequency of metastases, and depth of stromal invasion; peritoneal tumor involvement; microvessel density; lymph node metastases; and age.
- Postoperative radiation of patients with positive pelvic nodes should destroy microscopic residual disease in the pelvis and improve survival. To reduce bowel injuries, DiSaia recommends filling the pelvic basin with the redundant rectosigmoid.

- The irradiated patient experienced statistically significant decrease in sexual enjoyment, contrary to the surgically treated patient who has no significant change in sexual function.
- Mortality from cervical cancer in the United States is 3.4/100,000 female population (1991).
- Adequate follow-up is the key to detection of early recurrence: 35% of patients with invasive cervical cancer will have recurrent or persistent disease after therapy.
- Ninety-five percent of post-treatment ureteral obstruction is caused by progressive tumor.
- Weight loss, leg edema, and pelvic pain are indicative of recurrence.
- More than 75% of the recurrences are clinically evident in the first 2 years after therapy; frequent locations of recurrences are cervix, parametrium, and vagina. Lung and bone metastases are rare (2%).
- About half of all cancer deaths occur in the first year after therapy, 25% in the second year, and 15% in the third year, for a total of 85% by the end of the third year.
- Persistent or recurrent carcinoma of the cervix is a discouraging clinical entity with a 1-year survival rate between 10% to 15%.
- Recurrent disease can be treated with radical hysterectomy, radiation therapy, or chemotherapy (cisplatin) depending on the size and location of recurrence and the primary treatment. Result of chemotherapy has been poor.
- Bilateral ureteral obstruction from recurrent pelvic disease after primary surgical therapy should be considered for urinary diversion, followed by appropriate radiation therapy. Patients with bilateral ureteral obstruction following a full dose of pelvic irradiation have a dismal prognosis because 95% are due to recurrent tumor.
- Pelvic exenteration is the procedure of choice for carcinoma of the cervix recurrent or persistent within the pelvis after irradiation.
- One of the most serious postoperative complications of pelvic exenteration is small bowel obstruction. Mortality and morbidity related to pelvic exenteration usually occur within the first 18 months after surgery.
- The 5-year cumulative survival rate after pelvic exenteration varies from 20% to 62% (MD Anderson, 46%).
- Lymphomas of cervix are rare and best treated with radiation therapy and combination chemotherapy.
- Malignant melanoma of cervix is very rare, and the 5-year survival is very poor (40% stage I, 14% stage II).

QUESTIONS

Directions for Questions 1–57: Select the one best answer.

1. The prevalence of squamous cell carcinoma of the cervix is high in the following women *except:*
   A. women of lower socioeconomic groups
   B. women in whom first coitus occurs at an early age
   C. women who have multiple sexual partners
   D. women who have frequent sexual intercourse
2. Microinvasive carcinoma of the cervix, as defined by the Society of Gynecologic Oncologists, consists of:
   A. stromal invasion to 5 mm or less without confluent tongues and lymphatic or vascular invasion
   B. stromal invasion to 1 mm or less
   C. stromal invasion to 3 mm or less without lymphatic or vascular invasion
   D. stromal invasion to 2 mm or less
3. The overall incidence of pelvic node metastases in patients with carcinoma of the cervix invasive from 1 mm to 3 mm in the stroma is:
   A. 7%
   B. 3%
   C. 2%
   D. 1.2%
4. Consistent association of carcinoma of the cervix is found with the following factors *except:*
   A. use of oral contraceptives
   B. cigarette smoking
   C. early onset of sexual activity
   D. multiple sexual partners
5. The incidence of cervical cancer in the United States is approximately:
   A. 15 to 20/100,000/year
   B. 10 to 15/100,000/year
   C. 8 to 10/100,000/year
   D. 5 to 8/100,000/year
6. Of malignant tumors of the cervix, the proportion that are squamous cell carcinoma is:
   A. 90%
   B. 80%
   C. 70%
   D. 60%
7. The following are true of husbands of cervical cancer patients *except:*
   A. they had more sexual partners than controls
   B. they are heavy smokers
   C. they reported histories of condylomas, gonorrhea
   D. they had genital herpes
8. Symptoms of advanced disease in patients with carcinoma of the cervix include:
   A. pain in flank and legs, edema of lower extremities
   B. hematuria, rectal bleeding, or obstipation
   C. massive hemorrhage and uremia
   D. all of the above
9. The highest percentage of patients with carcinoma of the cervix is between:
   A. 25 and 35 years old
   B. 35 and 45 years old
   C. 45 and 55 years old
   D. 55 and 65 years old
10. "Barrel-shaped" lesion of the cervix refers to which gross lesion in the endocervical canal?
    A. infiltrating tumor
    B. ulcerative tumor
    C. exophytic tumor
    D. hemorrhagic tumor
11. The main route of spread of carcinoma of the cervix is:
    A. vaginal mucosa and lower uterine segment
    B. paracervical lymphatics and pelvic lymph nodes
    C. direct extension to adjacent structures (pelvic walls, bladder, rectum)
    D. all of the above

12. The proportion of patients with lymph node involvement in stage I carcinoma of the cervix is between:
    A. 5% and 10%
    B. 10% and 15%
    C. 15% and 20%
    D. 20% and 25%
13. The incidence of periaortic node metastasis in stage I carcinoma of the cervix is:
    A. 2%
    B. 4%
    C. 6%
    D. 8%
14. The following are true for adenocarcinoma of the cervix *except:*
    A. its incidence is approximately 10% to 15%
    B. it is a bulky lesion, often creating the barrel-shaped lesion
    C. it is best treated with surgery
    D. it recurs locally more often than squamous carcinoma
15. The following are true for neuroendocrine carcinoma of the cervix *except:*
    A. it is described as a small cell cancer
    B. it can be identified by light and electron microscopy and is indistinguishable from oat cell carcinoma of the lung
    C. it may be treated by radical hysterectomy with postoperative radiation therapy
    D. the prognosis for stage I disease is good
16. Glassy cell carcinoma of the cervix has the following features *except:*
    A. it is a poorly differentiated adenosquamous carcinoma
    B. it is infrequently diagnosed
    C. it has a good prognosis
    D. recurrences generally occur by 24 months
17. A patient with a tumor of the cervix infiltrating the medial left parametrium on clinical examination but found to involve the left pelvic side wall at laparotomy should be classified as having stage:
    A. Ib
    B. IIa
    C. IIb
    D. IIIb
18. A patient with carcinoma localized to the cervix has an IVP that shows unilateral hydronephrosis. She should be classified as having which stage?
    A. Ia_2
    B. Ib
    C. IIa
    D. IIIb
19. Diagnostic aids acceptable for determining a staging classification of cervical cancer are the following *except:*
    A. physical examination and routine radiographs
    B. lymphography and laparoscopy
    C. colposcopy, cystoscopy, and proctosigmoidoscopy
    D. IVP and barium studies of lower colon and rectum
20. The following examinations are not recommended for staging cancer of the cervix *except:*
    A. laparoscopy
    B. CT scan, MRI examinations
    C. IVP, barium enema
    D. lymphography and hysterography
21. Which of the following statements concerning the treatment of cancer of the cervix stages I and IIa is *false*?
    A. no significant difference was observed in survival rates of patients undergoing surgery alone as compared with patients receiving adjuvant postoperative radiation
    B. in stages I and IIa, comparable survival rates result from either surgery or radiation
    C. the advantage of radiotherapy is that it is applicable with few exceptions to all patients
    D. patients with cervical cancer in pregnancy, concomitant inflammatory disease of the bowel, or pelvic inflammatory disease should be treated with radiation therapy
22. Within the Rutledge extended hysterectomy classification system, which class of hysterectomy is the standard Meigs-Okabayashi radical hysterectomy?
    A. II
    B. III
    C. IV
    D. V
23. The standard Meigs-Okabayashi radical hysterectomy routinely includes all of the following *except:*
    A. radical excision of cardinal and uterosacral ligaments
    B. bilateral salpingo-oophorectomy
    C. bilateral pelvic lymphadenectomy
    D. en bloc resection of upper vagina
24. Radical hysterectomy and pelvic lymphadenectomy is appropriate primary therapy for all *except:*
    A. stage Ia_2 cervical cancer
    B. stage Ib cervical carcinoma
    C. some stage IIa cervical carcinoma
    D. stage Ia_1 cervical carcinoma
25. Advantages of a Rutledge class II hysterectomy over a class III include all *except:*
    A. higher chance of cure
    B. less devascularization of ureter
    C. preservation of bladder function
    D. less postoperative obstipation
26. Effective therapy of urinary retention after radical hysterectomy includes all *except:*
    A. Credé maneuver
    B. urethral dilation
    C. chronic intermittent self-catheterization
    D. chronic indwelling catheterization
27. The least radioresistant-listed tissue is:
    A. vagina
    B. rectum
    C. bladder
    D. ileum
28. True statements regarding the surgical staging of cervical carcinoma include all *except:*
    A. increases survival
    B. increases radiotherapy morbidity
    C. allows transposition of ovaries from area to be irradiated
    D. allows surgical methods to exclude small bowel from radiated fields

29. The *least* appropriate measure in reference to management of the lymphocyst is:
   A. prevention by routine use of suction drains and ligation of incoming lymphatic trunks or avoiding reperitonealization of the pelvic peritoneum
   B. nonintervention in the patient without ureteral obstruction
   C. operative marsupialization
   D. percutaneous aspiration
30. The most appropriate therapy for pelvic recurrence after surgery for cancer of the cervix is:
   A. supportive care only
   B. exenteration
   C. radiotherapy
   D. cisplatin-based combination chemotherapy
31. The following statements regarding pelvic radiotherapy are true *except:*
   A. interstitial brachytherapy may successfully substitute for intracavitary brachytherapy
   B. the addition of neoadjuvant chemotherapy to pelvic radiotherapy has increased response rates
   C. orthovoltage external beam radiotherapy is preferable to megavoltage radiotherapy
   D. some patients with periaortic metastases can be salvaged with extended-field external beam radiotherapy
32. True statements referent to cervical cancer in pregnancy include all *except:*
   A. there seems to be no detrimental effect of pregnancy on cancer
   B. the first-trimester patient should be treated as if nonpregnant
   C. pregnancy in the third trimester should be terminated through induction and vaginal delivery after confirmation of fetal viability, and appropriate therapy begun
   D. a modified radical (Rutledge class II) or a radical (class III) cesarean hysterectomy is often used
33. The following statements regarding suboptimal treatment situations are true *except*:
   A. postradiotherapy extrafascial hysterectomy should be performed on the patient with bulky low-stage disease
   B. excellent survivals are reported with early occult invasive carcinomas post-hysterectomy
   C. a high rate of complications results from radiotherapy of carcinoma of the cervical stump
   D. radical surgery is an effective alternative treatment for cervical stump carcinoma and for cervical carcinoma after inadvertent nonradical hysterectomy
34. The *least* important post-therapy poor prognostic factor is:
   A. high tumor grade
   B. large tumor volume/size
   C. deep stromal invasion
   D. extracervical extension
35. The following statements about epidemiology and natural history of cervical carcinoma are true *except:*
   A. the proportion of patients with stage I disease is increasing
   B. the proportion of patients with adenocarcinoma or adenosquamous carcinoma is increasing
   C. mortality from cervical carcinoma is decreasing
   D. advanced age is an independent poor prognostic risk factor
36. The following statements about recurrent cervical carcinoma are true *except:*
   A. 35% of treated patients will have recurrent disease post-therapy
   B. 85% of recurrences will occur before 3 post-treatment years
   C. persistence of tumor in the cervix beyond 4 weeks post-therapy is an ominous sign
   D. the majority of post-therapy recurrences are pelvic rather than extrapelvic
37. In reference to bony metastasis and cervical cancer, the following statements about treated patients are true *except:*
   A. bony metastasis at time of recurrence is evident in approximately 10% of patients
   B. bony metastasis at time of initial diagnosis is exceedingly rare
   C. at time of recurrence the prevalence of bony metastasis exceeds that at other sites
   D. the most common site of bony metastasis is the vertebral bodies
38. A Rutledge class I hysterectomy is appropriately included in the therapy for all of the following *except:*
   A. stage Ib carcinoma of the cervix
   B. stage I endometrial adenocarcinoma
   C. microinvasive carcinoma of the cervix
   D. stage IIa epithelial ovarian adenocarcinoma
39. When comparing radical surgery to radiotherapy for early invasive cancer of the cervix, the following statements are true *except:*
   A. recurrence rates post-treatment are similar
   B. mortality from therapy is greater with surgical management
   C. morbidity rates are similar
   D. cure rates are similar
40. Microinvasive adenocarcinoma of the cervix is a debatable entity, and many authors doubt its existence. However, using the 1994 FIGO staging of Ia_1 and Ia_2 and the works of Kaku, Ostor, and Schorage, one can conclude that there is:
   A. no recurrence in patients with tumor < 3 mm stromal invasion and < 7 mm horizontal spread with no LSI (lymph node invasion)
   B. no recurrence in patients with tumor < 5 mm stromal invasion and < 7 mm horizontal spread
   C. no recurrence in patients with < 5 mm/7 mm stromal invasion and spread with LSI
   D. no acceptable criteria for definition of adenocarcinoma of cervix
41. Recurrences of adenocarcinoma of cervix are strongly correlated with:
   A. lymph vascular involvement
   B. poorly differentiated lesion
   C. larger tumor size
   D. all of the above

42. The following comments regarding post-therapy cervical cancer patients are true *except:*
    A. survival is vastly compromised in the case of the gross "cut-through" hysterectomy
    B. postradiotherapy ureteral obstruction is usually secondary to treatment-associated fibrosis
    C. the patient with positive margins or lymph node metastasis probably should be offered post-surgery radiotherapy
    D. post-treatment sexuality is affected less by surgery than by radiotherapy
43. Recurrent squamous carcinoma of the cervix after initial therapy:
    A. is associated with a 1-year survival rate of 10% to 15%
    B. often may be associated with long-term survival if the recurrence is outside the initial radiotherapy treatment field
    C. always can be successfully treated with external beam irradiation if the initial therapy was radical hysterectomy
    D. often lends itself to successful reirradiation of pelvic recurrences if the recurrence is free of the bladder and rectum
44. Which of the following is true regarding chemotherapy of recurrent carcinoma of the cervix?
    A. since the introduction of modern chemotherapy, there is significant improvement in the survival rates of patients with recurrent cervical cancer
    B. the most active single agent in this setting is cisplatin
    C. combination chemotherapy with alkylating agents and cisplatin are associated with higher response rates than cisplatin used alone
    D. response rates of metastases to chemotherapy are the same regardless of the metastatic site in the body
45. Find the *incorrect* statement regarding the chemotherapy of recurrent cervical cancer:
    A. carcinoma of the cervix has limited sensitivity to cytotoxic drugs in the irradiated pelvis
    B. in the few responding patients the median duration of a response usually is long and associated with restoration of a patient's functional status
    C. there is difficulty in demonstrating an increase in survival in the treated patient population
    D. use of the most active agents is often compromised by coexistent renal compromise
46. Choose the following *true* statement regarding advanced cervical cancer:
    A. the optimum setting for chemotherapy for cervical cancer is in patients with small asymptomatic recurrences outside an irradiated field
    B. relief of pain is a main indication for chemotherapy in these patients
    C. a trial of cytotoxic drugs may be useful before scheduled pelvic exenteration to improve the chances of operability
    D. pelvic exenteration should be offered to patients with fixed pelvic recurrences who show no response to cytotoxic drugs
47. Compared with older patients, young patients with carcinomas of cervix:
    A. have a higher incidence of lymph node metastasis
    B. have a lower 5-year survival
    C. do better if they have high volume Ib and do poorly if they have advanced disease
    D. all of the above
48. For a patient with cervical cancer who has bilateral ureteral obstruction:
    A. decisions regarding urinary diversion are best made after radiation therapy, if the patient has received no treatment for her malignancy
    B. urinary diversion will often significantly complicate external beam radiation therapy
    C. urinary diversion should be seriously considered before planned radiation therapy
    D. antegrade placement of ureteral stents is reserved for patients not amenable to the construction of a urinary conduit
49. The patient with bilateral ureteral obstruction after radiation therapy:
    A. often will be found to have obstruction due to ureteral fibrosis
    B. may have significant prolongation of survival by palliative urinary conduit
    C. should be explored to confirm or rule out the presence of recurrence
    D. often can be managed with percutaneous placement of ureteral stents
50. Recent improvements in the use of pelvic exenteration as treatment for recurrent cervical cancer include:
    A. more liberal use of subtotal exenterations to improve a patient's functional status
    B. a broadening of indications for exenteration since patients with limited sidewall involvement often can be treated successfully
    C. the use of "wet colostomy" to eliminate a stoma
    D. the development of techniques for creation of a continent urinary reservoir
51. A candidate for pelvic exenteration:
    A. should not be explored if she has the symptom triad of unilateral leg edema, sciatica, and ureteral obstruction
    B. should have operability determined by pelvic examination, perhaps under anesthesia; fixation of the parametria and sidewalls rules out exploration
    C. for recurrent squamous carcinoma who has positive peritoneal washings should have the procedure aborted
    D. is more likely to have an aborted procedure due to intraoperative recognition of metastases with increasing age
52. Postoperative small bowel obstruction is a significant complication following pelvic exenteration. Which of the following statements concerning postexenteration small bowel obstruction is *not* true?
    A. when obstruction occurs, it is appropriately treated initially with conservative nonoperative therapy

B. since the site of anastomosis is away from the previously irradiated pelvis, prior irradiation has little effect on the incidence of postexenteration small bowel obstruction
C. the primary purpose of mobilization of the omentum at exenteration is to prevent adhesions to the denuded pelvic floor
D. the operative mortality of patients explored for postexenteration obstruction approaches 50%

53. After pelvic exenteration:
A. the most common cause of death is predominantly related to the urinary diversion
B. the most common cause of death is recurrent cancer
C. life-long urinary antisepsis probably has no effect on the incidence of pyelonephritis
D. urinary stones forming on stapled anastomoses are uncommon

54. According to DiSaia and Creasman, functional neovagina after pelvic exenteration should be performed using:
A. rectus abdominis myocutaneous graft
B. gracilis myocutaneous graft
C. isolated segment of bowel
D. split-thickness skin graft

55. Concerning pelvic exenteration:
A. most series report 5-year survival rates of greater than 60% if there are no nodal metastases
B. operative mortality remains around 15%
C. patients who were symptom-free before exenteration have a 2-year survival rate of greater than 60%
D. advanced patient age (65 years or more) at the time of exenteration is a relative contraindication to the procedure

56. The most common clinical feature of lymphoma of cervix or upper vagina is:
A. abnormal vaginal bleeding
B. vaginal mass
C. vaginal discharge
D. dyspareunia

57. Treatment of choice for cancer of the cervix with radiation is:
A. radiation alone
B. radiation followed with surgery
C. radiation therapy concomitant with cisplatin, fluorouracil, and hydroxyurea
D. radiation therapy with cisplatin alone

Directions for Questions 58–80: For each numbered item, select the letter of the most appropriate answer. Each letter may be used once, more than once, or not at all.

58–60. Match the following nodes involved in cervical cancer as:
A. primary nodal group
B. secondary nodal group
C. both
D. neither

58. Obturator and internal iliac nodes
59. Common iliac nodes
60. Sacral nodes

61–65. Match the following patients with the type of treatment. The patients have normal chest x-rays, IVPs, and laboratory tests.
A. conization or total hysterectomy
B. radical hysterectomy
C. radiation therapy
D. radical hysterectomy or radiation therapy

61. A 28-year-old patient with microscopic squamous cell carcinoma of the cervix that invades the stroma to a 2.5-mm depth and 6-mm width without vascular involvement.
62. A 40-year-old patient with squamous cell carcinoma of the cervix has stromal invasion to a 4-mm depth and 5-mm width without vascular involvement
63. A 45-year-old patient with squamous cell carcinoma of the cervix that invades the stroma to a 5-mm depth and 4-mm width. The patient has severe cardiac disease
64. A 30-year-old patient, 36 weeks pregnant, has a 2-cm invasive adenocarcinoma of the cervix
65. A 50-year-old patient has an adenocarcinoma of the cervix infiltrating the medial right parametrium

66–72. Match the stage of the cervical lesion with the microscopic or clinical findings:
A. stage Ia_1
B. stage Ia_2
C. stage Ib_1
D. stage Ib_2

66. Microscopic lesion 2 mm in depth and 6 mm in width
67. Microscopic lesion 3 mm in depth and 7 mm in width
68. Microscopic lesion 4 mm in depth and 7 mm in width
69. Microscopic lesion 4 mm in depth and 10 mm in width
70. Microscopic lesion 5 mm in depth and 7 mm in width
71. Malignant cervical growth 5 × 3 cm
72. Visible ulceration of cervix measuring 4 mm in depth and 7 mm in width microscopically

73–79. Match the following concepts with the appropriate method of radiotherapy administration:
A. Paris method
B. Stockholm method
C. Manchester method
D. all
E. none

73. Point A
74. Interstitial therapy
75. Point B
76. Two applications
77. Intracavitary therapy
78. Fletcher-Suit tandem and ovoids
79. Radium
80. Cesiump

ANSWERS

1. **D** page 53
There is no correlation of the prevalence of squamous cell carcinoma of the cervix with the frequency of sexual intercourse.

2. **C** page 54
In 1973 the Society of Gynecologic Oncologists defined microinvasion in cervical cancer as "a lesion which invades the stroma in one or more places to a depth of 3 mm or less below the base of the epithelium and in which lymphatic and vascular involvement is not demonstrated." The incidence of positive pelvic nodes is 0.2%. The treatment of this lesion is conization or total hysterectomy.
3. **D** page 56
The overall incidence of pelvic node metastasis based on 666 cases of carcinoma of the cervix invading the stroma from 1 to 3 mm is 1.2% (8 cases; Table 3–2).
4. **A** page 59
There is no consistent association between use of oral contraceptives and carcinoma of the cervix.
5. **C** page 59
The occurrence of cancer of the cervix is less frequent in Norway and Sweden and more frequent in underdeveloped countries than in the United States.
6. **A** page 62
About 85% to 90% of malignant lesions of the cervix are squamous cell carcinoma; 10% to 15% are adenocarcinomas.
7. **B** page 59
There is no known correlation between husbands who smoke and wives who develop cervical cancer, but smoking is one of the factors predisposing to cervical dysplasia.
8. **D** page 60
Pain referred to the flank or leg is secondary to involvement of ureter or of sciatic or obturator nerve. Rectal and bladder invasion produces hematuria and rectal bleeding. Extremity edema is due to lymphatic and venous blockage.
9. **C** page 60
Approximately 25% of patients with carcinoma of the cervix are between 45 and 55 years old, 15% are between 25 and 35 years old, 20% are between 35 and 45 years old, and 20% are between 55 and 65 years old (Fig. 3–6).
10. **C** page 60
The "barrel-shaped" lesion refers to an exophytic tumor arising within the endocervical canal and distending the cervical canal. Other types of gross lesions are infiltrating and ulcerating tumors.
11. **D** page 61
Carcinoma of the cervix spreads through the routes enumerated above. From the paracervical lymphatics, it invades the obturator, hypogastric, and external iliac nodes (collectively referred to as *pelvic nodes*).
12. **C** page 61
Lymph node involvement in stage I carcinoma of the cervix is between 15% and 20%, stage II is between 25% and 40%, and stage III is more than 50%.
13. **C** page 62
The incidence of positive periaortic nodes in carcinoma of the cervix stage I is 6.3%, stage II is 16.5%, and stage III is 8.6% (Table 3–5).
14. **C** page 64
The bulky, expansive nature of adenocarcinoma of the cervix and its more frequent local recurrence led many oncologists to advocate combined radiotherapy and surgery for its treatment. Also, remember that the lymphatic spread pattern of adenocarcinoma of the cervix is similar to that of squamous cancer except that it spreads by hematogenous route more frequently than squamous cancer.
15. **D** page 65
Neuroendocrine carcinoma of the cervix has a very poor prognosis. Among 14 stage Ib or IIa patients treated by radical hysterectomy and radiation by DiSaia and Creasman, all 14 have experienced recurrences.
16. **C** page 65
The prognosis of glassy cell carcinoma is also poor but more encouraging than that of neuroendocrine carcinoma. In some series, 5-year survival is as high as 50% for stage I disease. In 32 cases treated by radical hysterectomy by Lotocki, 5-year survival for Ib lesions was 45% (compared with 90% for squamous cell and 78% for adenocarcinoma).
17. **C** page 65
The staging of carcinoma of the cervix is clinical and should be done before surgery. When clinical staging was compared with surgical staging, mis-staging occurred on the magnitude of 22.9% in stage IIb disease and 64.4% in stage IIIb disease. Surgical staging, although more accurate, has failed to improve treatment results. This patient has stage IIb carcinoma of the cervix and should not be having a laparotomy.
18. **D** page 66
Obstruction of one or both ureters with a hydronephrosis or nonfunctioning kidney places the tumor in stage IIIb (although a tumor localized to the cervix is stage Ib).
19. **B** page 66
Lymphography and laparoscopy are not recommended for staging. Clinical staging is enhanced by the liberal use of rectovaginal examination.
20. **C** page 66
Of the listed examinations, only IVP and barium enema are acceptable for staging of cancer of the cervix. The other examinations are not uniformly available from institution to institution. Findings uncovered by CT scans or MRI can be used for planning therapy but not for changing clinical staging.
21. **D** page 72
Reasons for selection of radical surgery over radiation include cervical cancer in pregnancy, concomitant inflammatory disease of the bowel, previous irradiation therapy for other disease, presence of pelvic inflammatory disease, or an undiagnosed adnexal neoplasm.
22. **B** page 76
The class III hysterectomy is analogous to the standard Meigs-Okabayashi hysterectomy that is most commonly performed for stage I and stage II invasive carcinoma of the cervix (Table 3–10).
23. **B** page 75
Cervical cancer metastasis to the ovary is rare. Preservation of ovaries of women in their early to midreproductive years is safe, acceptable, and desirable in the presence of cervical tumors.

24. **D** page 75
Microinvasive cervical carcinoma (stage Ia_1), as defined by the Society of Gynecologic Oncologists (SGO) and by the American College of Obstetrics and Gynecology (ACOG), is best treated by nonradical means. The morbidity and mortality of radical procedures in this group outweigh the additional therapeutic benefits over nonradical treatment. Nonradical therapy (total hysterectomy, conization, or brachytherapy alone) is therefore the treatment of choice for this well-defined group. More extensive lesions should be treated radically (Table 3–10). For stage Ia_2 (3- to 5-mm depth, 7-mm width) some authors prefer radical surgery. However, if one is concerned about the 2% incidence of lymph node metastases, evaluation of nodes could be done by laparoscopy or retroperitoneal lymphadenectomy, followed by simple hysterectomy if nodes are negative. A less morbid effective treatment for CIS (CIN3) is cervical transformation zone ablation with cryosurgery, laser, electrocautery, or loop electrosurgical excision.
25. **A** page 75
For the carefully selected patient, the use of class II hysterectomy is not thought to affect survival differently from that of a class III hysterectomy. Preservation of a portion of the uterosacral ligament decreases the likelihood of rectal atony and obstipation. Preservation of the lateral cardinal ligament reduces blood loss, preserves some blood supply to the distal ureter, and allows retention of a significant portion of the bladder's innervation.
26. **B** page 77
After bladder denervation from cardinal ligament removal, sensory and motor function of the bladder are reduced. Increasing intravesical pressure (Valsalva and Credé maneuvers) is effective in patients with mild urinary retention. For the majority of patients with more severe or prolonged dysfunction, intermittent and chronic catheterization may be effective. Although in some postsurgery radical hysterectomy patients a condition of hypertonicity of the bladder and urethra exists, urethral dilation is not a commonly accepted therapy.
27. **D** page 80
In order of increasing radiosensitivity: small bowel (4000 to 4200 cGy), colon (5000 to 6000 cGy), rectum (6000 cGy), bladder (7000 cGy), and vagina/cervix (20,000 to 25,000 cGy).
28. **A** page 84
Wharton demonstrated high complication rates (25%) and high therapy-associated death rates (17%) in patients receiving surgical staging procedures and postsurgical radiotherapy. Though several patients with occult metastases were detected, none survived 5 years. Although beneficial in a few selected patients, the value of surgical staging in relation to 5-year survival has not been convincingly demonstrated. Adjunctive surgery such as bowel exclusion techniques and ovarian transposition can be added to transperitoneal surgical staging procedures to reduce postoperative radiotherapy-associated morbidity. Retroperitoneal surgery may provide useful staging information with less morbidity than transperitoneal techniques.
29. **D** page 78
Percutaneous aspiration of lymphocysts may predispose to abscess and should be avoided if possible. In general, the best management techniques are prevention and nonintervention. Surgical intervention is necessary in the patient with ureteral obstruction or who is excessively symptomatic and usually consists of marsupialization into the peritoneal cavity.
30. **C** page 93
Ten to twenty percent of patients develop tumor recurrence after surgical management. Recurrences cause dismal prognoses, leading to death in 85% of cases. Krebs suggested radiation therapy as the treatment of choice for patients with pelvic recurrences who did not have previous radiation therapy. The survival rate in that group of patients was 25%. In the rare patient already having undergone radiotherapy, evaluation for potentially curative exenteration or for palliative chemotherapy should be considered.
31. **C** page 82
High-energy external beam radiotherapy (megavoltage) is associated with deeper tissue penetration. Thus, a given tumor dose with megavoltage will radiate fewer superficial tissues than will orthovoltage. Fewer superficial complications such as ulceration, osteosclerosis, and fibrosis will follow. In general, the higher the voltage of a particle beam, the fewer the superficial complications.
32. **C** page 86
Note the authors' emphasis on achieving fetal *viability*, not maturity, before delivery of the patient with cervical cancer at 24 weeks' gestation or more. Viability—a function of gestational age vs. survival statistics for a particular population—should not be confused with maturity, which is determined by biochemical studies of the individual fetus. Vaginal delivery usually is discouraged because of the increased risk of maternal hemorrhage.
33. **A** page 87
The value and degree of morbidity of adjuvant extrafascial hysterectomy have not been clearly defined. Its postradiotherapy use in all patients with early stage bulky tumors is not recommended.
34. **A** page 88
The other listed factors have been found by many investigators to be poor prognostic factors, highly predictive of treatment failure. An additional poor prognostic factor is the presence of adenocarcinoma. Some recommend adjunctive postsurgical radiotherapy for factors such as these, and for capillary-like space involvement, but the benefit of additional therapy in these circumstances is not clearly established.
35. **D** page 88
Death rates for cervical carcinoma are higher with advanced age. A disproportionate number of the older (more poorly screened) population present with

advanced disease, accounting for this observation. When investigated as an independent prognostic factor and controlled for such factors as stage, age does not affect survival.

36. **C** page 90
Suit and Gallagher demonstrated that, after radiotherapy, nondividing cancer cells may persist for several months before they senesce and die. The authors recommend an interval of at least 3 months after treatment before evaluating the patient for persistent carcinoma.

37. **C** page 91
At time of recurrence, bony metastases are the third most common site of extrapelvic metastasis, occurring in about 10% of patients. Liver and lung metastases each occur in about 15% of these patients (Fig. 3–33).

38. **A** page 75
Patients with extensive localized carcinoma of the cervix (large stage Ib and IIa lesions, stage IIb, III, and IVa lesions) should undergo radiotherapy as their primary treatment (Table 3–10). The Rutledge class I hysterectomy is a standard extrafascial total hysterectomy and is appropriate therapy for many gynecologic disorders.

39. **B** page 88
No investigator has shown a clear advantage of radiotherapy over surgery (or vice versa) for early invasive carcinoma of the cervix. Prime determinants for the choice of therapy include psychology, sexuality, habitus, medical illnesses, and experience of the therapist.

40. **A** page 63
The term *microinvasive adenocarcinoma of the cervix* is appearing more frequently in the literature. Applying strict criteria of stage Ia_1 (3 mm/7 mm) with absence of LSI, one can use conservative therapy. Some authors are using tumor volume for simple hysterectomy.

41. **D** page 64
According to a study by Eifel at MD Anderson on 160 patients treated with different modalities, survival was strongly correlated with tumor size and grade. Patients with lesions that were 3 cm or smaller had a 90% survival rate. After 5 years, 45% of patients treated with radical hysterectomy had a recurrence.

42. **B** page 96
Ninety-five percent of the cases of postradiotherapy ureteral obstruction are secondary to persistent or recurrent cancer. Other common symptoms and signs of progressive cancer are buttock, pelvic, back, or leg pain; leg edema; and vaginal discharge or spotting.

43. **A** page 93
Recurrent squamous carcinoma following initial therapy has a dismal prognosis. Recurrences after initial radical hysterectomy for early carcinoma of the cervix are treated with radical radiation therapy, but the salvage rate is disappointing: only 10% to 15% of these patients are alive at 1 year. With rare exceptions, recurrences outside the initial field are usually indicators of disseminated cancer and are not amenable to curative local treatment. Reirradiation of a previously irradiated pelvis is associated with a high fistula rate and minimal, if any, salvage.

44. **B** page 94
Unfortunately, the management of disseminated cervical cancer has not improved significantly since the introduction of modern chemotherapy. The activity of all single chemotherapy agents is modest; cisplatin is the most active of these (Table 3–16).
There is no conclusive evidence that any cisplatin-containing combinations have higher response and survival rates than those when cisplatin is given alone, but combination cisplatin-containing regimens continue to be the standard with which new therapies are compared. A significant problem is the refractory nature of recurrent cervical cancer in a previously irradiated area; pulmonary metastases are much more likely to respond to chemotherapy than a recurrent pelvic mass.

45. **B** page 94
Statements **A, C,** and **D** are true. Cervical cancer is inherently refractory to most cytotoxic agents, and it has never been demonstrated conclusively that the use of these drugs results in prolonged survival of this population of patients. Despite isolated individual accounts of prolonged survival after therapy, most patients who respond do so for short periods with minimal restoration of functional status. Median duration of response is 3 to 7 months.

46. **B** page 97
The main indication for pelvic exenteration is isolated central recurrence in a previously irradiated pelvis. Operability is not improved by chemotherapy, and exenteration is unsuccessful as salvage therapy for chemotherapy failures. Relief of symptoms is the only widely accepted indication for using these drugs in patients with recurrent or advanced disease, and pain control is the most frequent symptom warranting a trial of chemotherapy. The use of cytotoxic drugs in a patient with a small symptom-free recurrence is controversial with little data to support its use.

47. **D** page 88
In a study by Rutledge, young patients with advanced disease (IIb and IIIb) did poorly, but those with stage Ib did better. However, in a study by Orlandi, 65 patients with stages Ib–IIa who were younger than 35 years of age and were treated by radical surgery had a higher incidence of lymph node metastases (46% vs. 24%) and a lower 5-year survival (65% vs. 76%) than those in the older group (n = 5199). This subject needs further study.

48. **C** page 96
The patient who has bilateral ureteral obstruction from untreated cervical cancer should be seriously considered for urinary diversion followed by appropriate radiation therapy. Placement of antegrade stents should be attempted first. When this is not successful, a urinary conduit should be constructed. The ease with which radiation can be delivered is actually facilitated when urinary diversion is performed before therapy.

49. **D** page 96
Less than 5% of patients with ureteral obstruction following radiation therapy for cervical cancer have ureteral fibrosis; the remainder have recurrent

malignancy. Despite this, all patients must be considered as possibly in this category until the presence of malignancy is proven. If recurrence is confirmed, there is no evidence to suggest that a "palliative" urinary conduit prolongs survival. Noninvasive imaging with percutaneous fine-needle aspiration should be used in preference to exploratory laparotomy to document recurrence. Ureteral stents often can be placed to provide some palliation; the route of placement (i.e., via the cystoscope or percutaneously) is based on the patient's site of obstruction.

50. **D** page 98
Complete exenteration is the treatment of choice for central recurrences following radiation therapy. Careful selection of operative candidates remains essential. Any patient with sidewall involvement is not a candidate for this procedure. Cogent objections have been raised regarding limited operations, such as anterior or posterior exenterations, because of the increased risk of incomplete resection. The wet colostomy is an outdated procedure with no current indications. Recent development of the continent reservoir is a distinct advance in patient rehabilitation.

51. **A** page 99
The triad of symptoms of unilateral leg edema, sciatica, and ureteral obstruction is pathognomonic of recurrent unresectable disease. The triad must be complete to be entirely reliable. Often resectability cannot be determined on pelvic examination. Laparotomy is often required in these patients, especially those with dense radiation fibrosis or previous pelvic inflammatory disease. Positive washings are predictive of unresectability in patients with recurrent cervical adenocarcinoma only, not squamous carcinoma. In a study by Miller, patients who underwent aborted exploration were younger (median age 49) than patients undergoing exenteration (median age 54).

52. **B** page 101
Small bowel obstruction is a major complication following exenteration. A major contributing factor is adherence of small bowel to the denuded irradiated pelvis. Mobilization of the omentum from its attachments on the transverse colon and stomach results in a fatty flap that can cover the pelvis. If a patient develops obstruction, conservative measures, including small bowel intubation and decompression, should be attempted. The operative mortality after reoperation in a patient with an exenteration is very high—as high as 50%!

53. **B** page 101
Cancer remains the most common cause of death following pelvic exenteration, but a significant portion of the long-term morbidity is related to the urinary diversion. Pyelonephritis is common and should be treated promptly and vigorously. Many believe that these patients should have long-term urinary antisepsis, perhaps for life. Ureteral stones may form on a nonadsorbable stapled anastomosis. Even though colic from the stones is not common, they may result in hematuria or ureteral obstruction.

54. **D** page 101
The authors prefer the more simple procedures requiring less time because pelvic exenteration is a very lengthy operation and, unfortunately, neovaginas are seldom used postoperatively.

55. **C** page 103
Among patients with symptomatic recurrence of cervical cancer before exenteration, the 2-year survival rate is reported as 47%. Among patients symptom-free before exenteration, the 2-year survival rate is 73%. Age greater than 65 is not a contraindication to surgery. In fact, recent survival data suggest these patients may do better than younger patients with similar disease. Operative deaths are decreasing and survival rates are improving, but most report 5-year survival rates of approximately 35% for patients undergoing the procedure (Table 3–19).

56. **A** page 104
Perren reviewed 77 cases of reticuloendothelial neoplasia of cervix or upper vagina and found that the most common clinical feature is vaginal bleeding (54%).

57. **D** page 84
Five landmark papers all reported significant improved survival for patients with cervical cancer when adjuvant chemotherapy is used in combination with radiation. The National Cancer Institute endorses this treatment.

58. **A** page 61
59. **B** page 61
60. **A** page 61

58–60. As described by Henriksen, the primary group of nodes involved in cervical cancer are the parametrial, paracervical, obturator, hypogastric (internal iliac), external iliac, and sacral nodes. The secondary group of nodes are the common iliac, inguinal, and periaortic nodes.

61. **A** page 56
This patient has a lesion that meets the criteria for microinvasive carcinoma of the cervix, as defined by the Society of Gynecologic Oncology. She has FIGO stage Ia_1. She could be treated with a conization (and close follow-up) or with a total hysterectomy.

62. **D** page 57
This lesion is a nonmicroinvasive FIGO stage Ia_2 cancer. The patient could be treated with a radical hysterectomy or with irradiation. Some authors prefer retroperitoneal lymphadenectomy and simple hysterectomy.

63. **C** page 57
The FIGO stage of this lesion is Ia_2. The patient should be treated with irradiation, since severe cardiac disease is a contraindication to surgery.

64. **D** page 86
The FIGO stage of this lesion is Ib_1. A cesarean section could be done, followed by radical hysterectomy or by irradiation.

65. **C** pages 69, 77
The FIGO stage of this lesion is IIb. The patient should be treated with irradiation, since surgery is contraindicated for stage IIb lesions.

66. **A** page 65
67. **A** page 65
68. **B** page 65
69. **C** page 65
70. **B** page 65
71. **D** page 65
72. **C** page 65
According to the new FIGO definition in 1994:
    a. Stage Ia_1 concerns lesions with stromal invasion up to 3 mm in depth and 7 mm in width. Stage Ia_2 concerns lesions with stromal invasion from 3.1 to 5 mm in depth and 7 mm in width.
    b. Lesions larger than these measurements are classified as Ib_1. A lesion localized to cervix and larger than 4 cm is classified as Ib_2. All gross lesions, even with superficial invasions, are classified Ib cancers.
    c. Survival of stages Ia_1 and Ia_2 approaches 99% and 97%, respectively. The incidence of lymph node metastasis is low (1% and 3%). Treatment is conservative: conization or simple hysterectomy.
73. **C** page 81
Point A, a dosimetry reference point usually associated with the Manchester method, is described as 2 cm superior to the lateral vaginal fornix and 2 cm lateral to the midline of the cervical canal. It is used to calculate dose to the parametrial tissues where the uterine artery approximates the ureter.
74. **E** page 83
All of the listed methods are intracavitary methods. Interstitial therapy involves insertion of radioactive material via direct penetration of tumor tissues.
75. **C** page 81
Point B is the reference point described as 3 cm lateral to point A. It is roughly analogous to, and used to calculate approximate dose to, the pelvic sidewall lymph nodes.
76. **C** page 81
The Manchester method, first described in 1938, is a combination of the two older techniques. The ovoids (colpostats) are adapted from the Paris method and the tandem is adapted from the Stockholm method. In most patients, adequate therapy and satisfactory morbidity occur with two placements. Since modified, it is the most widely used brachytherapy method in use for cervical cancer today.
77. **D** page 81
All are intracavitary methods of brachytherapy. They utilize preformed anatomic spaces in which to place radium or cesium applicators. Successful radiotherapy for cancer of the cervix involves a combination of brachytherapy techniques such as these, *plus* external beam radiotherapy.
78. **C** page 82
The Fletcher-Suit tandem and ovoids, commonly used for brachytherapy in the United States and Europe, are an afterloaded modification of the Manchester apparatus (Fig. 3–25).
79. **D** page 80
Radium was the first radioactive element used for therapy of cervical cancer, predating external beam radiotherapy by approximately 50 years. Each of the described methods originally used radium, although cesium seems to have identical antitumor effect and toxicity. Cesium is gaining favor because of its increased safety (does not emit radon gas), its improved handling (it is a metal rather than a powder), and storage/disposal and environmental concerns (markedly shorter half-life).
80. **D** page 80

chapter 4 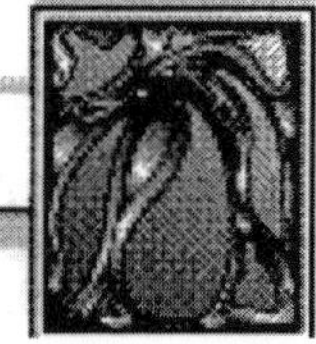

ENDOMETRIAL HYPERPLASIA/ESTROGEN THERAPY

KEY POINTS TO REMEMBER

- Endometrial hyperplasia results from prolonged, unopposed estrogenic stimulation of the endometrium.
- Anovulation and excessive endogenous or exogenous estrogens produce endometrial hyperplasia.
- Endometrial hyperplasia is classified as simple, complex, and atypical. Simple hyperplasia is characterized by a slight increase in the gland/stroma ratio with mild glandular crowding. Complex hyperplasia has more pronounced glandular crowding and complex glandular outlines. Atypical hyperplasia refers to significant glandular crowding with cytologic atypia. Cytologic atypia is the only important predictor of malignant potential and resistance to medical therapy.
- Simple and complex hyperplasias are more likely to be reversible with progestational therapy. They progress to carcinoma in 2% of cases. Atypical hyperplasia constitutes a significant risk for progression to carcinoma (8% to 29%).
- A symptom associated with hyperplasia or endometrial carcinoma is irregular or profuse uterine bleeding.
- Management of hyperplasia requires consideration of age of patient and type of hyperplasia: estrogen-progestin artificial cycles for the teenage girl and the childbearing woman, hysterectomy or progestin alone for the perimenopausal woman, hysterectomy for the postmenopausal woman. Resampling of the endometrium should be done every 3 to 6 months.
- Progesterone and synthetic progestins both have produced reversion of benign and atypical hyperplasia to an atrophic pattern. Their local effects are differentiation, maturation, secretion, epithelial metaplasia, and atrophy.
- Estrogen can be an etiologic agent in the pathogenesis of endometrial carcinoma (polycystic ovary syndrome/hormone-secreting tumors of ovary).
- In postmenopausal women, estrone makes up the largest amount of estrogen, resulting from the conversion of androstenedione. The postmenopausal ovary continues to secrete testosterone and androstenedione but almost no estrogen. The adrenal cortex is the almost unique source of plasma estradiol, estrone, progesterone, and 17-OH-progesterone, and the most important source of plasma dehydro–3-epiandrosterone. There is an increased incidence of endometrial cancer with the use of unopposed estrogen.
- Any risk associated with exogenous estrogen use can be abrogated by simultaneous progestin use.
- Six meta-analyses show no statistically significant increased risk of developing breast cancer with hormone replacement therapy (HRT). Mortality from all causes and mortality from breast cancer are reduced in estrogen replacement therapy (ERT) users compared with the rates in nonusers. Breast cancers in ERT users tend to be more well differentiated with a lower mitotic count, or S-phase fraction, and a smaller tumor size. This could be due to a direct estrogen receptor–mediated, growth-inhibitory effect of HRT on established breast tumors. A larger review of 51 studies worldwide, however, shows a very small increased risk of breast cancer in patients using HRT (0.6% in patients using HRT for 10 years).
- Estrogen replacement therapy is beneficial for women experiencing involuntary hot flashes, sweating, and symptoms attributable to atrophy of the vagina or urethra.
- There is an increased risk of deep venous thrombosis and pulmonary embolism in patients on HRT.
- Predominant evidence suggests that women who undergo postmenopausal HRT are at decreased risk for CHD (coronary heart disease). This benefit is limited to recent or current users. There is no net effect of HRT on recurrent CHD in women with CHD.
- HRT is beneficial for preventing and treating osteoporosis. Estrogen may inhibit osteoclast activity and increase proliferation of osteoblasts as well as collagen production.
- HRT may reduce the risk of colon and rectal cancer to 20%. Exogenous estrogen decreases secondary bile acid production, which may initiate or promote malignant changes in colonic epithelium. It also decreases serum levels of insulin-like growth factor–1, which is a mitogen for colorectal cancer.
- HRT may be given to patients with cancer of endometrium after total abdominal hysterectomy–bilateral salpingo-oophorectomy (TAH-BSO). Data reveal no trend in increased recurrence rate or poor outcome. The addition of progestin does not appear to be beneficial. HRT should be given within a few days after surgery.
- HRT can be given to breast cancer survivors to prevent ischemic heart disease and osteoporosis and to improve the quality of life, but the patient must be properly informed of the minimal risk of developing a new lesion.

No data indicate an increased risk of recurrent breast cancer in postmenopausal women receiving ERT.

- Estrogen therapy is begun with 0.625 mg of conjugated estrogen every day and cyclic progestin therapy (10 mg MPA) for 12 days, or with continuous estrogen-progestins (0.625 mg conjugated estrogen, 2.5 mg MPA). Daily ingestion of progestins relieves vasomotor symptoms in patients in whom estrogen is contraindicated.

QUESTIONS

Directions for Questions 1–28: Select the one best answer:

1. The most common cause of endometrial hyperplasia is:
   A. granulosa theca cell tumor
   B. Sertoli-Leydig cell tumor
   C. Anovulation
   D. Exogenous administered estrogens
2. The term *Swiss cheese hyperplasia* is equivalent to:
   A. simple hyperplasia
   B. complex hyperplasia
   C. atypical hyperplasia
   D. inactive endometrium with cystic changes
3. Correct statements concerning atypical adenomatous hyperplasia are the following *except:*
   A. it refers to the cytologic atypia in adenomatous hyperplasia
   B. these lesions have a great propensity for progression to adenocarcinoma
   C. they are often treated as carcinoma
   D. in case of severe atypical hyperplasia, the correct nomenclature is *carcinoma in situ*
4. The present classification of endometrial hyperplasia is the following:
   A. cystic hyperplasia, complex hyperplasia, and adenomatous hyperplasia
   B. adenomatous hyperplasia, complex hyperplasia, and atypical hyperplasia
   C. simple hyperplasia, complex hyperplasia, and atypical hyperplasia
   D. cystic hyperplasia, glandular hyperplasia, and adenomatous hyperplasia
5. Which is the most important predictor of malignant potential in endometrial hyperplasia?
   A. glandular crowding
   B. scarce stroma
   C. cytologic atypia
   D. glandular budding
6. Endometrial hyperplasia can be seen with the following ovarian tumors *except:*
   A. granulosa cell tumor
   B. theca cell tumor
   C. adrenal-like tumor
   D. polycystic ovary
7. Atypical endometrial cells detected in a Pap smear require the following evaluation:
   A. repeat Pap smear in 3 months
   B. colposcopy and endocervical curettage
   C. complete endometrial evaluation
   D. cervical biopsy and endocervical curettage
8. The risk of invasive cancer for patients with atypical hyperplasia is considered to be:
   A. 2%–5%
   B. 5%–10%
   C. 10%–30%
   D. 40%–50%
9. The morphologic feature that predicts the invasive potential in endometrial lesions is:
   A. crowding of glands
   B. budding of glands
   C. amount of necrosis
   D. cytologic atypia
10. Recommendations for therapy of endometrial hyperplasia are age dependent. The following statements about therapy are true *except:*
    A. the perimenopausal woman may be treated with surgery or progestins
    B. the postmenopausal woman should undergo hysterectomy unless strongly contraindicated
    C. hysterectomy is the treatment of choice for women of childbearing age
    D. the teenager should be treated with estrogen/progestin combinations
11. Statements regarding medical therapy of endometrial hyperplasia include all *except*:
    A. careful sampling of the endometrium is prerequisite
    B. medical induction of ovulation in women of childbearing age with endometrial hyperplasia is contraindicated
    C. progestins revert endometrial hyperplasia to an atrophic pattern a significant percentage of time
    D. use of progestins alone frequently results in irregular bleeding, anxiety, and noncompliance
12. Conditions associated with increased risk of development of hyperplasias and neoplasia of the endometrium include all *except:*
    A. endometriosis
    B. polycystic ovary syndrome
    C. obesity
    D. delayed menopause
13. The following statements regarding studies of the relationship between estrogen and endometrial cancer are true *except:*
    A. progestin use clearly seems to reduce the risk of developing endometrial cancer from estrogen use
    B. the major weakness in studies determining relative risk of estrogen users is that they are retrospective case-control studies
    C. population-based studies demonstrate rising endometrial cancer rates even in the absence of frequent estrogen use
    D. prospective blind studies implicated prolonged exogenous noninterrupted estrogen replacement as a causative factor for endometrial cancer
14. True statements regarding postmenopausal sex hormone production include all *except*:
    A. endometrial cancer patients seem to have higher levels of estrone than those without cancer
    B. the postmenopausal ovary produces a large proportion of total serum testosterone

C. postmenopausal endogenous estrogens and progestins originate from the adrenal cortex
D. adipose tissue converts androstenedione to estradiol

15. After menopause, most of the estrogens are derived from:
A. the ovary
B. peripheral conversions of testosterone from the ovary
C. peripheral conversion of androgens of adrenal origin
D. the adrenals

16. The use of current preparations of oral contraceptives has been associated with:
A. an increase in the incidence of breast cancer
B. an increase in the incidence of endometrial carcinoma
C. a 50% reduction in the incidence of endometrial carcinoma
D. an increase in the incidence of ovarian cancer

17. How many days of progestational therapy each month can eliminate adenomatous hyperplasia?
A. 6 to 8 days
B. 8 to 10 days
C. 10 to 12 days
D. 12 to 14 days

18. Concerning HRT and colorectal cancer, the following are true *except:*
A. there is a 20% decrease in risk of colon cancers in HRT users
B. there is also a decrease of 19% in rectal cancer
C. HRT acts by decreasing the production of bile acids
D. HRT increases serum level of insulin-like growth factor-1

19. The following statements concerning the use of estrogen replacement therapy (ERT) in postmenopausal women are true *except:*
A. ERT is beneficial for women having hot flashes and sweating
B. ERT raises blood pressure
C. ERT protects against heart disease
D. ERT prevents osteoporosis

20. Concerning ERT in patients with endometrial cancer, the following are true *except:*
A. ERT relieves symptoms of iatrogenic menopause
B. ERT should be given with progestin
C. many physicians feel more comfortable prescribing ERT for low-risk categories of endometrial carcinoma
D. there should always be a free hiatus of 2 years between therapy for endometrial carcinoma and the commencement of ERT

21. Surveillance of patients receiving exogenous estrogens consists of:
A. blood pressure measurements
B. breast and pelvic examinations
C. endometrial biopsy in case of abnormal bleeding
D. all of the above

22. Concerning estrogens and breast cancer, the following is true:
A. conclusive evidence exists that there is an increased risk of breast carcinoma in postmenopausal women taking estrogens
B. combined with estrogens, progestin may not provide protection against mammary malignancy
C. the use of estrogen with progestin is associated with an increased risk of breast cancer in middle-aged women
D. estrogens do not significantly increase the risk of breast cancer, and progestin may provide additional protection against breast cancer

23. The following are true concerning HRT *except*:
A. it effectively diminishes the risk of cardiovascular disease in 50- to 60-year-old women
B. it decreases HDL and increases LDL
C. it does not raise blood pressure
D. it has not been associated with increased incidence of stroke

24. In the 10-year double-blind study by Nachtigall to compare the effects of HRT on 84 postmenopausal patients and controls, the following results are found *except:*
A. improvement or no increase in osteoporosis
B. no difference in the incidence of myocardial infarction or uterine cancer
C. decreased incidence of cholelithiasis
D. lower incidence of breast cancer

25. The UCI study on HRT for patients with early stage endometrial carcinoma concluded that:
A. there is no increased recurrence rate
B. there is no increase in poor outcome
C. progestin should be given
D. all of the above

26. The authors suggest the use of HRT in breast cancer survivors because of the following reasons:
A. freedom from recurrent breast cancer can never be guaranteed without HRT
B. HRT prevents ischemic heart disease and osteoporosis
C. HRT provides relief of menopausal symptoms and improves the quality of life
D. all of the above

27. The estrogen that makes up the largest amount in a postmenopausal woman is:
A. estrone
B. estradiol
C. estriol
D. ethinylestradiol

28. Which hormone(s) is/are secreted by the postmenopausal ovary:
A. estradiol
B. estrone and progesterone
C. testosterone and androstenedione
D. 17-OH-progesterone

Directions for Questions 28–31: Match the types of endometrial hyperplasia (Fig. 4–1A–C) with their malignant potential.

29. No premalignant potential
30. 2% will progress to carcinoma
31. 29% will progress to carcinoma

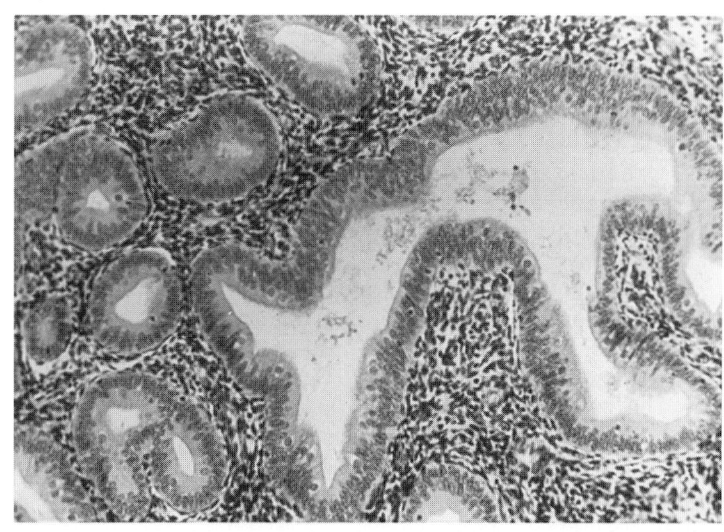

A

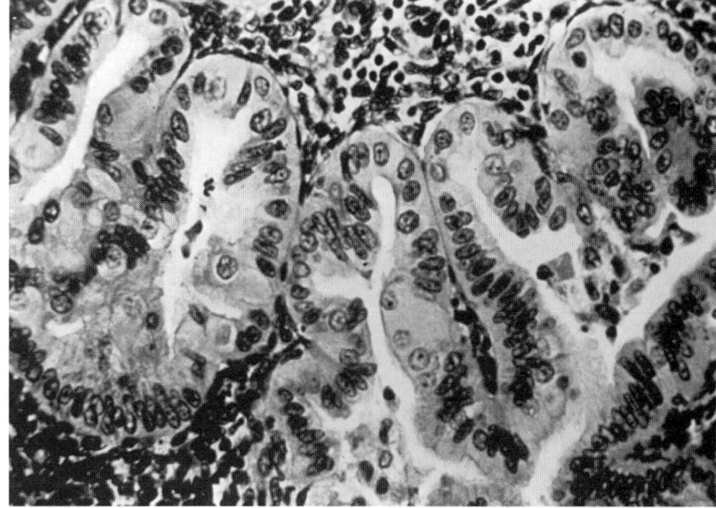

B

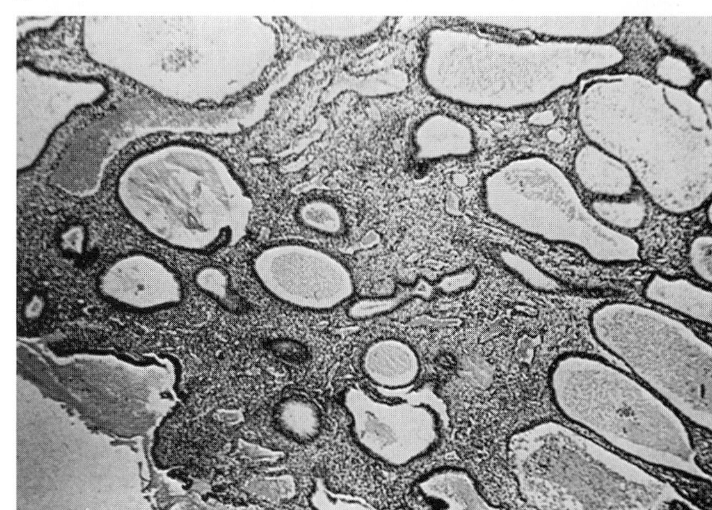

C

FIGURE 4–1.

ANSWERS

1. **C** page 113
Hyperplasia may result from exogenously administered estrogens or excessive estrogen produced by granulosa theca cell tumor, but the most common cause of hyperplasia is a succession of anovulatory cycles in teenage patients or in middle-aged perimenopausal patients. Sertoli-Leydig cell tumor produces testosterone and not estrogens.
2. **D** page 114
Swiss cheese hyperplasia describes inactive endometrium with cystic changes often observed in the endometrium of some menopausal women. It has no premalignant potential. This term is rarely used today.
3. **D** page 114
The term *carcinoma in situ* of the endometrium coined by Hertig is no longer used because it has no clinical implication different from *severe atypical hyperplasia*, which is the preferred term.
4. **C** page 114
The present classification suggested by the International Society of Gynecological Pathologists is simple hyperplasia, complex hyperplasia, and atypical hyperplasia. Endometrial hyperplasia without cellular atypia is classified as simple or complex hyperplasia, depending on the extent of glandular complexity and crowding. Endometrial hyperplasia with cellular atypia is classified as atypical hyperplasia, which can be mild, moderate, or severe.
5. **C** page 115
Cellular atypia is the important factor for distinguishing atypical hyperplasia from simple and complex hyperplasia. Whereas the malignant potentials of simple and complex hyperplasias are around 2%, the malignant potential of atypical hyperplasia is 8% to 29%.
6. **C** page 115
All listed ovarian tumors secrete estrogens except the adrenal-like tumor, which secretes testosterone.
7. **C** page 116
The finding of atypical endometrial cells requires a complete endometrial evaluation consisting of endometrial biopsy and/or hysteroscopy. Cherkis, studying 177 Pap smears with atypical endometrial cells, found adenocarcinoma, endometrial hyperplasia, and endometrial polyps in 20%, 11%, and 10% of the cases, respectively.
8. **C** page 115
The risk of progression of atypical hyperplasia to adenocarcinoma is considered to be 8% to 29% and the process may take 5 years or more. Only 2% of patients with nonatypical hyperplasia (simple or complex) progress to carcinoma.
9. **D** page 115
Only cytologic atypia is the important morphologic feature that distinguishes the simple and complex hyperplasias from atypical hyperplasia. The latter lesion is a precursor of endometrial carcinoma.
10. **C** page 18
In women of childbearing age, except for those with severely atypical hyperplasia, progestins or ovulation-inducing agents are the therapy of choice.
11. **B** page 118
Ovulation induction is an alternative to progestins in the medical management of endometrial hyperplasia. Careful sampling of the endometrium is a requisite, since a significant proportion of invasive cancers are not successfully diagnosed by simple biopsy alone.
12. **A** page 119, Table 4–3
Other conditions associated with endometrial neoplasia include family history, other neoplasms (breast, ovary), estrogen-secreting neoplasms (adrenal tumors, granulosa cell tumors, thecomas, and others), and unopposed exogenous estrogens in menopause.
13. **D** page 119
Prospective studies relating estrogen use to endometrial neoplasia have not been reported. In view of strong retrospective evidence implicating estrogen as a causative factor, such a study may be unethical. The retrospective evidence is from case-control studies, many of which have a large control selection bias.
14. **D** page 120
Androstenedione, which originates from the adrenal gland and the ovary, is converted to estrone in peripheral tissues, including adipose tissue.
15. **C** page 120
After menopause, most of the estrogens (estrone) are derived from peripheral conversion of androgens of adrenal origin (androstenedione) with only a small contribution by the ovary.
16. **C** page 121
The development of endometrial carcinoma has been associated with sequential OCAs, which were withdrawn from the market. Currently available combination preparations are associated with a 50% reduction in the incidence of endometrial carcinoma compared with the incidence in nonusers.
17. **D** page 121
It has been demonstrated that 12 to 14 days of progestational therapy each month can eliminate adenomatous hyperplasia.
18. **D** page 128
HRT decreases growth factor-1, which is an important mitogen associated with colon cancer.
19. **B** page 126
Unlike the effect of OCs in younger women, ERT among postmenopausal women does not raise blood pressure. There is also no increased incidence of stroke or cancer of the breast.
20. **D** page 129
ERT relieves symptoms of iatrogenic menopause: vaginal dryness, osteoporosis, insomnia, hot flushes, and so on. DiSaia and Creasman recommend the use of estrogen and progestin for replacement therapy in patients having endometrial carcinoma. For several years, they used only estrogen and noticed no difference in outcome. Many physicians prefer to give ERT to patients within low-risk categories of endometrial carcinoma, but these well-differentiated lesions are potentially most sensitive to the hormone manipulative therapy. The high-grade lesions that are most likely to recur are unlikely to respond to

exogenous estrogen or progesterone. There seems to be no consistent line of reasoning separating good candidates from poor candidates for this regimen.

The interval of 2 years between therapy and commencement of ERT is controversial. The data currently suggest no benefit in waiting. Eighty to ninety percent of all endometrial recurrences occur in the first 2 years after therapy. If the physician believes that waiting 2 years is necessary because of the adverse effect of estrogens, it seems illogical to submit the remaining 10% to 20% of patients to that increased risk, which can continue for 5 to 10 years. In 1990, ACOG recommended that estrogens could be used in women with a history of endometrial cancer for the same indication as for any woman but left the decision to the patient and her physician.

21. **D** page 132, Table 4–13
All the examinations should be performed every 12 months. The monitoring of blood pressure is of questionable value.
22. **D** page 123
Many studies indicate that menopausal estrogens neither protect against nor increase the risk of breast cancer. A 10-year double-blind study by Nachtigall detected 4 breast cancers in 84 placebo users and none in the 84 estrogen-progestin users. Progestin may provide additional protection against breast cancer as in endometrial cancer. Other studies (Stanford, 1995) confirmed that the use of estrogen with progestin does not appear to be associated with an increased risk of breast cancer in middle-aged women. Six meta-analyses of numerous studies concluded no or only a slight risk with prolonged use (15 years). Mortality rates of women taking estrogens at the time of breast cancer diagnosis are improved because of a low frequency of late-stage disease and better differentiated tumors.
23. **B** page 124
HRT increases HDL and decreases LDL, leading to a reduced risk in cardiovascular disease.
24. **C** page 127
Estrogen-treated patients had a higher incidence of cholelithiasis.
25. **D** page 129
In the UCI study, the authors recommended 0.625 mg of conjugated estrogens and 2.5 mg MPA and no hiatus between initial therapy and commencement of HRT. There should be good communication between physician and patient to understand the benefits/risk ratio.
26. **D** page 130
There is always a minimal risk of developing a new lesion in remaining breast tissue. The breast cancer survivor should be aware of the beneficial effects of HRT and should make her decision with her physician. The authors urge the abandonment of the practice of prohibiting the use of HRT in breast cancer survivors.
27. **A** page 120
Estrone, which makes up the largest amount of estrogen produced in the postmenopausal woman, is a result of peripheral conversion of androstenedione. There appears to be a greater conversion of androstenedione to estrone in endometrial cancer patients compared with healthy postmenopausal woman.
28. **C** page 120
The postmenopausal ovary continues to secrete substantial amounts of testosterone and androstenedione but virtually no estrogen. After menopause most of the estrogens are derived from peripheral conversion of androgens of adrenal origin with only a small contribution by the ovary.
29. **C** page 115
30. **A** page 115
31. **B** page 115
Inactive endometrium (**C**) has no propensity to degenerate into malignancy. According to a study of 170 patients by Kurman, 2% of patients with nonatypical simple or adenomatous hyperplasia (**A**) and 29% of women with atypical hyperplasia (**B**) progressed to carcinoma.

chapter 5 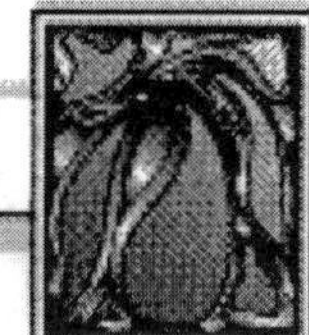

ADENOCARCINOMA of the UTERUS

Key Points to Remember

- Adenocarcinoma of the uterus is the most common gynecologic cancer and the fourth most common cancer in women. In 2000, approximately 361,000 women developed uterine cancer, with 6500 deaths.
- The median age for adenocarcinoma of the uterus is 61 years, with the largest number of patients between 50 and 59 years. Twenty to twenty-five percent will be diagnosed before menopause.
- Oral contraceptives and smoking reduce the risk of endometrial cancer.
- Factors associated with endometrial cancer are obesity, nulliparity, and late menopause. Diabetes and hypertension are often associated with endometrial cancer. Increased intake of ascorbic acid and beta-carotene (vegetables, fruits) is associated with a low risk of endometrial cancer.
- The relationship of endometrial cancer to unopposed estrogen is well documented. The addition of a progestin appears to be protective.
- Women on estrogens who develop endometrial cancer have a more favorable prognosis: lower stage and lower histologic grade. Survival is also better.
- Black women have a higher proportion of aggressive histologic types (clear cell, papillary serous) and a lower survival than white women. The reasons for these differences are unexplained.
- In the NSABP study, the benefit from tamoxifen is apparent: 121.3 fewer breast-related events per 1000 women treated with tamoxifen compared with 6.3 endometrial cancers per 1000 women.
- Patients taking tamoxifen have a higher incidence of endometrial thickness and endometrial polyps (megapolyps up to 12 cm). Tamoxifen-related endometrial cancers carry the same prognosis as the nontamoxifen group.
- Yearly endometrial sampling or ultrasound evaluation of patients receiving tamoxifen is not recommended at the present time.
- Postmenopausal bleeding, perimenopausal abnormal bleeding, and prolonged intermenstrual bleeding in obese young patients should be evaluated by endometrial biopsy to rule out malignancy. Routine use of endometrial biopsy as an office procedure is the first step for diagnosis because its accuracy is 90%. If it is negative, hysteroscopy is preferred.
- Measurement of endometrial stripe by US using the cutoff at 5 mm has a positive predictive value of 87% with specificity of 96% and sensitivity of 100% for endometrial abnormalities. US should not be used for evaluating endometrial thickness in women taking tamoxifen.
- Staging of endometrial carcinoma is surgical pathologic; 75% of patients present with stage I disease.
- Stage I: uterus; Ia: endometrium; Ib: less than one-half myometrium; Ic: more than one-half myometrium. Stage II: uterus and cervix; IIa: endocervical glandular involvement; IIb: stromal invasion. Stage III: serosa, adnexa, vagina, positive peritoneal cytology and positive pelvic or para-aortic nodes; IIIa: serosa, adnexa or positive cytology; IIIb: vaginal metastases; IIIc: metastases to pelvic or para-aortic nodes. Stage IV: bladder, bowel, or distant metastases; IVa: bladder or bowel mucosa; IVb: distant metastases.
- Grades: 1: well differentiated; 2: moderately differentiated; 3: poorly differentiated.
- Prognostic factors include histologic type (pathology), histologic differentiation, stage of disease, myometrial invasion, peritoneal cytology, lymph node metastasis, and adnexal metastasis.
- The most frequent histologic type is endometrioid adenocarcinoma (87%). Differentiation of adenocarcinoma (grades 1 to 3) is prognostically important. In adenocarcinoma with squamous differentiation, the differentiation of the squamous component is closely correlated with the differentiation of the glandular element, and the glandular element is a better predictor of outcome.
- Uterine papillary serous tumor is a highly aggressive carcinoma with early extrauterine disease and frequent lymph node metastasis. Five-year survival is around 23%. Clear cell carcinoma also has a worse prognosis, with 5-year survival around 44%.
- Recurrences correlate with grade of tumor, depth of invasion, location of tumor within the uterus, adnexal disease, cytology, and lymph node metastasis.
- Degree of histologic differentiation: recurrences in grade 1 occur in 4%, compared with 15% and 41% in grades 2 and 3, respectively. Survival in stage I is 92% in grade 1, compared with 87% and 74% in grades 2 and 3.
- The degree of myometrial invasion is a consistent indicator of tumor virulence. Positive peritoneal cytology is associated with decreased survival and progression-free interval. Patients with stage I disease have 10% of positive pelvic nodes and 5% of positive periaortic nodes. Occult metastases to the ovary occur in 10% of patients.
- Molecular biologic indices (DNA, ploidy, S-phase fraction, proliferative index, *HER2/neu* and *P53* gene

overexpression) are important prognostic factors, but they need standardization for clinical use.

- Capillary-like space involvement (CLS), tumor size, progesterone receptor–positive are also independent prognostic factors. There is a greater propensity for lymph node metastasis when disease is present in the lower uterine segment or in the cervix than when disease is limited to the fundus.
- The vaginal vault is not at high risk for recurrence and does not require radium or cesium treatment after surgery.
- In the GOG pilot study, only 25% of patients were determined to be at high risk and to require additional therapy. Seven percent of patients with intrauterine disease developed recurrences compared with 43% with extrauterine disease. With disease limited to the uterus, there is increased risk of recurrence if there are myometrial invasion, VIS, or positive washings.
- From surgical staging studies, one fourth of patients with clinical stage I have disease outside the uterus and only 24% of clinical stage II patients have disease in the cervix. Surgical staging accurately identifies the true extent of disease.
- Treatment of stage I, grade 1, endometrial carcinoma is extrafascial total abdominal hysterectomy and bilateral salpingo-oophorectomy (TAH-BSO) and peritoneal cytologic examination. If extensive disease is present in the uterus or outside the uterus, appropriate radiation, progestin, and/or chemotherapy are given.
- Preoperative radiotherapy appears to be of no benefit.
- Pelvic and periaortic node dissection should be added to TAH-BSO in case of deep myometrial invasion (> one third) and grades 2 and 3.
- Patients with stage I, grade 1 or 2 disease had 4% recurrence; those with grade 3 had 14% recurrence, all of the latter at distant sites.
- Postoperative irradiation should be considered in patients with deep myometrial invasion, grade 3 disease, positive nodes, positive surgical margins, and extrauterine disease.
- Simple TAH-BSO and pelvic and para-aortic lymphadenectomy may be adequate therapy for stage II disease (uterus and cervix). Postoperative irradiation is given depending on surgical pathologic findings.
- The benefit of lymphadenectomy is apparent; it is therapeutic, and survival appears to be improved. Patients undergoing multiple-site lymphadenectomy had a better survival rate than patients not undergoing lymphadenectomy (P = .0002). Patients in both low-risk and high-risk categories who had lymphadenectomies and no postoperative irradiation have a survival better than that of similar patients without lymphadenectomy but who received radiation therapy.
- Vaginal hysterectomy may be used for grade 1 endometrial carcinoma. It also can be performed in obese and poor surgical risk patients. Survival rates are comparable to those of the abdominal approach.
- Treatment of stage III or IV disease must be individualized: hormonal treatment or chemotherapy may be added to surgery and radiation.
- Recurrences in vaginal vault can be treated successfully with surgery, radiation therapy, or a combination of the two. Recurrences outside the vagina are treated with hormone therapy or chemotherapy.
- Prophylactic progestins for preventing recurrences are not of benefit to patients. Concerning progestin therapy, grade 1 lesions respond more frequently than poorly differentiated carcinomas. One third of patients with recurrent cancer have a positive receptor site to both estrogen and progesterone. Forty to ninety percent of receptor-positive respond to hormonotherapy compared with only 17% receptor negative. Progestin therapy may be administered in the form of DepoProvera, oral Provera, and megestrol acetate (Megace). GnRH and tamoxifen have been studied.
- Chemotherapy of metastatic disease with doxorubicin, cisplatin, and other cytotoxic drugs has a low response rate. Low estrogen or progesterone receptor values had a significantly greater response to combined cytotoxic therapy. With doxorubicin, only 10% of patients had a complete response rate lasting 7 months. With cisplatin, the mean duration of remission was 5 months. Total response was 22% for doxorubicin and 30% for doxorubicin and cyclophosphamide, with a median survival of 7 months in a GOG prospective study.
- Monitoring CA-125 levels of patients with advanced or recurrent disease may be helpful.
- Survival of patients with simultaneous endometrioid endometrial and ovarian carcinomas is excellent. This suggests that these patients have separate stage I primary tumors rather than a stage III metastatic endometrial carcinoma.
- Uterine papillary serous carcinoma is a highly aggressive carcinoma with a 5-year survival rate of 23%. Treatment should be intense in stage I with radical hysterectomy, bilateral pelvic lymphadenectomy, adjuvant pelvic irradiation, and four courses of cisplatin and epirubicin (Rosenberg regimen).
- Five-year survival for endometrial cancer.

Stage	a (%)	b (%)	c (%)
I	91	88	81
II	77	67	—
III	60	41	32
IV	20	5	—

- For stage I endometrial carcinoma, survival for grade 1 is 92%; grade 2, 87%; and grade 3, 74%.

QUESTIONS

Directions for Questions 1–37: Select the one best answer.

1. The most common gynecologic malignancy in American women is:
   A. ovarian cancer
   B. endometrial cancer
   C. cervical cancer
   D. vulvar cancer
2. Approximately what percentage of women will have endometrial adenocarcinoma before menopause?
   A. 5%–10%
   B. 10%–15%

C. 15%–20%
D. 20%–25%

3. Risk factors associated with endometrial cancer include the following *except:*
   A. obesity
   B. nulliparity
   C. late menopause
   D. DES exposure
4. The following are true concerning endometrial cancer *except:*
   A. the use of oral contraceptives decreases the risk of developing endometrial cancer
   B. cigarette smoking increases the risk of developing endometrial cancer
   C. diabetes mellitus and hypertension are frequently associated with endometrial cancer
   D. nulliparity, obesity, and late menopause are endometrial cancer risk factors
5. Upper body fat localization is a significant risk factor for endometrial cancer. The following findings are true *except:*
   A. women whose weight exceeds 78 kg have a 2.3 times risk of those weighing less than 58 kg
   B. upper body obesity (waist-to-height ratio) is a risk independent of body weight
   C. amount of body fat is associated with increased circulating levels of progesterone and sex hormone–binding proteins
   D. there is a strong inverse association between sitting height and risk of endometrial cancer
6. The following are true concerning estrogen users who develop endometrial carcinoma *except:*
   A. they have very favorable prognostic factors
   B. stage of disease and histologic grade are low
   C. clear cell carcinoma and adenosquamous carcinoma are frequent
   D. survival of estrogen-related endometrial cancer is much better than nonestrogen cancers
7. The first diagnostic step in a postmenopausal woman with uterine bleeding should be:
   A. Pap smear
   B. endometrial biopsy
   C. hysteroscopy
   D. endocervical curettage
8. The following is true concerning tamoxifen and endometrial cancer *except:*
   A. tamoxifen is being used in women with breast cancer as treatment and prophylaxis
   B. several cases of endometrial cancer and sarcomas have been reported in women taking tamoxifen
   C. tamoxifen, an antiestrogen, has some protection from osteoporosis and heart disease
   D. women taking tamoxifen are at higher risk for endometrial cancer
9. The following are true concerning tamoxifen and endometrial cancer *except:*
   A. there is a relationship between tamoxifen and adenocarcinomas of the endometrium
   B. the benefit from tamoxifen is apparent
   C. there is no increase in poor prognostic histology or tumor differentiation, compared with nontamoxifen endometrial carcinoma
   D. patients on tamoxifen should have a yearly sampling of the endometrium
10. A patient with endometrial carcinoma involving the cervical mucosa should be staged as:
    A. IIa
    B. IIb
    C. Ia
    D. III
11. Lymph node metastasis is high in patients with stage II endometrial carcinoma. According to a GOG study, the incidence of aortic node metastases in patients with cervical stromal invasion is:
    A. 0%
    B. 5%
    C. 10%
    D. 20%
12. Among the following molecular indices, which is the most independent prognosis factor concerning recurrences and cancer-related death in endometrial carcinoma?
    A. proliferative index
    B. S-phase fraction
    C. nondiploid pattern
    D. each of the above
13. What is the percentage of patients with clinical stage II endometrial carcinomas who have in fact surgical stage II?
    A. 10%
    B. 15%
    C. 20%
    D. 25%
14. A carcinoma that is confined to the corpus and has invaded more than half of the myometrium is staged as:
    A. IIa
    B. Ia
    C. Ib
    D. Ic
15. A tumor is limited to the endometrium. Histology shows adenocarcinoma with approximately 25% solid growth pattern. What is the stage and grade?
    A. Stage Ia grade 1
    B. Stage Ia grade 2
    C. Stage Ib grade 3
    D. Stage Ic grade 1
16. Which is the most frequently encountered stage of endometrial carcinoma?
    A. I
    B. II
    C. III
    D. IV
17. Prognostic factors in endometrial carcinoma include the following *except:*
    A. histologic type and differentiation
    B. stage of disease
    C. uterine size
    D. myometrial invasion and peritoneal cytology
18. Which is the most common histologic subtype in endometrial carcinoma?
    A. endometrioid adenocarcinoma
    B. adenoacanthoma

C. adenosquamous carcinoma
D. papillary adenocarcinoma

19. Which histologic subtype of endometrial carcinoma has the lowest 5-year survival?
A. adenoacanthoma
B. adenosquamous carcinoma
C. endometrioid carcinoma
D. clear cell carcinoma

20. Concerning histologic differentiation in endometrial cancer, the following are true *except:*
A. histologic differentiation is one of the most sensitive indicators of prognosis
B. as the tumor loses its differentiation, the chance of survival decreases
C. as the tumor becomes less differentiated, the chances of deep myometrial involvement increase
D. there is always a relationship between deep myometrial invasion and undifferentiated tumor

21. When the tumor is localized to the uterus, the following is/are true:
A. a tumor in the lower uterine segment has a higher incidence of pelvic metastases
B. a tumor in the lower uterine segment has a higher incidence of periaortic nodal metastases
C. stromal invasion of the cervix predicts a lower survival rate
D. all of the above

22. The following statements concerning peritoneal cytology and early-stage endometrial cancer are true *except:*
A. 2% of patients with negative cytologic test results develop recurrence
B. 5%–15% of patients will have positive peritoneal cytologic test results
C. 25%–30% of patients with positive cytologic test results have concomitant regional metastases
D. 30%–35% of patients with positive cytologic test results develop recurrence

23. The following statements referring to lymph node metastasis and endometrial cancer are true *except:*
A. 10% of patients with clinical stage I disease have pelvic lymph node metastasis
B. recurrence rates are significantly higher for patients with periaortic lymph nodes metastasis than for patients with pelvic lymph nodes metastasis only
C. 10% of patients with clinical stage I disease have periaortic lymph node metastasis
D. 35% of patients with clinical stage II disease have pelvic nodal metastasis

24. Of the following, one is *not* a poor prognostic factor:
A. adnexal metastasis
B. capillary-like space involvement
C. DNA euploidy
D. poor differentiation of tumor

25. True statements regarding therapy of the patient having endometrial cancer with one or more poor prognostic factors include all *except:*
A. the patient with low-stage disease and positive pelvic washings should be offered intraperitoneal ^{32}P
B. the majority of post-treatment recurrences occur outside the treated field external beam
C. radiotherapy should be administered in most cases
D. preoperative or postoperative radium or cesium brachytherapy should be administered in most cases

26. The following statements regarding radiotherapy and stage I endometrial cancer are true *except:*
A. vaginal vault recurrence negatively affects survival
B. irradiation of poorly differentiated tumors and superficial disease has minimal effect on survival
C. irradiation of deeply invasive tumors probably has minimal survival advantage
D. radiotherapy should be offered to the patient with nodal or other localized extrauterine disease

27. Suggested treatment for stage I adenocarcinoma of the endometrium is the following *except:*
A. for patients with stage I grade 1 tumor, surgery can be limited to TAH-BSO and peritoneal cytologic examination
B. patients with stage I grades 2 and 3 disease should have TAH-BSO, peritoneal cytologic tests, and pelvic and periaortic lymph node sampling
C. in patients with grade 3 disease and significant muscle involvement, postoperative irradiation or adjunctive progestins or chemotherapy should be considered
D. the hysterectomy should be intrafascial with removal of the upper vagina

28. Therapy for stage II carcinoma of the endometrium is the following *except:*
A. simple TAH-BSO, pelvic and periaortic lymphadenectomy
B. postoperative radiation therapy can be planned depending on surgical pathologic findings
C. if disease is limited to the uterus, postoperative radiation may not be necessary
D. adjunctive chemotherapy with doxorubicin decreases the incidence of recurrences

29. In stage II adenocarcinoma of the endometrium, surgery should be performed before radiation for the following reasons *except:*
A. radiation may not be needed
B. postoperative is as effective as preoperative irradiation therapy
C. if endocervical disease is found, radiation should always be given
D. "floaters" in the endocervical curettage specimen may be misconstrued as invasion of the cervix, which is not confirmed by histologic examination of the specimen

30. Recurrences of endometrial carcinoma are treated with:
A. surgery
B. radiation and surgery
C. hormones or chemotherapy
D. all of the above

31. The true statement concerning the use of progestins in recurrent adenocarcinoma of the uterus is:
A. progestins prevent recurrences
B. grade 3 recurrent tumor responds better than grade 1 tumor
C. progesterone receptor positive tumors are more hormonally responsive than progesterone receptor–negative tumors

D. median survival of responders to progestin therapy is 5 years

32. Progestin therapy for recurrent endometrial adenocarcinoma may be administered as:
A. DepoProvera
B. oral medroxyprogesterone (Provera)
C. megestrol acetate (Megace)
D. all of the above

33. Concerning the use of tamoxifen (TAM) in recurrent endometrial carcinoma, the following are true *except:*
A. TAM binds estrogen receptors and thereby blocks the access of estrogen into the nucleus
B. TAM can increase the number of progesterone receptors in vivo
C. TAM may induce endometrial cancer in some patients
D. the response rate to TAM is approximately 50%

34. Concerning chemotherapy of recurrent endometrial carcinoma, the following is true:
A. doxorubicin alone is the most effective agent
B. combination therapy is more effective
C. tumors with low estrogen or progesterone receptors have a higher response rate
D. the ideal therapeutic agent has not been found

35. Concerning simultaneous malignancies of the ovary and uterus, the following are true *except:*
A. ovarian involvement in endometrial cancer varies between 15% and 40%
B. in approximately one third of cases of endometrioid carcinoma of the ovary, endometrial carcinoma is also found
C. if metastasis is present, it is more common to go from the endometrium to the ovary rather than from the ovary to the endometrium
D. most common tumors are of the clear cell type

36. Concerning vaginal hysterectomy in adenocarcinoma of the uterus, the following are true *except*:
A. it may be used in all stages
B. it may be used in obese patients
C. it may be used in poor surgical risk patients
D. 5-year survival is around 90%

37. Surgical staging of endometrial carcinoma is very important because of the following reasons *except*:
A. it can more accurately identify the true extent of the disease
B. implications for therapy are great to prevent unnecessary treatment and to direct appropriate therapy
C. in clinical stage I disease, one fourth will have disease outside the uterus
D. in patients thought to have stage II disease, as many as 25% will have either less than stage II or extrauterine disease

Directions for Questions 38–50: For each numbered item, select the letter of the most appropriate answer. Each letter may be used once, more than once, or not at all.

38 – 42. Match the prognosis with the findings:
A. good prognosis
B. poor prognosis
C. unknown
D. neither (neutral)

38. Progesterone receptor positivity
39. Estrogen receptor positivity
40. Tumor size, <2 cm
41. Capillary-like space involvement
42. DNA aneuploidy

43–46. Match the stages of endometrial carcinoma
A. Stage Ib
B. Stage IIa
C. Stage IIb
D. Stage IIIb

43. Vaginal metastases
44. Invasion of less than half of myometrium
45. Cervical stromal invasion
46. Endocervical glandular involvement only

47–50. Match the letters (Figure Part **A, B,** or **C**) with the numbers (Fig. 5–1)

47. Highest estrogen and progesterone receptors contents
48. Highest probability of positive pelvic and aortic nodes
49. Surgery only
50. Surgery and irradiation

Answers

1. **B** page 137
Cancer of the uterine corpus is the most common gynecologic malignancy seen in American women today. It is the fourth most common cancer in women. It is three times more common than cancer of the cervix and 1.5 times more common than carcinoma of the ovary. It is one sixth as common as carcinoma of the breast.

2. **D** page 137
The median age of patients with carcinoma of the uterine corpus is 61 years with the largest number between 50 and 59 years. Twenty to twenty-five percent will be diagnosed before menopause.

3. **D** page 138
DES exposure is associated with adenosis and clear cell adenocarcinoma of the vagina and cervix. If a patient is nulliparous, obese, and reaches menopause at age 52 or later, there appears to be a fivefold increase in the risk of endometrial cancer over the patient who does not fulfill these criteria. Also upper body fat localization, which is related to lower serum hormone–bound globulin and higher endogenous production of non–protein-bound estradiol, is a risk factor for endometrial cancer.

4. **B** page 138
Cigarette smoking apparently decreases the risk of developing endometrial cancer. The greatest reduction in risk by smoking was in the heaviest women, but this advantage is outweighed by the increased risk of lung and cervical cancer and other major health hazards associated with cigarette smoking.

5. **C** page 138
The amount of body fat has been associated with decreased circulating levels of progesterone and sex hormone–binding proteins. With lower SHBP there is a higher endogenous production of non–protein-bound estradiol.

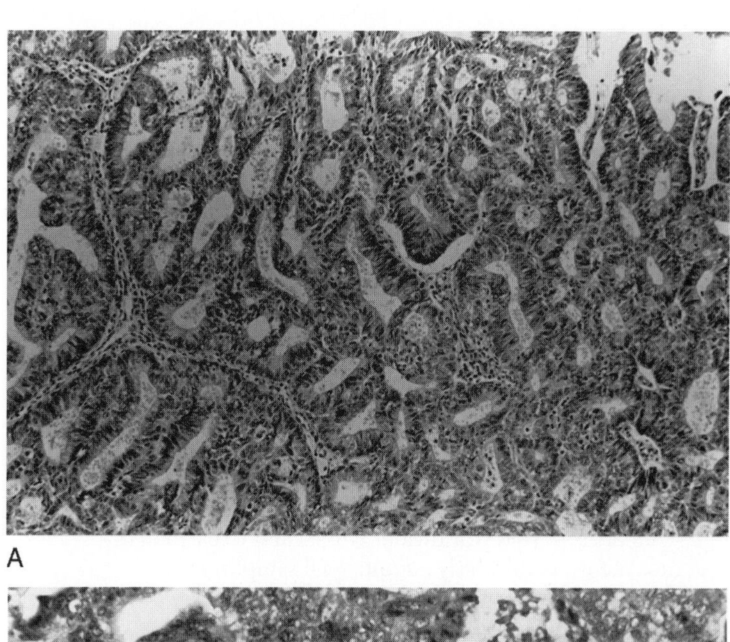

A

B

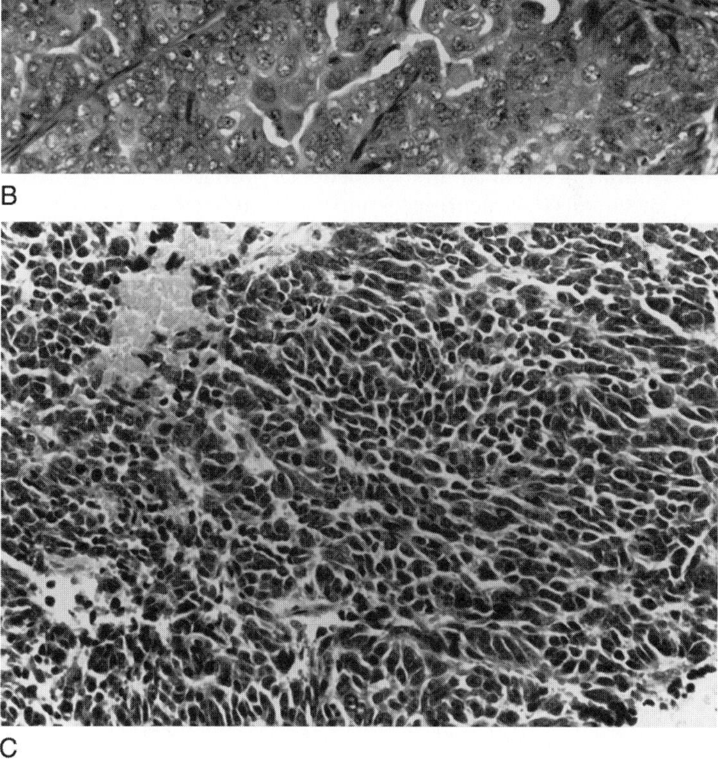

C

FIGURE 5–1. (Courtesy Dr. Gregory Spiegel.)

6. **C** page 139
   The poor prognostic histologic subtypes of endometrial adenocarcinomas such as clear cell carcinoma and adenosquamous carcinoma appear less frequently in estrogen users. Several studies also suggest that risk factors such as nulliparity and obesity are lower in estrogen users.

7. **B** page 141
Many endometrial carcinomas can be detected with office biopsy. If that result is negative and further evaluation is needed, hysteroscopy is advisable. Cytologic detection of endometrial cancer by Pap smear has been poor.
8. **D** page 140
The NSABP study suggests there may be a relative risk of 2.3 women developing endometrial cancer while on tamoxifen. However, the benefit of tamoxifen is apparent, considering there are 121.3 fewer breast-related events per 1000 women treated with tamoxifen compared with 6.3 endometrial cancers per 1000 women.
9. **D** page 140
With more than 3 million women in the United States having taken tamoxifen and only 250 endometrial cancers reported worldwide, DiSaia and Creasman do not recommend yearly endometrial sampling or ultrasound evaluation of the endometrium. The endometrium should be evaluated only if the patient is symptomatic.
10. **A** page 144
Extension of endometrial carcinoma to the cervix is stage II; endocervical glandular involvement is stage IIa: cervical stromal invasion is stage IIb (Table 5–3).
11. **D** page 154
Seventeen percent of patients with only endocervical glandular involvement had pelvic node metastases compared with 35% of those with cervical stromal involvement. None with glandular involvement only had aortic metastases compared with 23% of those with stromal invasion. This GOG study was based on 66 patients with stage II adenocarcinoma of the endometrium.
12. **A** page 155
Podratz noted in paraffin-embedded curettage specimens that recurrences and cancer-related deaths correlated with nondiploid pattern, S-phase fraction 9%, and proliferative index 14%. The latter was the most independent prognostic factor.
13. **D** page 151
A recent evaluation of 140 patients with clinical stage II cancers noted that only 35 (24%) in fact had surgical II disease.
14. **D** page 144
A carcinoma localized to the corpus is stage I; when the tumor is limited to the endometrium it is staged Ia; when it invades less or more than half of the myometrium, it is staged as Ib and Ic, respectively (Table 5–3).
15. **B** page 144
The tumor is limited to the endometrium and is staged Ia. Histology showing more than 5% but less than 50% solid growth pattern is grade 2 (moderately differentiated). Tumor differentiation is an important prognostic factor in endometrial carcinoma (Table 5–3).
16. **A** page 144
The distribution of endometrial carcinoma by surgical stage is the following: I, 73%; II, 11%; III, 13%; IV, 3% (Table 5–4).
17. **C** page 144
Prognostic factors in endometrial adenocarcinoma include histologic type, histologic differentiation, stage of disease, myometrial invasion, peritoneal cytology, lymph node metastasis, and adnexal metastasis. Uterine size is not a prognostic factor because the uterus can be enlarged by other benign pathologic conditions (leiomyoma, adenomyosis) or by multiparity.
18. **A** page 146
Endometrioid adenocarcinoma is the most common histologic subtype of malignancy in the endometrium. Eighty-seven percent of all adenocarcinomas are of this subtype.
19. **D** page 148
Clear cell carcinoma has the worse prognosis. Even with stage I disease, only 44% of patients survive 5 years.
20. **D** page 150 and Table 5–8
Exceptions can occur: a well-differentiated lesion can have deep myometrial invasion; a poorly differentiated lesion might have only superficial myometrial or endometrial involvement. Histologic differentiation is an important prognostic factor. The 5-year survival rate for surgical stage I, grades 1, 2, and 3 are 92%, 87%, and 74%, respectively.
21. **D** page 156
According to a study from the Gynecologic Oncology Group (GOG) on 621 clinical stage I patients, those with disease of the lower uterine segment have a higher incidence of pelvic lymph node metastases (16% vs. 8%) and periaortic nodal metastases (16% vs. 4%) than those with only fundal disease. Surwit also noted that patients with stromal invasion of the cervix have a lower 3-year survival rate than those with endocervical surface involvement (47% vs. 74%).
22. **A** page 152
Creasman's MD Anderson Cancer Center study reported recurrence in 10% of patients with clinical stage I disease and negative peritoneal cytologic findings. The GOG study demonstrated 6.5% recurrence with negative cytologic findings. Most investigators agree that a positive peritoneal cytologic finding is a poor prognostic factor; disagreement exists about whether or not it is an *independent* poor prognostic factor. Overall, in remembering some of the major poor prognostic factors in patients with clinical stage I disease, it may be beneficial to remember the rule of 10s: 10% will have positive pelvic nodes, 10% will have positive periaortic nodes, 10% will have positive cytologic findings, 10% will have adnexal involvement.
23. **B** page 154
DiSaia reported the long-term follow-up of stage I endometrial cancer patients whose nodes were surgically evaluated. Fifty-six percent of those with positive pelvic nodes had a recurrence vs. 59% of those with positive periaortic nodes, an insignificant difference.
24. **C** page 155
Podratz noted that recurrences and cancer deaths correlated with nondiploid pattern. Aneuploid tumor and high S-phase fraction were more common in advanced stages.

25. **D** page 157
In a GOG study of 621 surgically staged endometrial carcinoma patients and a study by Bond of 1703 patients, it was demonstrated that the vaginal vault was *not* a frequent area of recurrence (1% to 3.4% of patients), thus seriously questioning the validity of brachytherapy. Eighty to ninety percent of recurrences are outside of radiated fields. Several studies of radiotherapy and low-stage endometrial cancer show that external beam pelvic radiotherapy achieves good to excellent local control, but it does not seem to influence distant recurrences or survival.
26. **A** page 158
Studies of 621 patients by the GOG and 1703 patients by Bond suggest that the vagina is an infrequent site of recurrence, and vaginal recurrence does not appear to affect survival.
27. **D** page 160
The hysterectomy should be extrafascial. Removal of the upper vagina does not appear to decrease vault recurrences. If the disease is intrauterine only, patients with grade 1 or 2 disease had 4% recurrence; those with grade 3 and superficial disease had 14% recurrence. Surgery alone would be adequate treatment for these patients. In patients with grade 3 disease and significant muscle involvement, 40% recurrence was identified. In these patients postoperative irradiation and adjunctive hormonal therapy or chemotherapy should be considered.
28. **D** page 161
Primary surgery in the form of radical hysterectomy and pelvic lymphadenectomy had been acceptable therapy in the past for stage II adenocarcinoma of the uterus, but it appears that simple TAH-BSO and pelvic and periaortic node lymphadenectomy is adequate surgery today. There was no difference in recurrences in patients with high-risk stage I and occult stage II endometrial cancers receiving doxorubicin or not after surgery and irradiation (23% vs. 26%).
29. **C** page 162
Data from the surgical-pathologic study cited by DiSaia and Creasman might suggest that if only endocervical disease is found, patients do well with surgery alone. However, data from that limited study need further confirmation. Onsrud found that only 56% of cases originally recorded as stage II endometrial carcinoma were in fact stage II because of tumor cell "floaters" in the fractional curettage. Patients who were thus overdiagnosed had a survival rate similar to patients with stage I disease. A recent evaluation of 140 clinical stage II cancers noted that only 35 (24%) had surgical stage II disease.
30. **D** page 163
Recurrences in the vaginal wall can be treated successfully with surgery or radiation or a combination of the two. Hormonal treatment or chemotherapy may be the treatment of choice in many patients with recurrent carcinoma of the endometrium who had recurrences outside the vagina or who had radiation as part of their primary therapy.
31. **C** page 164
Progestins have been evaluated as adjunctive therapy in hopes of preventing recurrences. In three studies with medroxyprogesterone (MPA), there was no difference in survival between groups receiving MPA and groups receiving a placebo. In regard to response to progestins, grade 1 tumors have a higher objective response than grade 3: 51.7% vs. 15.5%. In a study by GOG on 420 patients with advanced or recurrent endometrial carcinoma treated with MPA, only 8% were complete responders. One half remained stable, and one half progressed. Median survival was 10.5 months.
Kauppila noted from five studies in the literature that 89% of progesterone receptor positive tumors were hormonally responsive compared to only 17% of progesterone receptor–negative tumors. The GOG noted that 40% of estrogen receptor–positive, progesterone receptor–positive tumors responded to progestins, compared to 12% of progesterone receptor–negative tumors.
32. **D** page 164
Progestin therapy may be administered in several ways. DiSaia and Creasman prefer medroxyprogesterone (DepoProvera) 400 mg IM at weekly intervals. Oral medroxyprogesterone (Provera) in the range of 150 mg/day and megestrol acetate (Megace) 160 mg/day are other recommended progestins. Progestins are continued indefinitely if an objective response is obtained. If progression of disease is noted, progestins should be discontinued and chemotherapy considered.
33. **D** page 165
Combined results of several small studies noted a response rate of 22% (complete response 8%) in 257 patients. These studies suggest that grade 1 lesions are more responsive than other grade tumors.
34. **D** page 166
In the GOG report, Thigpen noted that 37% of patients with advanced or recurrent cancer had an objective response to doxorubicin alone. The response lasted only 7 months. Experiences at MD Anderson with cisplatin had an objective response of 42% of patients, but the mean duration of remission was 5 months. A large prospective GOG study composed of 336 patients with advanced or recurrent adenocarcinoma treated with doxorubicin with or without cyclophosphamide found a total response of 30% and 20%, respectively. Kauppila noted that patients with low estrogen or progesterone receptor values had a significantly greater response rate to combined cytotoxic therapy than patients with higher receptor values.
35. **D** page 166
Most common tumors are of the endometrioid type. Most studies suggest that most of the synchronous ovarian and corpus carcinomas are independent primary tumors. The survival of these patients is excellent if they are stage I. In many instances, adequate treatment is surgery only (TAH-BSO with adequate surgical staging).

36. **A** page 163
Massi and coworkers described 180 patients treated with vaginal hysterectomy and obtained a 90% 5-year survival. Patients were stage I, obese, and poor surgical risk.
37. **D** page 162
Seventy-five percent of clinical stage II will have either less than stage II or extrauterine disease (stage III). In a retrospective review at Norwegian Radium Hospital, Onsrud has found that 56% originally recorded as stage II endometrial cancer were in fact stage II. In another study in the United States on 140 clinical stage II patients, only 24% had surgical stage II disease.
38. **A** page 155
Creasman found progesterone and estrogen receptor positivity to be independent favorable prognostic factors.
39. **A** page 155
See above answer.
40. **A** page 155
Schink demonstrated metastasis in 6% of patients in clinical stage I disease in tumors less than 2 cm in size. Rates of metastasis ranged up to 40% with larger tumors.
41. **B** page 155
Hanson demonstrated recurrence rates of 2% for capillary-like space–negative patients and 44% if positive. A GOG study associates capillary-like space involvement with 27% and 19% of pelvic and para-aortic metastases, respectively, compared with 7% and 3% occurrence with no capillary-like space involvement.
42. **B** page 154
Britton demonstrated an increased risk of recurrence in aneuploid tumors 3.5 times that of euploid (diploid) tumors.
43. **D** Table 5–3, page 144
44. **A** Table 5–3, page 144
45. **C** Table 5–3, page 144
46. **B** Table 5–3, page 144
47. **A** page 165
Figure 5–1*A*, *B*, and *C* represent a well-differentiated (grade 1), a moderately differentiated (grade 2), and a poorly differentiated (grade 3) adenocarcinoma of the uterus, respectively. According to Creasman, 70% of grade 1 tumors have estrogen and progesterone receptors. Fifty-five percent of grade 2 and 41% of grade 3 tumors have estrogen and progesterone receptors (Table 5–21).
48. **C** page 156
Grade 3 tumors have 18% positive pelvic nodes and 11% positive aortic nodes; grade 1 tumors have 3% and 2%, respectively (Table 5–14).
49. **A** page 160
50. **C** page 160
In stage I grade 1 cancer, because of the low incidence of lymph node metastasis (2%), deep muscle invasion (4%), and recurrence (4%), TAH-BSO and peritoneal cytologic examination are considered to be adequate treatment. However, in stage I grade 3 cancer, with its high incidence of lymph node metastasis (27%), deep muscle invasion (39%), and recurrence (42%), one could probably justify postoperative external irradiation to the pelvis and consider adjunctive progestins or chemotherapy.

chapter 6 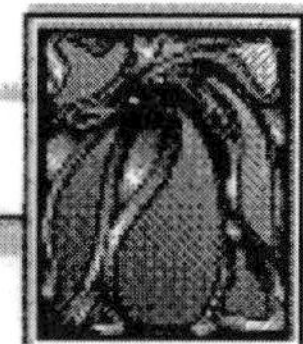

SARCOMA of the UTERUS

Key Points to Remember

- Sarcomas of the uterus are rare and constitute 3% to 5% of all uterine tumors.
- Classification of uterine sarcomas by GOG: leiomyosarcomas, endometrial sarcomas, mixed homologous müllerian sarcomas (carcinosarcoma), mixed heterologous müllerian sarcomas (mixed mesodermal sarcoma), and other uterine sarcomas.
- The incidence of sarcoma of the uterus is 1.7/100,000 women aged 20 years or older. The mean age of patients with leiomyosarcoma (LMS) is the mid–50s, 10 years younger than patients with endometrial stromal sarcoma (ESS) and mixed mesodermal sarcomas (MMS).
- Leiomyosarcoma (LMS) and mixed mesodermal sarcoma (MMS) were more common in black women than in white women.
- Pain, rapidly enlarging abdominal mass, and menorrhagia or perimenopausal bleeding are the most frequent complaints. A large polypoid mass protruding through the dilated cervix may be seen. A history of pelvic irradiation is noted in 5% to 10% of patients with sarcoma.
- MMS is the most common uterine sarcoma. Staging of uterine sarcomas is adopted from the staging of endometrial adenocarcinomas.
- Cellular myoma and bizarre leiomyomas are benign and contain less than 5 MF/10 HPF on histologic evaluation.
- Although other criteria are sometimes used, the diagnosis of leiomyosarcoma is based on the number of mitoses per 10 HPF: more than 10 MF/10 HPF or 5 to 9 MF/10 HPF with cellular atypia. Lymph node metastasis occurs in 4% of leiomyosarcomas. Sixty-three percent of patients experience recurrence with most of these at distant sites. Leiomyosarcomas prefer the hematogenous route of metastatic spread with involvement of regional and distant sites. Surgical stage is the most important prognostic factor in LMS in addition to age, grade, mitotic index, and DNA ploidy of tumor. Premenopausal patients have a better 5-year survival rate (63.6%) than postmenopausal patients (5.5%).
- Mixed müllerian sarcomas are aggressive tumors. Sixty percent of patients have disease outside the uterus at the time of original diagnosis. Thirty-five percent of stage I tumors have pelvic lymph node metastasis. Hematogenous spread to the lung and liver is common. According to a recent GOG study, heterologous elements did not affect the frequency of node metastases but did have an effect on survival (median PFI of 22.7 months compared with 62.6 months with the homologous MMS). Poor outcome correlates with deep myometrial invasion and extent of tumor outside the uterus. Five-year survival for stage I was 58%; stage II, 33%; stage III, 13%; and stage IV, 0%. Pelvic recurrence is common within the first 12 to 18 months after surgery. Metastatic sites may be pure carcinoma in some patients.
- Endolymphatic stromal myosis (ESM) is a low-grade sarcoma that requires surgery for treatment only but may recur after a long interval, even with stage I disease.
- Endometrial stromal sarcoma has a more aggressive course with frequent metastases and poor survival. It is distinguished from ESM by having 10 or more mitoses per 10 HPF.
- Adenosarcoma of the uterus is an unusual tumor with low malignant potential. Myometrial invasion is associated with a high risk of recurrence. Pure heterologous uterine sarcomas are rare. Rhabdomyosarcoma is the most common, followed by chondrosarcoma and osteosarcoma.
- Primary treatment of uterine sarcomas consists of total abdominal hysterectomy and bilateral salpingo-oophorectomy with selective pelvic and periaortic lymphadenectomy. A positive peritoneal cytologic specimen has a poor prognosis. Radiation treatment seems ineffective in increasing the survival rate. Adjunctive chemotherapy has proved of no benefit.
- Median survival in months: LMS 20.6, MMT-HO 62.6, MMT-HE 22.7.
- According to a Phase III GOG study, recurrent, persistent, or advanced disease can be treated with ifosfamide and mesna with or without cisplatin with 29% complete responders and 18% partial responders. Cisplatin and doxorubicin have resulted in 60% to 70% response in MMT. The Yale group treated 42 patients with MMT with a combination of etoposide, cisplatin, and doxorubicin and achieved a 2-year survival of 92% in stages I and II and 33% in advanced disease.
- Recurrences of ESM are treated with high-dose progestins.

Questions

Directions for Questions 1–14: Select the one best answer.

1. Sarcomas of the uterus constitute what percent of uterine tumors?
   A. 1%–2%
   B. 3%–5%
   C. 6%–8%
   D. 10%–15%

2. Classification of uterine sarcomas by the Gynecologic Oncology Group (GOG) includes:
   A. leiomyosarcoma, endometrial stromal sarcoma, mixed homologous and mixed heterologous müllerian sarcomas
   B. stromal sarcoma, leiomyosarcoma
   C. rhabdomyosarcoma, mixed müllerian tumors, carcinosarcoma
   D. chondrosarcoma, osteosarcoma, carcinosarcoma
3. Frequent symptoms and signs in patients with uterine sarcomas are:
   A. menorrhagia and polypoid mass
   B. abdominal mass and pain
   C. rapidly enlarging uterus and nausea
   D. abdominal pain and ascites
4. The most important histologic criterion of malignancy in smooth muscle tumors is:
   A. more than 10 mitotic figures per 10 high power fields (10/HPF)
   B. more than 10 mitotic figures per 1 high power field (1/HPF)
   C. cytologic atypia
   D. vascular involvement
5. In addition to the low mitotic count and surgical stage, which are the other favorable prognostic factors in a leiomyosarcoma?
   A. premenopausal status of the patient
   B. low grade of the tumor
   C. confinement of the tumor to a myoma
   D. all of the above
6. Of the factors listed below, which is *least* predictive of poor outcome in patients with clinical stage I mixed müllerian sarcoma?
   A. large uterine size
   B. presence of heterologous, rather than homologous, elements
   C. presence of occult extrauterine disease
   D. deep myometrial invasion
7. Choose the false statement regarding mixed müllerian sarcoma and leiomyosarcoma:
   A. the overall incidence of mixed müllerian sarcoma greatly exceeds that of leiomyosarcoma
   B. the risk of nodal metastases and the risk of death are greater for the leiomyosarcoma patient
   C. heterologous elements in a mixed müllerian sarcoma portend a more grave prognosis than if absent
   D. the risk of recurrence depends on histologic type
8. Choose the one true statement regarding endometrial stromal sarcoma:
   A. survival of patients with endometrial stromal sarcoma is improved over that of patients with leiomyosarcoma and other sarcomas
   B. endolymphatic stromal myosis is a high-grade variant of endometrial stromal sarcoma
   C. mitotic count may not be an independent prognostic factor for endometrial stromal sarcoma
   D. progestin therapy is contraindicated in endometrial stromal sarcoma
9. The following statements regarding therapy of uterine sarcomas are true *except:*
   A. total abdominal hysterectomy, bilateral salpingo-oophorectomy, and selective pelvic/periaortic lymphadenectomy are the mainstay of therapy
   B. radiotherapy does not improve survival
   C. radiotherapy reduces the risk of pelvic recurrence
   D. radiotherapy alone should be considered for the patient with disease confined to the uterus
10. The primary treatment for sarcomas of the uterus should be:
    A. radiation therapy
    B. chemotherapy
    C. radiation therapy followed by surgery
    D. surgery
11. Using surgery and radiation, which uterine sarcoma in stage I has the highest 5-year survival rate?
    A. mixed mesodermal sarcoma
    B. leiomyosarcoma
    C. endometrial stromal sarcoma
    D. none has 5-year survival advantage
12. The best adjunctive therapy for sarcomas of the uterus is:
    A. doxorubicin or VAC
    B. radiotherapy
    C. methotrexate
    D. no proven adjuvant therapy
13. The best therapy for recurrent uterine sarcoma is:
    A. doxorubicin
    B. doxorubicin and DTIC (dimethyl triazeno-imidazole carboxamide)
    C. VAC
    D. ifosfamide-mesna
14. The following are true for uterine sarcomas *except:*
    A. in stage I disease there is no significant difference between surgery and surgery plus irradiation in LMS, MMT, ESS
    B. patients treated with only radiation fare worse
    C. treatment of recurrences or advanced MMT with ifosfamide and mesna with and without cisplatin results in 50% of complete (30%) and partial (20%) responses
    D. doxorubicin is shown to prolong survival

ANSWERS

1. **B** page 173
   Sarcomas of the uterus are rare and constitute only 3% to 5% of all uterine tumors.
2. **A** page 174, Table 6–2
   The GOG classification groups sarcomas into four main histologic categories because the majority of sarcomas belong to those groups. The Ober classification is more complete and categorizes these tumors by their cell type and site of origin. Using the Ober system, the sarcomas can be pure or mixed and homologous or heterologous.
3. **B** page 174
   An abdominal mass or pain is a frequent complaint or finding with uterine sarcomas. Other symptoms include vaginal bleeding, a polypoid mass through a

dilated cervix, or a rapidly enlarging uterus. Associated clinical findings include obesity and hypertension in a third of the patients and a history of pelvic irradiation in 5% to 10% of patients with sarcoma.

4. **A** page 175
Taylor and Norris believe that mitotic count is extremely important. If more than 10 MF/10 HPF are present, the tumor is a leiomyosarcoma and the prognosis is grave. Intravascular disease and disease outside the uterus are also poor prognostic signs.
5. **D** page 177
All the cited prognostic factors stressed by many authors (Silverberg, Dinh, Nordal, Vardi) are favorable for a long survival.
6. **A** page 178
A trend to poorer survival is noted in patients with a large uterus, advanced age, or previous pelvic irradiation. The remaining listed prognostic factors seem to be *strong* predictors of poor outcome.
7. **B** pages 178
The median survival for LMS is 20 months compared with 22 in MMT-HE and 62 in MMT-HO (Table 6–5).
8. **C** page 179
Although Kempson and Bari noted poorer survival rates in patients with endometrial stromal sarcoma with higher mitotic counts, they did not show this to be an *independent* prognostic factor. A later Mayo Clinic study, in fact, demonstrated extent of disease, size of primary tumor, and tumor grade were important prognostic indicators; mitotic count and DNA pattern were not.
The survival of patients with ESS is no better than those with other sarcomas. Endolymphatic stromal myosis ESM is a low-grade variant of ESS. Progestins are often used as palliative or adjunctive therapy for ESM.
9. **D** page 179
Patients treated with radiotherapy alone do significantly worse than those treated with surgery alone or surgery plus radiotherapy (Table 6–6).
10. **D** page 179
The preferred treatment of sarcomas is primarily surgery. A peritoneal washing is performed before total abdominal hysterectomy and bilateral salpingo-oophorectomy. Selective pelvic and periaortic lymphadenectomy is also performed. The authors do not postoperatively treat patients who have disease limited to the endometrium or superficial myometrium.
11. **C** page 180, Table 6–6
Based on 24 patients with stage I disease treated with surgery and radiation, endometrial stromal sarcoma had the highest 5-year survival rate of 88%, followed by leiomyosarcoma (75%) and mixed mesodermal sarcoma (48%).
12. **D** page 181
Although the development of a good systemic therapy is needed, to date it appears that "proven" adjuvant therapy is anecdotal at best. In a prospective, randomized study by the GOG using doxorubicin on 156 patients, no benefit was found in using doxorubicin as an adjuvant therapy for the treatment of uterine sarcomas. Adjuvant irradiation increases the rate of pelvic control but has not produced an increase in overall survival.
13. **D** page 182
Half of patients with stage I uterine sarcoma and 90% with stages II–IV disease will develop a recurrence. Effective therapy for recurrent disease is needed but not yet found. Hannigan reported on 39 patients with recurrent disease treated with doxorubicin alone or in combination with other chemotherapeutic agents and found a median survival of 7.2 months and a response rate of 10.3%. He also reported on 74 patients treated with VAC and found a response rate of 28.9% with a 15% probability of survival at 5 years. In a GOG protocol using doxorubicin and cyclophosphamide, the response rate was 19% and the median survival 10.9 months. A comparable group of patients given doxorubicin alone displayed essentially identical response rates and survival. Ifosfamide and mesna with or without cisplatin are evaluated in a recent GOG study. On 130 evaluable patients, there have been 29% CR and over 18% PR. This over 50% response is encouraging. Cisplatin and doxorubicin have shown activity against MMT also.
14. **D** page 182
Van Rijswyk reviewed 28 studies and noted that in the adjuvant setting, doxorubicin has not been shown to prolong survival.

chapter 7 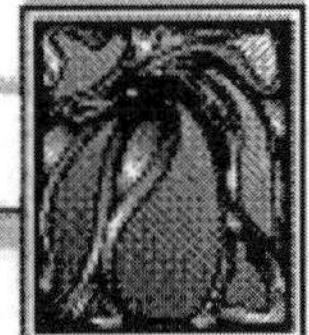

GESTATIONAL TROPHOBLASTIC NEOPLASIA

Key Points to Remember

- *Gestational trophoblastic neoplasia* (GTN) is the term commonly applied to choriocarcinoma and related tumors. GTN is recognized today as the most curable gynecologic malignancy.
- GTN represents a derangement in development of the conceptus, associated with unregulated trophoblastic proliferation and invasion with the propensity for hematogenous metastasis.
- The incidence of hydatidiform mole is 1/1000 pregnancies in the United States and 2/1000 in Japan.
- A significant increase in the incidence of mole was seen in women 15 years old or younger and 40 years of age or older.
- Deficiency of animal fat and fat-soluble vitamin carotene may contribute to this disease.
- Women with a previous hydatidiform mole have more than 10 times the risk of having another mole compared with women who have never had one. The risk is 1 in 76 pregnancies for a second mole after the first mole and increases to 1 in 6.5 pregnancies in women who already have had two moles.
- Symptoms of mole consist of vaginal bleeding, nausea and vomiting, preeclampsia in the first trimester, abnormal uterine size, theca lutein cysts, and hyperthyroidism (rare).
- The combination of theca lutein cysts with uteri that are large for gestational age results in an extremely high risk for malignant sequelae of GTN and required subsequent therapy (57%).
- Diagnosis is made with measurement of hCG and use of ultrasound.
- Complete hydatidiform mole results from the fertilization of an "empty egg" by a single sperm carrying 23 chromosomes. This haploid set of chromosomes reduplicates to give a 46 karyotype. The usual 46 XX is a result of the doubling of the paternal set of chromosomes. Rarely, in 10% of cases, an empty egg may be fertilized by two sperms, X and Y, and the complete mole has an XY chromosomal pattern that is derived paternally. A normal karyotype (46 XX) is present in 90% of complete moles. Twenty percent of patients with complete moles will develop malignant sequelae.
- Partial hydatidiform mole consists of placenta and fetus. The karyotype is triploid, which results from fertilization of a normal egg by dispermy (69 XXX, XXY, or XYY). The usual clinical diagnosis of partial mole is missed abortion or incomplete abortion. A partial mole is a pathologic diagnosis. Only 3.5% of patients with partial mole developed persistent disease, and 0.6% developed metastatic disease.
- Oral contraceptive pills can be given immediately after suction curettage. Primary hysterectomy may be selected if the patient does not desire fertility.
- Follow-up of molar pregnancy should be done with serum beta-hCG determinations at 1- to 2-week intervals until there are two normal determinations. Oral contraceptives should be used for 6 to 12 months after normal titers. Regular pelvic examinations and chest radiographs should also be performed. Subsequent pregnancies may occur after 6 months of a normal hCG determination.
- The average time for beta-hCG to reach undetectable levels is 73 days after evacuation, with half the patients having undetectable levels at 8 to 9 weeks.
- Eighty percent of patients with molar pregnancy will go into spontaneous remission after evacuation.
- In patients with gestational trophoblastic neoplasia, 50% had hydatidiform mole, 25% had normal pregnancies, and 25% had an abortion or an ectopic pregnancy.
- Patients who have elevation or plateaued hCG levels as determined by two weekly hCG levels during follow-up should receive chemotherapy.
- FIGO staging of trophoblastic tumors: Stage I: uterus; II: outside uterus but restricted to genital structures; III: lungs; IV: all other metastatic sites. Add a if there are no risk factors, b if there is 1 risk factor, or c if there are 2 risk factors. Risk factors include hCG higher than 100,000 mIU/mL and duration of disease longer than 6 months from last pregnancy.
- Phantom hCG syndrome (pseudohypergonadotropinemia) refers to persistent mild elevations of hCG. This led to treatment with cytotoxic chemotherapy when there is no true GTN present. To exclude this syndrome, the laboratory should demonstrate dilutional parallelism in the hCG results and the presence of hCG in both serum and urine samples.
- Treatment of nonmetastatic trophoblastic disease consists of methotrexate with folinic acid rescue or actinomycin D. Therapy should be continued until negative hCG titers are reported. A remission is defined as three consecutive normal weekly hCG titers. Contraception should be used for at least 6 months after remission. Treatment of nonmetastatic GTN has been 100% successful. Ninety-seven percent of those who wish to get pregnant actually conceive, and 86% have at least one live birth.

- Treatment of good prognosis metastatic trophoblastic neoplasia consists of methotrexate or actinomycin D, as discussed above. If there is resistance to both drugs, MAC (methotrexate, actinomycin, Cytoxan) or MBP (modified Bagshawe protocol) should be used. Primary or secondary hysterectomy may be performed on certain patients. The follow-up should be similar to that for patients receiving chemotherapy. Sustained remission may be observed in all patients.
- Poor-prognosis metastatic neoplasia consists of patients who have brain or liver metastases, serum beta-hCG higher than 40,000 mIU/mL, unsuccessful prior chemotherapy, or symptoms (antecedent pregnancy) longer than 4 months.
- Liver metastases carry a worse prognosis than brain metastases.
- Multiple-agent chemotherapy (MAC, EMA-CO) and multiple-modality approach (radiation, surgery, chemotherapy) should be used on poor-prognosis patients. Regression is around 80%. The primary treatment of poor-prognostic disease should be continued until three consecutive weekly serum beta-hCG levels have been obtained. Two to four cycles of consolidation chemotherapy should be delivered after initial normalization of beta-hCG for decreasing the risk of relapse.
- Recurrence occurs in 2.1% of nonmetastatic GTN, 5.4% of metastatic good-prognosis GTN, and 21% of metastatic poor-prognosis GTN. These cases are treated with a multimodality approach. Surgery is combined with EMA-CO (etoposide, actinomycin, methotrexate, vincristine, cyclophosphamide) or BEP (bleomycin, etoposide, cisplatin) or ICE (ifosfamide, etoposide, cisplatin). The cure rate reaches 80%. Tumor regression as noted on chest radiographs lags behind the hCG response.
- Placental site trophoblastic tumor (PSTT) is rare and may be found after abortion, mole, or normal pregnancy. The tumor is composed of intermediate trophoblast. It is diffusely positive for HPL, only focally positive for hCG. Treatment of PSTT is hysterectomy. The response of metastatic disease to chemotherapy is short-lived, and the mortality rate is 15% to 20%.
- Pregnancy outcomes in women with molar pregnancies are no different from outcomes of other women.
- Standard chemotherapy protocols in the treatment of GTN have minimal impact on the subsequent ability to reproduce.
- Patients who are pregnant with a coexistent normal pregnancy and GTN are at increased risk for hemorrhage and paraneoplastic medical complications (HELLP, PIH, ARDS).
- Survivors of successful treatment of GTN are at increased risk for myeloid leukemia, colon cancer, and breast cancer when the survival exceeds 25 years.

QUESTIONS

Directions for Questions 1–39: Select the one best answer.

1. The incidence of hydatidiform mole in the United States is:
   A. 1 in 120 pregnancies
   B. 1 in 77 pregnancies
   C. 1 in 5000 pregnancies
   D. 1 in 1000 pregnancies
2. Spontaneous regression occurs in what percentage of hydatidiform moles?
   A. 80%–85%
   B. 60%–65%
   C. 50%–55%
   D. 40%–45%
3. Effects of maternal age, parity, and gestational age on hydatidiform mole are the following *except:*
   A. there is an increase in the incidence of mole in women 15 years old or younger and 40 years old or older
   B. the greatest relative risks are in women 50 years of age or older
   C. age and parity affect the clinical outcome of an individual with hydatidiform mole
   D. gestational age at the time of diagnosis of the hydatidiform mole does not appear to influence subsequent sequelae
4. Nutritional factors may have an effect on the incidence of hydatidiform mole. A prevalence of which vitamin deficiency is found in locations with high incidence of hydatidiform mole?
   A. vitamin A
   B. vitamin B
   C. vitamin C
   D. vitamins D and K
5. The most frequent symptom(s) of hydatidiform mole is (are):
   A. nausea and vomiting
   B. vaginal bleeding
   C. manifestations of hyperthyroidism
   D. acute respiratory distress
6. The best diagnostic technique to identify a hydatidiform mole is:
   A. ultrasound
   B. quantitative beta-hCG
   C. amniography
   D. uterine arteriography
7. The most frequent karyotype of complete hydatidiform mole is:
   A. XY
   B. XX
   C. XXX
   D. XYY/XO
8. The usual karyotype of partial mole is:
   A. XY
   B. XX
   C. XXY or XYY
   D. XYY/XO
9. Follow-up of hydatidiform mole after evacuation consists of the following *except:*
   A. beta-hCG determination every 1 to 2 weeks until negative two times, then bimonthly for 1 year
   B. contraception for 1 year
   C. physical examination, including pelvic examination, every 2 weeks until remission, then every 3 months for 1 year; chest radiograph should be done initially and repeated if hCG level rises
   D. prophylactic chemotherapy for 6 months

10. Method of choice for evacuation of a hydatidiform mole:
    A. hysterotomy
    B. hysterectomy
    C. suction curettage
    D. oxytocin (Pitocin) evacuation
11. Hydatidiform mole precedes malignant disease in what proportion of patients?
    A. 10%
    B. 20%
    C. 50%
    D. 75%
12. Poor-prognosis metastatic GTN includes the following factors *except:*
    A. high pretreatment hCG titer
    B. disease evident less than 4 months from antecedent pregnancy
    C. significant prior chemotherapy
    D. brain or liver metastasis
13. The minimum workup for those with the initial diagnosis of GTN includes all *except:*
    A. pelvic ultrasound
    B. chest radiograph
    C. pretreatment hCG titer
    D. hematology and chemistry screens
14. Under the 1991 FIGO staging system for trophoblastic tumors, the patient with choriocarcinoma metastatic only to the vagina and with neither of two risk factors is classified as stage:
    A. Ib
    B. Ic
    C. IIa
    D. IIb
15. A patient has choriocarcinoma metastatic only to lung. Both risk factors are present. The proper FIGO stage is:
    A. IIIc
    B. IVa
    C. IVb
    D. IVc
16. Choose the factor from the WHO scoring system that is given the highest risk score:
    A. prior single-drug chemotherapy
    B. antecedent pregnancy resulting in hydatidiform mole
    C. liver metastasis
    D. 12 months from last pregnancy
17. Choose the type of antecedent pregnancy that is given the lowest risk score in the WHO GTN scoring system:
    A. spontaneous abortion
    B. elective abortion
    C. term pregnancy
    D. hydatidiform mole
18. Appropriate first-line therapy for nonmetastatic GTN includes all *except:*
    A. methotrexate
    B. cisplatin
    C. 5-FU
    D. actinomycin
19. The major reason for the increasing popularity of high-dose methotrexate with leucovorin rescue over standard therapy with methotrexate alone is:
    A. lower relapse rate
    B. increased ease of administration
    C. increased efficacy (higher response rates)
    D. decreased toxicity
20. The factor that would not necessarily dictate a change in treatment for nonmetastatic GTN undergoing first-line chemotherapy is:
    A. plateau of hCG titer
    B. rising hCG titer
    C. appearance of new metastases
    D. persistence of mass
21. Appropriate statements regarding the use of hysterectomy in patients with GTN limited to the uterus include all *except:*
    A. hysterectomy may be considered for primary therapy (primary hysterectomy)
    B. hysterectomy should be considered for chemoresistant disease in the uterus (secondary hysterectomy)
    C. hysterectomy should be performed in most patients (primary hysterectomy)
    D. hysterectomy should be performed for the patient who has failed two types of chemotherapy (tertiary hysterectomy)
22. Proper management of the patient undergoing chemotherapy for nonmetastatic GTN includes all *except:*
    A. brief intervals between treatments
    B. continuation without interruption of drug until titer has definite downward trend
    C. dose reduction with severe oral/gastrointestinal ulceration or granulocytopenia
    D. oral contraception, if not contraindicated
23. Choose the *false* statement in regard to remission of nonmetastatic GTN:
    A. childbearing may be allowed at any time during remission
    B. remission is defined as three consecutive normal hCG titers
    C. 100% of patients can enter remission
    D. 90% of patients can enter remission with preservation of the uterus
24. True statements relevant to the treatment and follow-up period include all *except:*
    A. second-line therapy is needed in up to one third of patients
    B. second-line therapy should be used if hCG titers plateau or rise
    C. hCG titers should be monitored at least monthly for 6 months, then bimonthly for an additional 6 months after remission
    D. hCG titers should be monitored monthly until remission
25. Patients with metastatic GTN are categorized as poor prognosis when the following are present *except:*
    A. brain or liver metastasis; serum beta-hCG 40,000 mIU/mL
    B. unsuccessful previous chemotherapy

C. symptoms (antecedent pregnancy) longer than 4 months
D. antecedent abortion

26. Patients with good-prognosis metastatic GTN are treated with:
    A. methotrexate or actinomycin D
    B. MAC (methotrexate, actinomycin D, chlorambucil)
    C. modified Bagshawe protocol, or hysterectomy
    D. all of the above
27. The best treatment for poor-prognosis metastatic GTN is:
    A. chemotherapy and radiation therapy
    B. chemotherapy
    C. chemotherapy and primary surgery
    D. chemotherapy and secondary surgery
28. Which metastases carry the worse prognosis?
    A. brain metastases
    B. liver metastases
    C. vaginal metastases
    D. lung metastases
29. Factors responsible for treatment failures in poor prognosis metastatic GTN are:
    A. extensive disease
    B. inadequate initial treatment
    C. failure of presently used chemotherapy protocols in advanced disease
    D. all of the above
30. Recurrences in poor prognosis metastatic disease are in the order of:
    A. 2%
    B. 5%
    C. 20%
    D. 50%
31. Minimal therapy for placental site trophoblastic tumor (PSTT) should be:
    A. dilation and curettage
    B. hysterectomy
    C. chemotherapy with methotrexate
    D. radiation
32. The two risk factors used in FIGO staging for trophoblastic tumors are:
    A. serum hCG > 100,000 mIU/mL and duration of disease > 6 months from termination of the antecedent pregnancy
    B. serum hCG > 100,000 mIU/mL and prior chemotherapy for known GTT
    C. serum hCG > 100,000 mIU/mL and placental site trophoblastic tumor
    D. serum hCG > 100,000 mIU/mL and previous normal pregnancy
33. EMA-CO chemotherapy includes all *except:*
    A. methotrexate
    B. etoposide; actinomycin D
    C. vincristine, cyclophosphamide
    D. doxorubicin (Adriamycin)
34. Compared with women who never have a hydatidiform mole, women with a previous molar pregnancy have how many times the risk of having another mole?
    A. 2 times
    B. 3 times
    C. 5 times
    D. 10 times
35. According to a recent study by the Boston Group, the classic symptoms of complete mole are changing. Which remains the most common symptom?
    A. vaginal bleeding
    B. excessive uterine size
    C. preeclampsia
    D. anemia
36. What is the percentage of complete hydatidiform mole having a 46 XY chromosomal pattern?
    A. 2%–5%
    B. 6%–10%
    C. 11%–15%
    D. 16%–20%
37. What percentage of partial mole develops persistent disease and metastatic disease?
    A. 4%
    B. 10%
    C. 15%
    D. 20%
38. According to Berkowitz, the following symptoms are at high risk for persistent GTT *except:*
    A. serum hCG > 100,000 mIU/mL
    B. excessive uterine size
    C. prominent theca lutein cyst
    D. degree of anemia
39. Surgery has an important role in primary and recurrent disease. The use of surgery is indicated in the following cases *except:*
    A. primary hysterectomy combined with chemotherapy in a multigravida
    B. secondary hysterectomy for recurrent disease in the uterus with no evidence of extrauterine disease
    C. pulmonary wedge resection of pulmonary metastases in patients with disease in the pelvis
    D. pulmonary wedge resection of a solitary nodule with no evidence of disease and persistent elevated hCG

Directions for Questions 40–45: For each numbered item, select the letter of the most appropriate answer. Each letter may be used once, more than once, or not at all.

40–43. Match the following:
    A. complete hydatidiform mole
    B. partial hydatidiform mole
    C. both
    D. neither

40. 20% malignant degeneration
41. Triploidy
42. Beta-hCG
43. CA–125

44–45. Match the types of chemotherapy concerning the risk of secondary cancer following treatment of GTN:
    A. Risk increases
    B. Risk decreases
    C. No risk

44. Multiple-agent chemotherapy
45. Single-agent therapy

ANSWERS

1. **D** page 186
In the United States hydatidiform mole occurs in 1 of 1000 pregnancies. It is more frequent in the Far East, where the incidence is 2 of 1000 pregnancies.
2. **A** page 191
Spontaneous regression occurs in 80% to 85% of hydatidiform moles, compared with 96% of partial moles.
3. **C** page 186
Age and parity do not appear to affect the clinical outcome of an individual with hydatidiform mole.
4. **A** page 186
Berkowitz suggested that a deficiency of animal fat and fat-soluble vitamin carotene may contribute to hydatidiform mole. A prevalence of vitamin A deficiency corresponds to geographic locations where there is a high incidence of this disease.
5. **B** page 186
Vaginal bleeding is present in 97% of complete moles. Nausea and vomiting are reported in almost one third of patients. Preeclampsia in the first trimester of pregnancy occurs in only 12% of patients. Clinical manifestations of hyperthyroidism occur in less than 1% of patients. Acute respiratory distress is thought to be due to trophoblastic pulmonary embolization. Uterine size excessive for gestational age is found in 50% of patients with moles. Fifteen percent of patients with intact hydatidiform mole have enlarged theca lutein cysts of the ovary.
6. **A** page 188
Ultrasound is the technique of choice and is extremely accurate. Combined use of ultrasound and quantitative measurement of hCG correctly identifies hydatidiform mole in 89% of patients on first examination by the gynecologic oncology group at Yale University.
7. **B** page 189
Usually a complete hydatidiform mole has a 46 XX karyotype (90%), rarely 46 XY. There is fertilization of an "empty egg" by a single sperm carrying 23 chromosomes. The usual 46 XX is a result of the doubling of the paternal set of chromosomes; the 46 XY is derived from two sperms: one X and one Y chromosome.
8. **C** page 190
Partial mole usually has a triploid karyotype. A normal egg is usually fertilized by dispermy (which can carry either sex chromosome), resulting in 69 chromosomes with a sex configuration of XXX, XXY, or XYY. The usual clinical diagnosis of a partial mole is missed abortion or incomplete abortion. A partial mole is a pathologic diagnosis. Although the malignant transformation is much less frequent after a partial mole than after a complete mole, hCG titers should be monitored after evacuation of all molar pregnancies.
9. **D** page 192
Chemoprophylaxis reduces the incidence of persistent trophoblastic disease in patients at high risk, but it increases tumor resistance and morbidity. Prophylactic chemotherapy for all patients with hydatidiform mole is not indicated because 80% of patients with hydatidiform mole will go into spontaneous remission and require no therapy. Chemotherapy on the contrary, should start immediately if the hCG titer rises or plateaus during follow-up or if metastases are detected at any time.
10. **C** page 191
Suction curettage is the method of choice for evacuation of a mole. A primary hysterectomy may be selected as the method for evacuation if the patient does not desire more pregnancies. The role of hysterotomy is extremely limited unless major hemorrhage is present. Even if hysterectomy is used, patients must be observed closely.
11. **C** page 193
Of patients with malignant trophoblastic disease, the antecedent gestational event is hydatidiform mole in 50% of cases, normal pregnancy in 25% of patients, and abortion or ectopic pregnancy in 25%.
12. **B** page 195
The NCI, Hammond, WHO, and FIGO classification systems acknowledge that short duration of disease is a good prognostic factor for the patient with metastatic disease (Tables 7–3 and 7–4).
13. **A** page 196
Initial evaluation of the patient with GTN includes history and physical examination, chemistry and hematology screens, pretreatment hCG titer, and chest radiographic examination. If any of these are abnormal or suspicious, brain CT, pelvic ultrasound, and/or liver scan is recommended by the authors. A study at Duke University using the above plan in 324 women with GTN revealed 100% sensitivity and 63% specificity at detecting metastases.
14. **C** page 195
Stage I: disease is confined to the uterus. Stage II: disease has extended from the uterus but involves genital structures only. With any of the four stages, if neither of the two high-risk factors (serum hCG >100,000 mIU/mL or disease longer-than-6-month duration) are present, it is subclassified as "a" (Table 7–4).
15. **A** page 195
Disease metastatic to lungs as the only identified site outside of genital organs requires classification as stage III. If both risk factors are present, it is subclassified as "c." If one risk factor is present, it is subclassified as "b." If neither risk factor is present, it is subclassified as "a" (Table 7–4).
16. **D** page 195
All experts agree that prognosis is inversely related to the length of time from pregnancy to identification of the presence of GTN. In the WHO scoring system, 12 months or more is given a risk score of four. The remaining listed factors are given a risk score of two or less.
17. **D** page 195
Hydatidiform mole is given a risk score of 0, abortion is given a risk score of 1, and term pregnancy is given a risk score of 2 (Table 7–3).
18. **B** page 196
Methotrexate and actinomycin are the drugs classically used for initial therapy of nonmetastatic GTN in North America and Europe. In Asia 5-FU is a

prominent part of GTN therapy. Sung demonstrated a 93% remission rate for choriocarcinoma with 5-FU and a 1.4% recurrence rate. Cisplatin is infrequently used with low-risk disease, although it may be effective with poor-prognosis disease.

19. **D** page 197
The major advantage that high-dose methotrexate and leucovorin seem to have over standard methotrexate is (1) decreased toxicity and (2) the need for fewer courses of methotrexate to achieve remission. There is no widespread evidence yet to conclusively demonstrate a higher response or lower relapse rate with high-dose therapy.
20. **D** page 197
Each of the first three choices implies persistently viable or reproducing tumor cells resistant to the chosen therapy. This should lead to a change in treatment. Although a mass may persist on examination or radiograph, it might not be composed of viable cells and should not be used as the sole factor to determine therapy (Table 7–7).
21. **C** page 198
The majority of women with GTN are young and of relatively low parity. In view of the high success rates, low mortality, and acceptable morbidity of medical therapy, an attempt at preservation of fertility is feasible in most patients.
22. **B** page 197
Chemotherapy should be continued at 7- to 10-day intervals until the hCG titer is normal.
23. **A** page 197
The authors' practice is to recommend contraception for 1 year of remission. Many authors now think that 6 months of normal titers are sufficient. Pregnancy may then be allowed. Subsequent reproduction is generally unchanged by the chemotherapy used for nonmetastatic GTN.
24. **D** page 197
hCG titers should be monitored *weekly* until remission (three subsequent weekly normal titers) when they may become less frequent. Frequent pelvic examinations are recommended during the follow-up period.
25. **D** page 198
It is suggested by the Southeastern Trophoblastic Disease Center that patients who had an antecedent term pregnancy (and not abortion) and developed GTN should be placed in the poor-prognosis category. Patients with metastatic GTN and without the first three enumerated conditions are considered as good prognoses.
26. **D** page 199
Methotrexate is considered by many as the drug of choice for patients with good prognosis metastatic GTN. If resistance to methotrexate occurs, patients are switched to dactinomycin. If resistance to both drugs develops, patients should be started on a multiple-agent protocol such as MAC or modified Bagshawe protocol consisting of hydroxyurea, dactinomycin, vincristine, methotrexate, cyclophosphamide, folinic acid, and doxorubicin (CHAMOMA). Hysterectomy may be performed if future fertility is not desired. The remission rate approaches nearly 100%, although more courses of chemotherapy may be required.
27. **A** page 200
With chemotherapy and radiation therapy the remission rate is around 87%. The remission rate for all poor prognosis metastatic GTN is 66% (Table 7–16), and the recurrence rate is 20%. (Table 7–18).
28. **B** page 200
Liver metastases appear to carry a worse prognosis than brain metastases. Liver metastases are usually associated with widespread metastases. A recent literature review indicates that 38% of patients with liver metastases achieve remission, in contrast to 58% with brain metastases.
29. **D** page 201
Lurain et al. noted all three factors as being responsible for treatment failures.
    a. Many patients had extensive disease at the time of initial treatment: 23% were dead within 1 month of diagnosis.
    b. At the Brewer Trophoblastic Disease Center, the cure rate was 94% with patients treated at the Center vs. 55% with patients treated elsewhere. It is therefore extremely important that patients who fall into the high-risk category have proper consultation and referral to an institution with expertise in this disease.
    c. Before MAC was used in high-risk patients, there was a 39% cure, compared with 90% remission with the multiple-agents regimen. Secondary chemotherapy yields very poor results: not a single remission with second-line chemotherapy has been noted at the Brewer Trophoblastic Disease Center.
30. **C** page 203
Recurrences in nonmetastatic, good-prognosis metastatic, and poor-prognosis metastatic GTN are 2.1%, 5.4%, and 21%, respectively (Table 7–18).
Remission rate after treatment is 100%, 100%, and 66%, respectively (Table 7–19). Total remission rate is 92% for GTN, the most curable of all gynecologic malignancies.
31. **B** page 204
PSTT is an indolent variant of choriocarcinoma. Hysterectomy should be the minimal therapy for PSTT. The hCG is often low even with metastases and therefore is a poor predictor of prognosis. Patients with metastatic disease apparently do not respond to chemotherapy as do patients with GTN.
32. **A** page 195
Risk factors affecting staging include serum hCG 100,000 mIU/mL and duration of disease greater than 6 months from termination of the antecedent pregnancy. The other factors should be considered and noted in reporting.
33. **D** page 202
Newlands first reported a large experience with EMA-CO in poor-prognosis GTN. It differs from the standard MAC regimen by (1) adding etoposide and vincristine to the standard dactinomycin and cyclophosphamide and (2) increasing the dose of

methotrexate and adding folinic acid rescue. It has shown the best balance to date of high survival (85%) and lower treatment mortality/morbidity, although regimens adding cisplatin show promising results in early studies.

34. **D** page 186
Women with a previous mole have more than 10 times the risk of having another mole compared with women who have never had one. This risk increases if a patient had more than one mole.
35. **A** page 186
The Boston Group compared symptoms in complete mole from 1988–1993 to those seen in 1965–1976. Vaginal bleeding was still the most common symptom but occurred in only 84% vs. 97%. Excessive uterine size, preeclampsia, and hyperemesis occurred in 28%, 1.3%, and 8% compared with 51%, 27%, and 26%, respectively. Anemia was present in 5% of recent patients compared with 54% of older group patients.
36. **B** page 190
About 6% to 10% of complete moles have a 46 XY chromosomal pattern, derived paternally, resulting from the fusion of an "empty egg" with two sperms X and Y.
37. **A** page 190
From nine published reports of 1125 patients with incomplete mole, 3.5% and 0.6% developed persistent disease and metastatic disease, respectively.
38. **D** page 190
The three first answers are symptoms of marked trophoblastic growth, and patients are at high risk for persistent GTT. Degree of anemia has no relationship with persistent disease.
39. **C** page 204
Resection of pulmonary disease is unnecessary in the majority of patients. The Duke University experience on 32 patients treated with primary hysterectomy and 28 patients with secondary hysterectomy for recurrent disease showed a regression rate of 100% and 83%, respectively.

MATCHING

40. **A** page 190
Spontaneous regression occurs in 80% of patients with complete mole.
41. **B** page 189
Partial moles usually have a triploid karyotype that is the result of fertilization of a normal egg by dispermy.
42. **C** page 191
After evaluation, follow-up should be done with serum beta-hCG for complete or partial mole.
43. **D** see page 329.
CA-125 is used for diagnosis and follow-up of ovarian cancer.
44. **A**
45. **C**
The risk is significantly increased for myeloid leukemia, colon, and breast cancer when the survival exceeds 25 years in patients receiving multiple chemotherapy. The risk is not increased in patients treated with a single agent. Leukemias develop only in patients who receive etoposide plus other cytotoxic drugs.

chapter 8

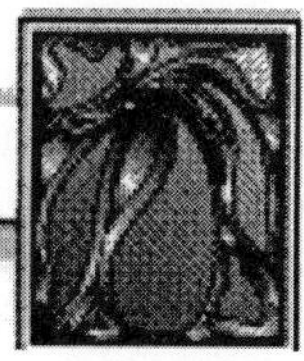

INVASIVE CANCER of the VULVA

KEY POINTS TO REMEMBER

- Cancer of the vulva accounts for 5% to 8% of all female genital malignancies.
- Vulvar cancer appears most frequently in women between 65 and 75 years old; a study at MD Anderson Hospital reported that about 15% occurs in women younger than 40 years old.
- The majority (86%) of all vulvar cancers are squamous in origin.
- Long-term pruritus or a lump or mass on the vulva is present in 50% of patients.
- Biopsy should be done on all suspicious lesions of the vulva.
- The cause of cancer of the vulva is unknown; the correlation with HPV is not as strong as that with VIN.
- Approximately 70% of cancer of the vulva arises on the labia.
- The four histologic types of cancer of the vulva behave similarly and use the lymphatic route for initial metastases (squamous, melanoma, sarcoma, adenocarcinoma).
- The superficial inguinal nodes are the primary nodal group and serve as sentinel nodes of the vulva. The deep femoral nodes are secondary nodal recipients with the Cloquet's node, which is the last node of the deep femoral group (Cloquet's node is absent in 54% of cases).
- A deep femoral lymphadenectomy does not require removal of the fascia lata because the deep femoral nodes are always situated within the openings in the fascia at the fossa ovalis and no lymph nodes are distal to the lower margin of the fossa ovalis under the fascia cribrosa.
- Clinical significance of lymphatics from the clitoris directly to the deep pelvic nodes appears to be minimal: it is unusual to find positive pelvic nodes, even when the clitoris is involved.
- The incidence of positive inguinal and pelvic nodes increases with the size of tumor (20.7% for T1 lesion [<2 cm in diameter], 44.8% for T2 lesion [>2 cm in diameter]), the grade of the tumor, the depth of invasion, and the involvement of vascular spaces. With stages III and IV lesions, the incidence of inguinal node metastases is 53% and 90%, respectively.
- Verrucous carcinoma, a variant of squamous cell carcinoma, is locally invasive but nonmetastasizing. Wide excision with tumor-free margins should be the therapeutic aim.
- Staging of invasive cancer of the vulva is based on surgical-pathologic evaluation:

  Stage 0: Carcinoma in situ (CIS), intraepithelial carcinoma
  Stage I: tumor smaller than 2 cm confined to vulva or perineum
  Ia: tumor smaller than 2 cm, stromal invasion less than 1.0 mm
  Ib: tumor smaller than 2 cm, stromal invasion more than 1 mm
  Stage II: tumor larger than 2 cm confined to vulva or perineum—no nodal metastasis
  Stage III: tumors any size with spread to lower urethra or vagina or anus, and/or unilateral regional lymph node metastasis
  Stage IVa: tumor invades upper urethra, bladder mucosa, rectal mucosa, pelvic bone, and/or bilateral lymph node metastasis
  Stage IVb: any distant metastasis, including pelvic lymph nodes
- Sentinel node biopsy is under evaluation; it is not 100% accurate.
- Management of invasive cancer of the vulva consists of radical vulvectomy and bilateral inguinal lymphadenectomy. Unilateral lesion can be treated with ipsilateral inguinal lymphadenectomy. Pelvic lymph node irradiation is recommended for patients with positive inguinal nodes.
- Other management alternatives have been proposed: radical vulvectomy combined with elective node irradiation for stages I and II (Daly and Million); surgical extirpation of lymph nodes and combination of external and interstitial irradiation in case of advanced disease (Boronow); preoperative chemoirradiation before surgery, exenteration and radical vulvectomy (Cavanagh); and cryovulvectomy (Concalver).
- Operative mortality of radical vulvectomy is 1% to 2%. Complications are wound breakdown (50%) and lymphedema of the lower extremities (69%).
- Corrected 5-year survival rate is 90% in stages I and II disease, 75% for all stages of vulvar cancer. Regardless of the stage, if nodes are negative, the survival rate is 96%; if positive nodes are present, it drops to 66%.
- Eighty percent of recurrences occur in the first 2 years after therapy. Half of the recurrences are local and near the site of the primary lesion and can be treated successfully with local excision and interstitial radiation, with a salvage rate of 40%. Distant recurrences are treated with cisplatin and have a 30% response rate.

- The International Society for the Study of Vulvovaginal Diseases (ISSVD) defines microinvasive carcinoma of the vulva: a squamous carcinoma having a diameter of less than 2 cm with a depth of invasion of less than 1 mm. Vascular space involvement by tumor excludes the lesion from this definition (stage Ia). Large excision without lymphadenectomy is the recommended treatment. Node metastasis is nearly nil.
- The depth of invasion is measured from the epidermal-stromal junction of the most superficial adjacent dermal papilla to the deepest point of invasion. If depth of invasion is 3 mm, there is a 4.8% node metastasis; if 5 mm, there is a 11.4% node metastasis.
- DiSaia suggests a novel and conservative approach for lesions smaller than 1 cm and focal invasion less than 5 mm using the inguinal nodes as sentinel nodes. Groin recurrence or death approaches zero.
- Paget's disease of the vulva is rare and presents as a hyperemic and thickened lesion. Underlying adenocarcinoma is unusual. Adequate biopsy specimens and fine needle aspiration of the subcutaneous masses (guided by palpation) should be performed for diagnosis. Treatment of intraepithelial Paget's disease consists of large excision with negative margins. Recurrences are frequent. Patients in whom an underlying apocrine adenocarcinoma is associated with Paget's disease are treated by radical vulvectomy and inguinal lymphadenectomy.
- Melanoma, second most common invasive cancer in the vulva, is rare and often localized at the labia minora and clitoris. Median age of patients is 65. Prognosis is related to size, depth of invasion (Clark's classification or Breslow's or Chung's methods), and histologic growth pattern (superficial spreading vs. nodular). Clark's staging—level I: in situ melanoma; level II: papillary dermis; level III: papillary dermis to reticular dermis; level IV: reticular dermis; level V: subcutaneous fat. Treatment consists of radical local excision with 2-cm margins for thin lesions (<7 mm) and 4-cm margins for thick lesions. Lymphadenectomy is more prognostic than therapeutic. Lymph node metastases increase with depth of invasions: level I: 0%; level II: 10%; level V: 29%. Five-year survival is 100% with lesions that are less than 1.5-mm thick, 65% with lesions 1.5 to 4 mm, and 25% with lesions larger than 4 mm (Breslow method). Ten-year survival associated with Clark's levels I, II, III, IV, V is 100%, 100%, 83%, 65%, and 23%, respectively.
- Sarcoma of the vulva is rare and is treated with radical vulvectomy and bilateral inguinal lymphadenectomy.
- Therapy consists of radical vulvectomy and inguinal lymphadenectomy. Five-year survival is 84%.
- Adenocarcinoma of the Bartholin's gland is rare. Any enlargement in the Bartholin's gland area in a postmenopausal woman should be investigated. Half of all carcinomas are squamous.
- Treatment of adenoid cystic carcinoma of the Bartholin's gland is wide excision with ipsilateral inguinal lymphadenectomy.
- Basal cell carcinoma of the vulva is treated by local excision.

QUESTIONS

Directions for Questions 1–41: Select the one best answer.

1. Cancer of the vulva accounts for what percentage of all gynecologic malignancies?
   A. 10%
   B. 8%
   C. 15%
   D. 20%
2. The average age of women with cancer of the vulva is between:
   A. 35 and 45 years
   B. 45 and 55 years
   C. 55 and 65 years
   D. 65 and 75 years
3. The most frequent histologic type of cancer of the vulva is:
   A. squamous
   B. melanoma
   C. sarcoma
   D. adenocarcinoma
4. The following is true concerning verrucous carcinoma of vulva *except:*
   A. it is a type of epidermoid carcinoma
   B. it is distinguished from ordinary condyloma by the absence of fibrovascular cores
   C. it is best treated with radiotherapy
   D. it seldom metastasizes to lymph nodes
5. Symptoms present in more than 50% of patients with invasive vulvar cancer include:
   A. bleeding
   B. discharge and pruritus
   C. bleeding and pruritus
   D. pruritus and a mass
6. The most common type of HPV DNA found in invasive carcinoma of the vulva is:
   A. 6
   B. 11
   C. 16
   D. 18
7. The most common location of invasive carcinoma of the vulva is:
   A. labium majora
   B. labia minora
   C. clitoris
   D. perineum
8. The most frequent sign or symptom of vulvar cancer is:
   A. pruritus
   B. pain
   C. bleeding
   D. ulceration
9. The lymphatic spread of vulvar carcinoma is the following:
   A. superficial inguinal (femoral) nodes, iliac nodes, obturator nodes
   B. superficial inguinal (femoral) node, deep femoral nodes, pelvic nodes
   C. pelvic nodes, para-aortic nodes
   D. deep femoral nodes, pelvic nodes, superficial inguinal nodes

10. The Cloquet's node is:
    A. the most proximal node of the deep femoral group
    B. the node nearest to the superficial epigastric vein
    C. the superficial inguinal node above the Camper fascia
    D. the most proximal node of the external iliac group
11. Which nodes can serve as the sentinel lymph nodes of the vulva?
    A. Cloquet's node
    B. superficial inguinal (femoral) nodes
    C. deep femoral nodes
    D. obturator nodes
12. The incidence of lymph node involvement in a T1 vulvar lesion (≤ 2 cm in diameter) is approximately:
    A. 5%
    B. 10%
    C. 15%
    D. 20%
13. When the inguinal nodes are positive for metastatic disease, what percentage of pelvic nodes are involved?
    A. 10%
    B. 15%
    C. 20%
    D. 25%
14. Special features concerning verrucous carcinoma of the vulva are the following *except:*
    A. it is a variant of squamous carcinoma
    B. there is a lack of histologic malignant features
    C. the correct treatment is radical vulvectomy and bilateral inguinal lymphadenectomy
    D. it is locally invasive but nonmetastasizing
15. What is the percentage of contralateral positive groin nodes in tumors of the vulva between 3 and 5 mm thick?
    A. 0%
    B. 1%
    C. 2%
    D. 3%
16. A 1.5-cm tumor of the vulva with stromal invasion of 0.9 mm is classified as FIGO stage:
    A. Ia
    B. Ib
    C. IIa
    D. IIb
17. Prognostic factors of invasive squamous cell carcinoma of the vulva include:
    A. size of lesion
    B. grade of tumor
    C. depth of invasion and vascular space involvement
    D. all of the above
18. The incidence of positive pelvic nodes in case of metastases to inguinal nodes is:
    A. 10%
    B. 15%
    C. 20%
    D. 25%
19. In patients with positive inguinal nodes, DiSaia and Creasman recommend:
    A. pelvic lymph node dissection
    B. pelvic lymph node irradiation
    C. pelvic exenteration
    D. aortic lymph node irradiation
20. The initial procedure most surgeons perform on a patient with invasive carcinoma of the vulva is:
    A. radical vulvectomy and bilateral inguinal lymphadenectomy
    B. radical vulvectomy, bilateral inguinal lymphadenectomy, and pelvic lymphadenectomy
    C. simple vulvectomy
    D. radical vulvectomy and elective node irradiation
21. True statements related to the morbidity and mortality of radical vulvectomy and lymphadenectomy include all *except:*
    A. advanced age is a contraindication to surgical management
    B. current mortality is 1% to 2%
    C. complications occur in most patients
    D. the most frequently encountered complication is delayed healing
22. Common complications after radical vulvectomy and lymphadenectomy include:
    A. incisional breakdown
    B. inguinal lymphocyst
    C. lower extremity lymphedema
    D. all of the above
23. True statements in regard to survival of patients with carcinoma of the vulva include all *except:*
    A. 5-year survival should approach 90% for stages I and II disease
    B. 5-year survival with negative lymph nodes is greater than 90%
    C. 5-year survival with positive inguinal nodes is approximately 75%
    D. 5-year survival with positive pelvic nodes is approximately 20%
24. True statements relative to recurrent vulvar carcinoma include all *except:*
    A. more than 80% of recurrences occur within 2 years of primary therapy
    B. more than half of recurrences are local and at the site of the original lesion
    C. 40% of patients with local recurrence may be salvaged
    D. 20% of patients with nodal metastasis may be salvaged
25. The following statements in regard to early vulvar carcinoma are true *except:*
    A. high-grade tumors correlate with a higher risk of nodal metastasis
    B. combined studies demonstrate a risk of nodal positivity of 5% with a 3-mm depth of tumor invasion
    C. lymph and vascular space involvement are associated with a higher risk of nodal metastasis
    D. combined studies demonstrate a risk of nodal positivity of 12% with a 5-mm depth of tumor invasion
26. The definition of early invasive carcinoma of the vulva (stage Ia) proposed by the International Society for the Study of Vulvar Disease includes all *except:*
    A. squamous histology
    B. 3 cm or less diameter
    C. 1 mm or less invasion
    D. absence of vascular space involvement

27. The authors proposed a conservative therapy for those with early carcinoma of the vulva. Their current criteria for those who may successfully be treated by this conservative method include all *except:*
    A. squamous histology
    B. 2 cm or less diameter
    C. 5 mm or less invasion
    D. absence of vascular space involvement
28. Major differences between the authors' conservative surgical procedure and the standard radical vulvectomy/lymphadenectomy include:
    A. unilateral lymphadenectomy (if lateral disease) through separate incision
    B. resection of primary lesion with hemivulvectomy (wide local excision) rather than vulvectomy
    C. removal of superficial and deep inguinal (femoral) lymph nodes for frozen section
    D. usual preservation of clitoris
29. Paget's disease of the vulva can be misdiagnosed as:
    A. basal cell carcinoma
    B. Bartholin's gland adenocarcinoma
    C. squamous cell carcinoma
    D. CIS of vulva or melanoma
30. Paget's disease without underlying adenocarcinoma is treated by:
    A. wide local excision
    B. laser vaporization
    C. simple vulvectomy
    D. radical vulvectomy and inguinal lymphadenectomy
31. Paget's disease associated with an underlying adenocarcinoma is treated by:
    A. wide local excision
    B. laser vaporization
    C. simple vulvectomy
    D. radical vulvectomy and inguinal lymphadenectomy
32. The location of most vulvar melanomas is:
    A. labia majora
    B. labia minora and clitoris
    C. perineum
    D. vestibule
33. According to Clark's staging classification, a melanoma that extends through the basement membrane into the papillary dermis is staged as level:
    A. I
    B. II
    C. III
    D. IV
34. Concerning melanoma of the vulva, the following are true *except:*
    A. prognosis is related to lesion size and depth of invasion of the lesion
    B. histologic growth patterns influence survival
    C. there is 100% survival in patients with lesions less than 1.5 mm in thickness
    D. lymphadenectomy in melanoma is therapeutic
35. Concerning sarcoma of the vulva the following are true *except:*
    A. it is a rare lesion occurring in a younger group of patients
    B. histologic grade appears to be the most important factor in prognosis
    C. therapy is radical vulvectomy and bilateral inguinal lymphadenectomy
    D. in low-grade lesions, therapy is the same because they often recur
36. The most frequent type of Bartholin's gland carcinoma is:
    A. squamous
    B. adenomatous
    C. adenoid cystic
    D. adenosquamous
37. True statements concerning Paget's disease of the vulva include the following *except:*
    A. there are two types of lesions: one intraepithelial and one with an underlying adenocarcinoma
    B. gross lesions show hyperemic areas with white coating
    C. Paget's cells contain intracytoplasmic mucin
    D. treatment is radical vulvectomy and inguinal lymphadenectomy
38. The second most common cancer occurring in the vulva is:
    A. squamous cell carcinoma
    B. adenocarcinoma
    C. melanoma
    D. sarcoma
39. Clark's and Breslow's classifications of melanomas are based on:
    A. size of lesion
    B. depth of lesion
    C. growth pattern
    D. presence or absence of inguinal node metastasis
40. The most important factor in prognosis of sarcoma of the vulva is:
    A. histologic grade of the sarcoma
    B. size of the lesion
    C. type of sarcoma
    D. age of the patient
41. Diagnosis of the lesion of the vulva in Figure 8–1 is:
    A. Basal cell carcinoma of the vulva
    B. Paget's disease of the vulva
    C. verrucous carcinoma of the vulva
    D. squamous cell carcinoma of the vulva

Directions for Questions 42 – 50: For each numbered item, select the letter of the most appropriate answer. Each letter may be used once, more than once, or not at all.

42–45. Match the following tumors of the vulva with their stage:
    A. Stage I
    B. Stage II
    C. Stage III
    D. Stage IV

42. A 1-cm tumor of the labium majus with one femoral lymph node metastasis
43. A 3-cm tumor of the perineum without lymph node metastasis
44. A 2-cm tumor of the clitoris involving the lower urethra with bilateral inguinal metastasis
45. A 2-cm tumor of the labium minus without lymph node metastasis

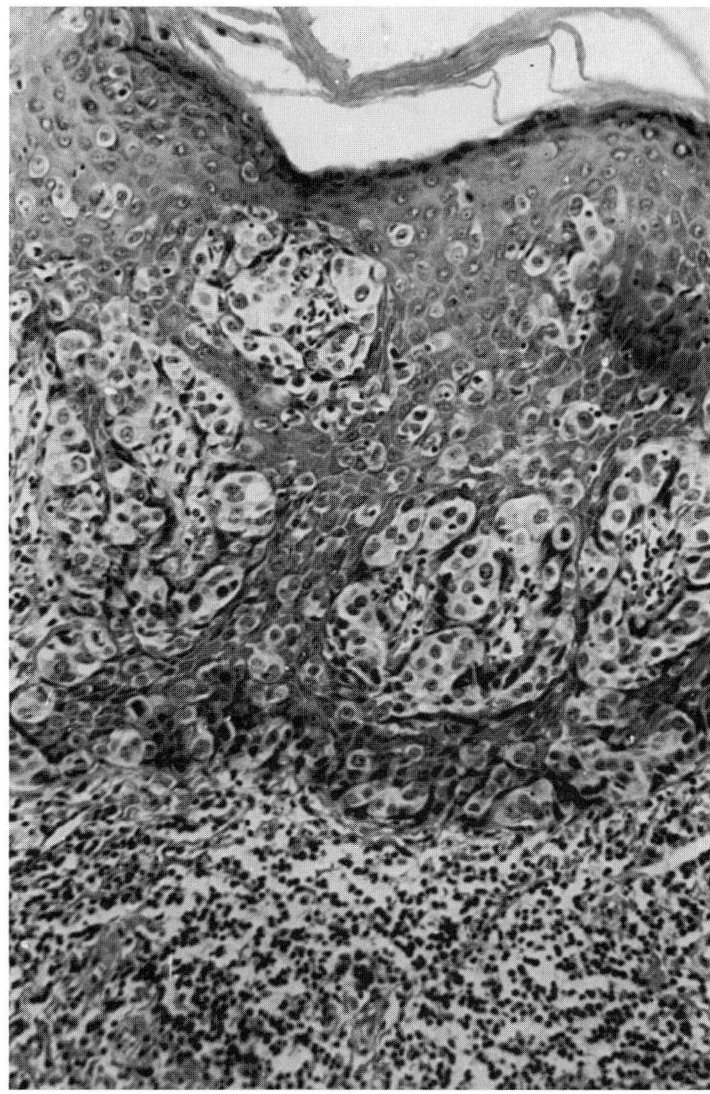

FIGURE 8–1.

46–49. Match the type of vulvar cancer with the adequate treatment:

A. large excision
B. wide excision and ipsilateral lymphadenectomy
C. radical vulvectomy *and* inguinal lymphadenectomy
D. wide local excision *or* radical vulvectomy with inguinal lymphadenectomy

46. Basal cell carcinoma of the vulva
47. Adenoid cystic carcinoma of Bartholin's gland
48. Squamous cell carcinoma of Bartholin's gland
49. Paget's disease of the vulva
50. Stage I, Clark's level I melanoma of the vulva

ANSWERS

1. **B** page 211
According to Green, the incidence of cancer of the vulva continues to increase, associated with the increased rise in the average age of the female population. From 1927 to 1961 it accounted for 5% of all gynecologic malignancies; it has now increased to 8%.
2. **D** page 211
Vulvar cancer most frequently affects women between 65 and 75 years of age (30% to 35% of cases). In the MD Anderson hospital series, 15% of all vulvar cancers occurred in women younger than 40 years.
3. **A** page 211
The incidence of squamous cell carcinoma of the vulva is 86% of vulvar neoplasms. Melanoma of the vulva is the second most frequent vulvar cancer (5%).
4. **C** page 213
Radiotherapy is contraindicated in the treatment of verrucous carcinoma of the vulva because of its ineffectiveness and its possible instigation of a more aggressive behavior. Surgical excision is the main treatment.
5. **D** page 212
Long-term pruritus and a mass of the vulva are present in more than 50% of patients with invasive vulvar cancer.

6. **C** page 213
HPV 16 DNA was found in 10 of 21 invasive carcinomas of the vulva, according to DiSaia and Creasman. The correlation is not as strong as that with VIN.
7. **A** page 213
Labia majora are the most frequent site of cancer of the vulva.
8. **A** page 212
Pruritus and vulvar mass are found in 45% of patients with vulvar cancer. Pain, bleeding, and ulceration are observed in 23%, 14%, and 14% of patients, respectively.
9. **B** page 214
Lymphatic drainage of the vulva begins with a meshwork of fine vessels covering the labia majora and labia minora and is always limited to an area medial to the genitocrural fold. These vessels merge into three or four collecting trunks that course toward the mons veneris and then change direction and terminate in ipsilateral or contralateral superficial inguinal nodes in the medial upper quadrant group. The superficial nodes drain into the deep femoral nodes and from there to the pelvic nodes.
10. **A** page 214
Cloquet's node is the most proximal node of the deep femoral group and is located just beneath Poupart's ligament. It is the last node involved before drainage into the deep pelvic nodes occurs. According to Borgno, this node is absent in 54% of his 100 inguinal lymphadenectomy specimens.
11. **B** page 214
Most authors agree that superficial inguinal nodes are the primary nodal group for the vulva and can serve as the sentinel lymph nodes of the vulva.
12. **D** page 215
Morley has shown that the incidence of lymph node involvement in a T1 lesion (<2 cm in diameter) of the vulva is approximately 20%; in a T2 lesion (>2 cm but limited to the vulva) it is more than doubled to 44%.
13. **D** page 218
The pelvic nodes are positive approximately 25% of the time when the inguinal nodes have metastatic disease. In turn, approximately 20% of patients with positive pelvic nodes will survive 5 years or more. DiSaia and Creasman recommend pelvic node irradiation therapy for patients with positive inguinal nodes.
14. **C** page 215
The proper treatment of verrucous carcinoma is wide excision with tumor-free margins. Verrucous carcinoma rarely metastasizes to lymph nodes or other organs. Radiotherapy is contraindicated because of its ineffectiveness and its possible instigation of more aggressive behavior by the tumor.
15. **C** page 218
For tumors less than 2 cm, the percentage of positive contralateral groin node is 0%, for tumors between 3 and 5 mm, it is 1.9%. Ipsilateral groin nodes are positive in 6.8% for less than 2-mm tumors and in 20.4% for tumors between 3 and 5 mm (Homesley).
16. **A** page 217
According to the new 1995 FIGO staging, stage Ia represents a lesion 2 cm or less in size with stromal invasion no greater than 1 mm. Since there is a very low incidence of nodal metastasis, large excision is the treatment. There are no stages IIa and IIb, only stage II, which represents a lesion of the vulva more than 2 cm in greatest dimension without nodal metastasis.
17. **D** page 218
Size of lesion, grade of tumor, depth of invasion, and presence of vascular and lymphatic involvement correlate with the incidence of lymph node metastasis.
18. **D** page 218
Pelvic nodes will be positive approximately 25% of the time when the inguinal nodes have metastatic disease. Approximately 20% of patients with positive pelvic nodes will survive 5 years or more.
19. **B** page 218
Pelvic lymph node irradiation is recommended for patients with positive inguinal nodes. Pelvic node dissection in conjunction with inguinal node dissection definitively increases morbidity in patients with cancer of the vulva, who are often elderly and medically infirm.
20. **A** page 218
Most surgeons limit the initial procedure to radical vulvectomy and bilateral superficial and deep inguinal node dissection. Pelvic lymph node dissection is not done routinely because the deep pelvic nodes are essentially never involved with metastatic disease when the more superficial inguinal nodes are uninvolved. If the presence of tumor is documented in the inguinal lymph nodes, a pelvic lymphadenectomy is one option for therapy on the involved side. Because of the increased morbidity of pelvic lymphadenectomy, DiSaia and Creasman recommend pelvic lymph node irradiation in those cases. Simple vulvectomy is infrequently done in case of cancer of the vulva. Radical vulvectomy with elective node irradiation is advocated by Daly and Million but has been performed only in a small number of patients. Radiotherapy has not been used widely for vulvar cancer because of technical difficulties and irradiation vulvitis.
21. **A** page 220
The procedure is frequently performed on patients in their eighth to tenth decades with surprisingly low morbidity and mortality. Mortality has been reduced from 20% in the earliest series to 1% to 2%. More than 85% of patients exhibit some form of delayed incisional healing.
22. **D** page 220
Lymphocyst is the least common of the listed morbidities; it is best treated as any other lymphocyst—with preventive measures and nonintervention. It usually resolves spontaneously. Delayed incisional healing occurs in up to 85% of patients, with incisional breakdown occurring in more than 50%. Sixty-nine percent of patients report significant lymphedema.
23. **C** page 224
Five-year survival for the patient with positive inguinal lymph nodes is approximately 40% (Table 8–8). In addition to stage and presence of positive lymph nodes, other factors relating to survival

include number of positive lymph nodes and bilaterality of metastases.

24. **D** page 224
Simonsen reported a 40% salvage rate for patients with local disease and 8% for patients with nodal metastasis at time of recurrence. Salvage therapy for recurrent vulvar carcinoma includes surgery and/or irradiation.

25. **A** page 225
In early vulvar carcinoma, there does not appear to be a definitive correlation between tumor differentiation and nodal metastasis or survival, whereas increasing depth of invasion and vascular space of involvement increases the risk of nodal metastasis. This is in contrast to more advanced carcinoma, in which tumor grade does correlate with nodal metastasis.

26. **B** page 226
The ISSVD has attempted to define a subcategory of vulvar carcinoma with essentially a 0% chance of nodal metastasis, which may thus be treated conservatively. Their definition of early invasive carcinoma of the vulva includes choices A, C, and D, and lesions 2 cm or less in diameter.

27. **D** page 228
The authors' criteria for choosing patients eligible for conservative surgical management does not address presence or absence of vascular space involvement. Squamous lesions 2 cm or less in diameter (T1) and up to 5 mm of invasion are included. In patients so treated, 1 of 50 patients had nodal metastases and died of the disease; the 5 local recurrences were successfully treated with re-excision. This approach uses the superficial inguinal nodes as sentinel nodes in the treatment.

28. **C** page 228
The conservative procedure practiced by the authors begins with removal of the superficial and deep regional lymph nodes on the ipsilateral side of the lesion. A frozen section is performed. If nodal metastasis is detected, a classic radical vulvectomy and complete bilateral inguinal lymphadenectomy is performed. If no nodal metastasis is present, a radical wide local excision of the primary lesion with 3-cm margins is performed.

29. **D** page 230
Misdiagnosis of CIS or melanoma has been made for Paget's disease of the vulva. Sufficient tissue for histologic evaluation and special stains eliminate this confusion and readily identify an underlying adenocarcinoma.

30. **A** page 231
Wide local excision to include the entire lesion is sufficient for the treatment of intraepithelial Paget's disease. Surgical margins should be free of tumor. Recurrences are common even when the surgical margins do not contain neoplastic cells. Some surgeons have abandoned the use of frozen section surgical margins for this reason.

31. **D** page 231
Patients in whom an adenocarcinoma is identified in association with Paget's disease of the vulva should be treated with radical vulvectomy and inguinal lymphadenectomy. If metastases are present in the lymph nodes, the prognosis is guarded.

32. **B** page 233
Most vulvar melanomas are located on the labia minora or clitoris.

33. **B** page 233, Table 8–13
Prognosis of melanoma is related to size of the lesion and depth of invasion. With levels I and II, a wide local excision may be adequate treatment. If the disease is intraepithelial (level I), cure should be close to 100%. Ten-year survival rates associated with Clark's level II, III, IV, and V tumors were 100%, 83%, 65%, and 23%, respectively.

34. **D** page 234
The role of lymphadenectomy in melanomas is more prognostic than therapeutic. It is rare that a patient with positive inguinal nodes has a long-term survival.

Histologic growth patterns also influence survival: 5-year survival for superficial spreading and nodular melanomas were 71% and 38%, respectively.

Using the Breslow's micrometer measurement method, Jamarillo and Day reported 100% survival in patients with lesions less than 1.5 mm in thickness, 65% to 70% survival in patients with lesions 1.5 to 4.0 mm, and 25% to 35% survival in patients with lesions greater than 4 mm. Since prognosis is directly related to invasion, there is a recent tendency to be more conservative. Melanomas at Clark's levels I and II are treated by DiSaia and Creasman with large excision; III, IV, and V are treated with radical vulvectomy and inguinal and femoral lymphadenectomy.

35. **D** page 235
Wide local excision should be considered in the low-grade lesions, because nodal involvement is rare.

36. **A** page 235
Almost half of Bartholin's gland carcinomas are squamous. Prognosis is good if lymph node metastasis is not present.

37. **D** page 230
Therapy for the two types of Paget's disease of the vulva is different: large excision with free margins for intraepithelial Paget's disease and radical vulvectomy with inguinal lymphadenectomy for Paget's disease with underlying adenocarcinoma. There are also two other forms of Paget's disease: minimally invasive (<1 mm) and invasive Paget's disease.

38. **C** page 232
Melanoma is the second most common cancer occurring in the vulva. This malignancy is still rare and probably arises from a junctional or a compound nevus.

39. **B** page 233
Clark's and Breslow's classifications of melanomas are based on depth of the lesion.
According to Clark's staging classification:
- Level I refers to in situ melanoma
- Level II melanoma extends into the papillary dermis
- Level III melanoma fills the papillary dermis and extends to the reticular dermis
- Level IV melanoma invades the reticular dermis
- Level V extends to the subcutaneous fat

Breslow's technique is more simple and relies on micrometer measurement. The lesions are classified according to their thickness: less than 1.5 mm in thickness, between 1.5 and 4 mm, and greater than 4 mm. Survival is related to thickness.

40. **A** page 235
The histologic grade of the sarcoma appears to be the most important factor in prognosis. An undifferentiated rhabdomyosarcoma has a poor prognosis; a well-differentiated leiomyosarcoma has a better prognosis.
41. **B** page 231
The figure represents Paget's disease of the vulva with characteristic large cells with clear cytoplasm found singly or forming acini in the epidermis (Paget's cells).
42. **C** page 217
Although the tumor is small (<2 cm), metastasis in one femoral lymph node changes the stage from I to III.
43. **B** page 217
Without lymph node metastasis, the tumor is in stage II because it is larger than 2 cm.
44. **D** page 217
Involvement of the lower urethra alone classifies the tumor as stage III. Bilateral inguinal metastasis classifies the tumor as stage IV.
45. **A** page 217
This is the largest size of the tumor (2 cm) without inguinal metastasis to be classified as stage I.
46. **A** page 236
47. **B** page 236
48. **C** page 235
49. **D** page 232
50. **A** page 233
When performing wide local excision, the margins should be free of tumor. Basal carcinoma should be distinguished from basosquamous cell carcinoma, which should be treated like a squamous cell carcinoma of the vulva.

Adenoid cystic carcinoma of the Bartholin's gland is a rare entity manifested by frequent local recurrences and slowly progressive disease, including pulmonary metastasis.

The 5-year survival of patients with Bartholin's gland carcinoma, including all histologic types and all stages, was 84%, as reported by Copeland, on 36 patients.

Depending on the type of Paget's disease, wide local excision is performed for intraepithelial Paget's; radical vulvectomy and bilateral inguinal lymphadenectomy are the treatment for Paget's with underlying adenocarcinoma.

Level I melanoma of vulva is treated by large local excision (margins 2 cm).

chapter 9 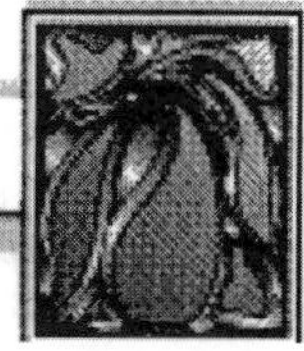

INVASIVE CANCER of the VAGINA and URETHRA

KEY POINTS TO REMEMBER

- Primary cancer of the vagina is very rare (1.5% to 2% of genital malignancies). Age incidence is between 35 and 90 years.
- Secondary carcinoma of the vagina is seen more frequently, mostly from extension of cervical cancer.
- Primary cancer of the vagina is generally squamous cell carcinoma (85%). Lesions predominate in the upper third and on the posterior wall of the vagina.
- Most frequent symptoms are vaginal discharge and irregular bleeding. Urinary symptoms are common.
- The Pap smear is effective in detecting vaginal cancer in an asymptomatic patient. DiSaia suggests that smears should be done every 2 to 3 years, even in patients who had hysterectomies for benign disease.
- The lymphatic system of the vagina is complex: the upper vagina drains into the iliac nodes, and the distal vagina drains into the lymph nodes of the femoral triangle. Lesions in the upper vagina metastasize similar to those of carcinoma of the cervix (obturator, iliac, and hypogastric lymph nodes); lesions in the lower vagina are similar to those of cancer of the vulva (inguinal and femoral nodes).
- FIGO staging of carcinoma of the vagina is clinical. Stage 0: carcinoma in situ; stage I: vaginal wall; stage II: subvaginal tissue; stage III: pelvic wall; stage IV: (1) IVa is mucosa of bladder and rectum, or beyond pelvis, and (2) IVb is distant organs.
- In situ carcinomas are treated almost exclusively with surgery. Invasive carcinomas are treated with radiotherapy (74%), surgery (32%), and chemotherapy (12%). Surgery is used most often for stage I tumors, particularly for those in the upper vagina.
- Radiation therapy must be tailored to the stage and extent of disease: external irradiation of 4000 to 5000 cGy followed with vaginal ovoid or interstitial implant of 6000 to 8000 cGy. Tumors of the distal one third of the vagina are best treated by radical inguinal lymphadenectomy before radiation therapy. Patients who have lesions of the upper one third of the vagina after hysterectomy should be given an "open implant." Incidence of complications after radiation therapy is low. Serious complications occur in 10% of patients (rectovaginal fistulae, severe rectal bleeding requiring diversion).
- Five-year relative survival rate was 96% for stage 0, 73% for stage I, 58% for stage II, and 36% for stages III and IV.
- Most recurrences appear locally within 2 years of primary therapy (51% overall recurrence rate) and are treated with ultraradical surgery (exenteration). Prognosis is grave (30 of 33 patients died within 8 months). Cisplatin gives disappointing results.
- Carcinoma in situ is treated by wide local excision. Thirty percent of intraepithelial lesions progress to invasive cancer if left untreated. Superficially invasive squamous cell carcinoma of the vagina (<2.5 mm from the surface) can be treated with local excision.
- As of 1992, 594 cases of vaginal and cervical clear cell adenocarcinomas were reported. Maternal history of positive DES or chemically related estrogen was 2 in 3. Age at diagnosis ranged from 7 to 42 years, with a peak frequency at 19 years. Patients 15 years old and younger appeared to have more aggressive carcinoma than those 19 years of age and older.
- In all cases of clear cell adenocarcinoma, DES was begun before the 18th week of pregnancy. The risk of development of carcinoma in DES-exposed females has been estimated to be 0.14 to 1.4/1000. There is no correlation of dose and duration of treatment with the incidence of malignancy. Abnormal bleeding is the initial symptom in most patients, but 20% are asymptomatic.
- Adenosis has been found accompanying vaginal clear cell adenocarcinoma in nearly all cases.
- Surgery and radiation are effective in the treatment of clear cell adenocarcinoma of the vagina. The incidence of lymph node metastases is high: 16% in stage I and 30% in stage II. The optimal therapy for clear cell carcinoma of the cervix and vagina has not been established.
- Radical hysterectomy with upper vaginectomy and pelvic lymphadenectomy is the recommended therapy for tumor confined to the cervix or upper vagina. Radiation is used for more extensive tumors and lesions of the lower two thirds of the vagina.
- Five-year survival is 80%: stage I 91%, stage II 82%, and stage III 37%.
- Nineteen percent of patients had recurrences of clear cell adenocarcinoma within 3 years after primary tumor treatment (60% in pelvis, 36% in lungs, and 20% in supraclavicular nodes). Patients should have a prolonged follow-up because some recurrences may occur up to 7 years after initial therapy. Surgery and irradiation have been effective in some cases; chemotherapy results have been disappointing.
- Malignant melanoma of the vagina constitutes less than 0.5% of all vaginal malignancies. Surgery remains the

treatment of choice. Overall survival rate is 15%. Elective lymph node dissection is recommended only for level III–V lesions. Recurrences develop in the pelvis and lung. The interval to recurrence is usually less than 1 year, and survival from point of recurrence averages 8 months.

- Spindle cell sarcomas of the vagina (leiomyosarcoma, fibrosarcoma) are very rare and are treated with local excision in cases of well-differentiated tumors.
- Sarcoma botryoides of the vagina, which predominately affects children, is treated with conservative surgery and adjuvant chemotherapy (vincristine, dactinomycin, and cyclophosphamide).
- Endodermal sinus tumor of the vagina occurs in infants younger than 2 years of age and is treated with surgery and chemotherapy. The survival is poor (25% alive at 2 years).
- Primary carcinoma of the urethra is rare. Most cases are squamous and are treated with radiotherapy (interstitial irradiation) after inguinal lymphadenectomy. Overall 5-year survival is 65% (71% for patients with anterior urethral carcinoma and 50% for patients with posterior carcinoma).

QUESTIONS

Directions for Questions 1–33: Select the one best answer.

1. The most frequent location of cancer of the vagina is:
   A. lower third, posterior wall
   B. middle third, anterior wall
   C. upper third, posterior wall
   D. lateral walls
2. The most frequent malignant neoplasm of the vagina is:
   A. secondary carcinoma from cancer of the cervix
   B. primary squamous cell carcinoma
   C. adenocarcinoma
   D. melanoma
3. The most frequent histologic type of primary carcinoma of the vagina is:
   A. melanoma
   B. adenocarcinoma
   C. squamous cell carcinoma
   D. sarcoma
4. Comparing a total number of genital malignancies, the incidence of vaginal cancer is approximately:
   A. 3%
   B. 5%
   C. 8%
   D. 10%
5. True statements concerning the use of Papanicolaou smear in detecting vaginal cancer in patients who had undergone prior hysterectomies for benign diseases are the following *except:*
   A. the Pap smear is effective in detecting vaginal cancer in asymptomatic women
   B. Bell and Benedet reported that 35% and 19% of their patients, respectively, with cancer of the vagina had previous hysterectomy
   C. considerations of cost-effectiveness should be considered for advising the use of the Pap smear
   D. Pap smear should be done every year in patients with prior hysterectomies
6. The most frequent symptom of invasive vaginal cancer is:
   A. vaginal bleeding
   B. bloody vaginal discharge
   C. dysuria
   D. tenesmus
7. Diagnostic studies required in carcinoma of the vagina include the following *except:*
   A. chest radiographic examination
   B. intravenous pyelogram (IVP)
   C. cystoscopy and proctoscopy
   D. lymphangiogram and barium enema
8. Stage II squamous cell carcinoma of the vagina should be treated with:
   A. radical vaginectomy and pelvic node dissection
   B. simple vaginectomy and femoral node dissection
   C. external irradiation followed by interstitial implant
   D. external irradiation only
9. Serious complications after irradiation therapy for carcinoma of the vagina occur in 10% of patients and include the following *except:*
   A. intestinal obstruction
   B. rectal stenosis
   C. rectovaginal fistulae
   D. severe rectal bleeding
10. The treatment of advanced primary vaginal carcinoma that provides the highest survival rates is:
    A. external beam therapy and brachytherapy
    B. interstitial and intracavitary therapy
    C. radical surgery
    D. external beam therapy
11. Best treatment as suggested by DiSaia and Creasman for vulvovaginal cancer is:
    A. pelvic exenteration
    B. large excision
    C. radiation therapy
    D. surgical resection of the groin nodes followed by radiation therapy
12. True statements relative to recurrent carcinoma of the vagina include all *except:*
    A. 50% of patients will develop recurrence
    B. cisplatin-based chemotherapy is the treatment of choice for recurrent disease
    C. 40% of those with recurrent carcinoma respond to treatment
    D. 80% of recurrences occur in the pelvis
13. In reference to early invasive squamous carcinoma of the vagina, choose the therapy favored by the authors:
    A. brachytherapy
    B. external beam therapy plus brachytherapy
    C. wide local excision/partial vaginectomy
    D. radical vaginectomy
14. The proper management for the post-treatment pelvic radiotherapy patient with abnormal vaginal cytologic findings is:
    A. repetition of physical examination and Pap smear in 4 months
    B. topical 5-FU

C. cryotherapy
D. physical examination, and colposcopic-directed biopsies

15. Appropriate treatment of vaginal intraepithelial neoplasia (VAIN) after pelvic radiotherapy includes all *but:*
A. cryotherapy
B. local excision
C. laser vaporization
D. topical 5-FU

16. Proper therapy for vulvovaginal cancer includes all *except:*
A. exenteration
B. radiotherapy
C. radical surgery plus radiotherapy
D. inguinal lymphadenectomy followed by radiotherapy

17. True statements relative to the age of patients with clear cell genital adenocarcinoma include all *except:*
A. the youngest patient was age 7
B. most patients were born after 1945
C. the peak frequency was at age 19
D. the oldest patient was age 34

18. True statements relative to the link between in utero DES exposure and clear cell adenocarcinomas include all *except:*
A. DES exposure is more closely linked with vaginal, rather than cervical, clear cell adenocarcinoma
B. 60% of clear cell adenocarcinoma is vaginal; 40% is cervical
C. the estimated risk to the DES-exposed female is less than 1 in 1000
D. the risk of development of genital malignancy was proportional to the maternal dose of DES

19. Analysis of data from the DESAD (National Collaborative Diethylstilbestrol Adenosis) Project reveals all *except:*
A. in utero DES exposure is a carcinogenic event
B. an inherited genetic factor may be the predisposing factor
C. a viral role in clear cell adenocarcinoma is suggested
D. the survival rate of oral contraceptive users with clear cell carcinoma is higher than that of nonusers

20. The following true statements in regard to invasive squamous carcinoma of the vagina include all *except:*
A. the incidence of serious complications from standard therapy is 10%
B. the prognosis for lower vaginal lesions is worse than that for upper vaginal lesions
C. overall survival approximates 50%
D. 90% of patients will experience cystitis or proctitis during radiation therapy

21. Choose the true statement relative to clear cell carcinoma of the vagina:
A. 100% are associated with adenosis
B. there is a predilection for occurrence in the lower vagina
C. occurrence of lymph node metastasis is rare
D. the neoplasm is usually deeply invasive

22. True statements regarding therapy of lower genital clear cell carcinoma include all *except:*
A. radical hysterectomy, vaginectomy, and pelvic lymphadenectomy are the preferred therapy for patients with cervical or upper vaginal disease
B. for stage I vaginal lesions, local therapy is less effective than conventional therapy
C. radiotherapy is recommended for extensive or lower vaginal lesions
D. exenteration is used for central pelvic recurrence or postradiotherapy persistence

23. Five-year survival rate of patients with stage I clear cell adenocarcinoma of the cervix and vagina is:
A. 91%
B. 80%
C. 58%
D. 37%

24. Concerning recurrences of clear cell carcinoma of the vagina, the following are true *except:*
A. surgery and radiation have been effective in the control of pelvic recurrences in some cases
B. recurrences occur in the pelvic area and rarely in the lungs
C. chemotherapy results are disappointing
D. there is no objective response with progestational agents

25. Concerning primary adenocarcinoma of the vagina, the following are true *except:*
A. it can arise from vaginal adenosis
B. it can arise from foci of endometriosis
C. it can arise from Gartner's duct remnants
D. therapy for these adenocarcinomas is radical vaginectomy and pelvic node dissection

26. Pelvic and abdominal cancers that give rise to most common vaginal metastases are:
A. carcinomas of ovary and fallopian tubes
B. carcinomas of colon and rectum
C. cervical and endometrial carcinomas
D. renal cell neoplasms

27. The percentage of patients with recurrence of clear cell adenocarcinoma of the vagina is approximately:
A. 30%
B. 25%
C. 19%
D. 10%

28. The most frequent location of melanoma of the vagina is:
A. upper one third of the vagina, anterior wall
B. lower one third of the vagina, anterior wall
C. upper one third of the vagina, posterior wall
D. lower one third of the vagina, posterior wall

29. The treatment of choice for melanoma of the vagina is:
A. surgery
B. radiation
C. chemotherapy
D. combination of A, B, and C

30. Choose the characteristics of vaginal sarcomas that predict recurrence after surgery:
A. tumors larger than 3 cm with more than 10 mitotic figures (MF) per 10 high-power fields (HPF)

B. tumors larger than 5 cm with more than 5 MF/10 HPF
C. tumors larger than 3 cm with more than 5 MF/10 HPF
D. tumors larger than 5 cm with more than 10 MF/10 HPF

31. True statements concerning sarcoma botryoides of the vagina (rhabdomyosarcoma) are the following *except:*
A. it predominantly afflicts children
B. it is usually multicentric and arises in the anterior wall of the vaginal apex
C. the best treatment is radical vaginectomy and hysterectomy
D. the best treatment is chemotherapy followed by conservative surgery

32. The best treatment for endodermal sinus tumor of the vagina is:
A. radical surgical therapy
B. radiation therapy
C. chemotherapy (vincristine, dactinomycin, and cyclophosphamide [VAC])
D. surgery plus VAC, with or without radiation therapy

33. The treatment of choice for urethral cancer is:
A. local excision
B. local excision and chemotherapy
C. inguinal lymphadenectomy and interstitial irradiation
D. chemotherapy and irradiation

Directions for Questions 34–42: For each numbered item, select the letter of the most appropriate answer. Each letter may be used once, more than once, or not at all.

34–35. Match the lymphatic drainage of the vagina with the appropriate lymph nodes.
A. common internal iliac nodes and external iliac nodes
B. femoral nodes
C. both
D. neither

34. Distal vagina
35. Upper vagina

36–38. Match each described tumor with its appropriate FIGO stage:
A. I
B. II
C. III
D. IV

36. A 3-cm tumor in the lower vagina, encroaching the symphysis pubis
37. A 1-cm lesion in the upper vagina limited to the mucosa
38. A 2-cm lesion in the left lateral vagina involving the subvaginal tissue but free from pelvic walls; an IVP is normal

39–42. Match the type and location of cancer of vagina with the type of treatment:
A. external radiation and interstitial implant
B. interstitial radiation therapy
C. inguinal lymphadenectomy followed by external irradiation and interstitial implant
D. "open implant" and pelvic radiotherapy

39. Cancer of the upper third of the vagina after hysterectomy
40. Small carcinoma of the vagina
41. Cancer of the distal one third of the vagina
42. Stages III and IV carcinomas of the vagina

ANSWERS

1. **C** page 241
Primary cancer of the vagina occurs frequently in the upper third (55%). The middle third and lower third of the vagina account for the location of approximately 13% and 32% of primary carcinoma, respectively. Lesions predominate on the posterior wall of the vagina, although in recent reports by Manetta there is no real predominance of a posterior site.
2. **A** page 241
Secondary carcinoma of the vagina is more frequently seen than primary cancer. Metastatic cancer in the vagina can come from cervix, endometrium, ovary, urethra or bladder, rectum, and malignant trophoblastic disease.
3. **C** page 241
Primary cancer of the vagina is often of squamous histologic type (85%). Adenocarcinoma represents 6% of primary vaginal cancers.
4. **A** page 242
Based on nine studies of 44,432 patients with genital malignancies, the incidence of vaginal cancer ranges from 1.2% to 3.1%.
5. **D** page 242
DiSaia and Creasman recommend that Pap smears should be done every 2 to 3 years in patients with prior hysterectomies. Annual screening should be performed for cancer of the cervix in the patient without hysterectomy. This recommendation is a compromise for cost-effectiveness.
6. **B** page 242
Vaginal discharge, often bloody, is the most frequent symptom. Postmenopausal bleeding is also the initial symptom in many patients with invasive lesions. Dysuria or tenesmus denotes extension of the tumor to urethra or bladder and rectum.
7. **D** page 243
Lymphangiogram and barium enema are optional but helpful diagnostic studies. Barium enema is indicated for patients suspected of diverticulitis.
8. **C** page 245
Squamous cell carcinoma of the vagina stage II has been treated primarily by radiotherapy consisting of external irradiation in a dose of 4000 to 5000 cGy followed with vaginal ovoids and an intrauterine tandem or with an interstitial implant. Radical vaginectomy and pelvic lymphadenectomy are used for stage I tumors in young patients.
9. **A** page 247
Rectal stenosis, rectovaginal fistulae, and severe rectal bleeding requiring diversion occur in 10% of patients. Thirty-five percent of patients have cystitis or proctitis during or after radiation therapy, but symptoms often resolve spontaneously.

10. **A** page 245
The preferred method of radiotherapy for invasive carcinoma of the vagina is similar to that for carcinoma of the cervix: external beam radiotherapy and interstitial or intracavitary brachytherapy.
11. **D** page 249
The authors prefer treatment plans that preserve the bladder and rectum. They agree with Boronow, who recommends surgical extirpation of the inguinal nodes with a combination of external and interstitial irradiation for control of the central lesion. Boronow obtained a 5-year survival rate of 75%.
12. **B** page 248
Radiation is the treatment of choice in patients not having received prior radiation. However, since most patients with recurrence have already undergone radiotherapy, they are not eligible for more. Only patients found eligible for exenteration may be cured; this is the treatment of choice for appropriate patients who had previously undergone radiotherapy. Cisplatin-based chemotherapy is most favored for patients with recurrence who have had radiotherapy and are not eligible for exenteration. It should be viewed only as potentially palliative in view of the limited frequency and duration of response.
13. **C** page 249
The authors favor local surgical treatment based on its efficacy and better ability to preserve vaginal function. Radiation is an appropriate alternative in some patients. Brachytherapy alone (intracavitary or interstitial therapy) is all that is usually necessary, because the risk of nodal metastasis (and thus the need for external beam therapy) in early squamous cell carcinoma is low.
14. **D** page 249
Atypical vaginal cytology after pelvic radiotherapy is commonly noted. There is a tendency to attribute this to "radiotherapy changes." An MD Anderson Hospital study demonstrates that a significant proportion of patients will have developed intraepithelial neoplasia, 30% of which will progress to invasive cancer if untreated. These patients should undergo immediate evaluation by examination, colposcopy, and biopsies.
15. **A** page 249
The authors feel that surgical excision, laser vaporization, or topical 5-FU are appropriate treatments for postradiotherapy VAIN. Cryotherapy is rarely used in the vagina.
16. **B** page 249
Radiotherapy alone is not felt to be sufficient therapy for vulvovaginal carcinoma. Various types of surgery, with and without radiotherapy, are thought to have high success rates with low morbidity.
17. **D** page 250
The registry maintained by Herbst has attempted to access all North American females with genital clear cell adenocarcinoma. The data demonstrated that this entity was rarely seen before 1945 and that the peak of 31 cases occurred in 1975. Ninety percent of the patients were over the age of 14 years at diagnosis. The oldest patient was 42 years old.
18. **D** page 250
Neither dose nor duration of maternal DES treatment was correlated with the risk of developing clear cell adenocarcinoma.
19. **A** page 251
Examination of DES data from the DESAD Project has failed to prove that DES is a carcinogen. It may be a teratogen, however, and the teratogenic effect may increase susceptibility to malignancy. Other hypotheses thought to be possible were those of seasonal viral exposures and inherited genetic factors. A higher proportion of clear cell carcinoma patients using oral contraceptives had lower stages, accounting for the increased survival noted in this group.
20. **D** page 247
As many as 35% of patients will experience cystitis or proctitis during or shortly after therapy.
21. **A** page 252
Clear cell adenocarcinoma of the vagina is not seen without concomitant adenosis. There is a predilection for occurrence in the upper and anterior vagina. The incidence of nodal metastasis is comparatively high: approximately 16% in stage I and 30% or more in stage II. This neoplasm tends to remain superficial.
22. **B** page 252
Of 219 stage I vaginal clear cell carcinomas in the Herbst registry, 20% received local therapy and 80% received conventional radical therapy (radiotherapy or radical surgery). Five- and 10-year survival was equivalent.
23. **A** page 253, Table 9–8
Five-year survival for patients with clear cell adenocarcinoma of the vagina and cervix stage I is 91%, stage IIa of the cervix is 80%, and stage II of the vagina is 82%.
24. **B** page 253
A higher proportion of clear cell adenocarcinomas of the vagina metastasize to the lungs and supraclavicular area than do squamous cell carcinomas of the vagina and cervix. In a study on 346 patients by Herbst, 58 patients (19%) had recurrences: 60% in the pelvis, 36% in the lungs, and 20% in the supraclavicular lymph nodes. Prolonged follow-up is important because some recurrences have occurred 7 years after initial therapy.
25. **D** page 254
Therapy for these adenocarcinomas is presently analogous to that for their squamous counterpart: irradiation or surgery combined with irradiation, depending on the location of the tumor.
26. **C** page 241
Most common vaginal metastases are from lesions of cervical and endometrial origin.
27. **C** page 253
Among 346 patients analyzed by Herbst, 20 were never free of disease and 19 died at the time of the report. Fifty-eight patients (18.8%) had recurrences, and most of these were diagnosed within 3 years after primary tumor treatment.

28. **B** page 254
Melanoma of the vagina is located predominantly in the lower one third of the vagina, commonly on the anterior wall.
29. **A** page 254
Surgery remains the treatment of choice of melanoma of the vagina. Neoplasms that involve the lower third of the vagina are treated with radical vulvectomy/vaginectomy and inguinal and pelvic node dissection. Neoplasms that involve the upper two thirds of the vagina require some form of exenteration.
Radiation therapy in general has not proved to be effective; chemotherapy is also disappointing. The overall survival rate for vaginal melanoma is about 15%.
Dissection of lymph nodes that are clinically negative for melanoma of the vagina, urethra, and vulva continues to be controversial and seems to be more of prognostic than of therapeutic benefit. DiSaia and Creasman found Clark's and Breslow's classifications of skin melanomas very useful in prognosticating mucosal tumors. They perform lymph node dissection only for levels III to V lesions.
30. **C** page 255
Tavassoli and Norris reported only 5 recurrences among 60 patients with smooth muscle tumors of the vagina. The tumors were all greater than 3 cm with more than 5 MF/10 HPF. Local excision with free margins was the treatment of choice when the tumor was well-differentiated and well-circumscribed.
31. **C** page 256
A combination of vincristine, dactinomycin, and cyclophosphamide (VAC) appears to be very effective in rhabdomyosarcoma of the vagina and results in a marked reduction in tumor size when the drug combination is used as initial therapy, permitting more conservative surgery.
32. **D** page 256
A combination of chemotherapy with and without radiation therapy following conservative surgical excision can be effective in controlling endodermal sinus tumor of the vagina.
33. **C** page 256
Interstitial irradiation to the central lesion followed by dissection of inguinal lymph nodes is the therapy for urethral cancer recommended by the authors.
Discovery of lymph node metastases should be followed by pelvic irradiation. Unlike vulvar cancer, the role of radiotherapy for urethral cancer is substantial.
34. **C** page 243
The distal or lower vagina is drained by a lymphatic network that ends in the regional lymph nodes of the femoral triangle (femoral nodes) and from there to the pelvic nodes (external iliac nodes).
35. **A** page 243
The lymphatic trunks of the upper vagina drain into the most dorsal group of iliac nodes represented by the common iliac and hypogastric nodes.
36. **C** page 243
A tumor with involvement of the symphysis pubis is classified as stage III.
37. **A** page 243
Stage I is composed of carcinomas limited to the vaginal mucosa.
38. **B** page 243
A carcinoma that affects the subvaginal tissue but has not extended into the pelvic wall is considered as being in stage II.
39. **D** page 246
An "open implant" should be considered in patients with cancer of the upper half of the vagina after hysterectomy. The laparotomy offers opportunity for the creation of an omental carpet and for effective dosimetry, thus diminishing complications. Open implants are never done alone; they are done after whole pelvic radiotherapy.
40. **B** page 245
Interstitial radiation therapy alone can be used to treat small carcinomas of the vagina. A minimum of 6000 to 7000 cGy should be delivered to the neoplasm.
41. **C** page 245
Cancer of the distal one third of the vagina frequently metastasizes to inguinal nodes. A radical inguinal dissection should be done before external irradiation and interstitial implant.
42. **A** page 245
Stages III and IV of the vagina are treated initially with 5000 cGy external radiation for 5 to 6 weeks. After receiving 5000 cGy, the patient should be re-examined for an additional 1000 to 2000 cGy external radiation to reduced fields. An interstitial implant is needed for residual tumor.

chapter 10 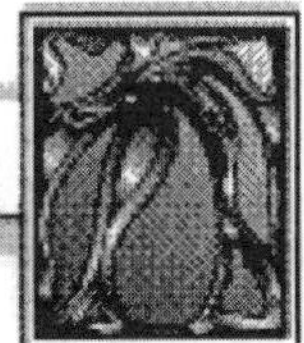

THE ADNEXAL MASS and EARLY OVARIAN CANCER

KEY POINTS TO REMEMBER

- Five to ten percent of women in the United States will undergo a surgical procedure for a suspected ovarian neoplasm during their lifetime. Thirteen to twenty-one percent of these women will be found to have ovarian cancer.
- Age is probably the most important factor in determining the potential for malignancy.
- Functional cysts are the most common clinically detectable enlargements of the ovary during the reproductive years (follicular cysts, theca lutein cysts, corpus luteum cysts).
- Only 20% of all ovarian neoplasms are pathologically malignant. The most common benign cystic neoplasms of the ovary are serous and mucinous cystadenomas and cystic teratomas. Benign solid tumors of the ovary are usually of connective tissue origin (fibromas, thecomas, or Brenner tumors).
- Any mass larger than 10 cm in diameter should be surgically explored. Laparoscopy should be used cautiously in the presence of any mass with clinical or ultrasonographic characteristics suggestive of malignancy.
- True functional cysts of the ovary regress in a 4-to 6-week follow-up period of observation. All persistent adnexal enlargement must be considered malignant until proved otherwise.
- An elevated CA-125 is associated with a malignancy less than 25% of the time in patients younger than 50 years of age and 80% of the time in patients older than 50 years of age. Only 50% of patients with stage I epithelial cancer of the ovary will have an elevated CA-125. CA-125 values in excess of 300 U/mL are usually associated with malignancy even in patients younger than 50 years.
- All patients scheduled for operative laparoscopy for an adnexal mass should also consent to laparotomy if malignancy is uncovered.
- Serous cystadenomas are more common than the mucinous type and harbor psammoma bodies. Bilaterality may be found in 10% of patients.
- Mucinous cystadenomas may become huge (100 to 200 lb), may perforate, and may initiate pseudomyxoma peritonei, the treatment of which is primarily surgical. There is essentially no significant incidence of bilaterality.
- Brenner tumors can arise from diverse sources (surface epithelium, rete ovarii, ovarian stroma); most are benign except for some rare cases of malignancy. Treatment is excision.
- Benign cystic teratomas (dermoid cyst) are often bilateral (10% to 25%). The management is cystectomy in patients who desire fertility.
- Fibromas are benign and are sometimes associated with Meigs' syndrome.
- Abdominal pain and abdominal mass are the two frequent symptoms in children with adnexal mass.
- In a study by Van Winter on 521 adnexal masses in infancy, childhood, and adolescence, 64% were non-neoplastic and 36% were neoplastic. Only 8% of neoplastic lesions were malignant. Germ cell tumors are the most frequent.
- During the postmenopausal years, the presence of a palpable ovary must alert the physician to the possibility of an underlying malignancy.
- Ten to fifteen percent of patients with a palpable postmenopausal ovary who are subjected to oophorectomy have a malignant neoplasm. However, the most common finding is a benign ovarian lesion (fibroma, Brenner tumor). In the postmenopausal woman, cysts larger than 5 cm in diameter have a high probability of malignancy, especially when they are associated with a high serum CA-125.
- Borderline malignant epithelial ovarian neoplasms occur more frequently in the younger population, with a 10-year survival rate of 95% for stage I lesions. Recurrence may occur 10 to 20 years after therapy in a few patients.
- Treatment of borderline or low-malignant-potential tumors (LMP) should strive to extirpate the tumor completely. If the disease is unilateral, salpingo-oophorectomy should be done, with exploration of the other ovary, peritoneal cytologic examination, and partial omentectomy. If the disease is extensive, total abdominal hysterectomy with bilateral salpingo-oophorectomy and radical excision of the involved peritoneum is recommended. In addition, selected pelvic and aortic lymphadenectomy should be done in more advanced disease. Survival of advanced borderline lesions is still appreciable (stage III).
- Measurement of DNA content and nuclear morphology may provide important prognostic information in patients with borderline ovarian tumors, information that can help clinicians consider chemotherapy for biologically aggressive lesions. Invasive implants are associated with a poor outcome compared with that in the noninvasive group. Kurman suggests considering SBL tumors with invasive implants and micropapillary types as carcinomas because of their poor prognosis.

- Combined 5-year survival rate for stages I and II epithelial cancer of the ovary varies from 50% to 70% and from 40% to 50% respectively. These disappointing rates are due to unsuspected metastases: aortic node metastasis in 10% and omentum microscopic metastasis in 4.7% of patients with stages I and II disease. Thirty percent of patients with stage I or II ovarian carcinoma have free-floating cancer cells in the pelvis or paracolonic spaces.
- In young women, the definitive treatment for stage Ia ovarian cancer may be unilateral salpingo-oophorectomy and sampling of the omentum and pelvic and periaortic nodes. Incidence of microscopic metastases in the opposite ovary is approximately 12%. Mucinous and endometrioid lesions fare better than serous lesions. Recurrence rate is 7%. Multivariate analysis shows that tumor grade, presence of dense tumor-associated adhesions, and large-volume ascites were the only three significant independent prognostic factors.
- Optimal requirements for conservative management in epithelial ovarian cancer stage Ia are well-differentiated tumor; young woman of low parity; normal pelvis free of adhesions; no invasion of capsule, lymphatics, or mesoovarium; negative findings from peritoneal washings; negative results from omental biopsy and evaluation of opposite ovary; and excision of residual ovary after completion of childbearing.
- FIGO staging of early stage ovarian carcinoma:
  - Stage I: disease limited to ovaries
    - Ia: one ovary, no ascites, no surface involvement, capsule intact
    - Ib: both ovaries, no ascites, no surface involvement, capsule intact
    - Ic: either Ia or Ib with ascites containing malignant cells, or positive peritoneal cytology, capsule ruptured, or surface involvement
  - Stage II: disease involving one or both ovaries with pelvic extension
    - IIa: extension to tubes or uterus
    - IIb: other pelvic organs or pelvic sidewall
    - IIc: either IIa or IIb with ascites containing malignant cells, or positive peritoneal cytology, capsule ruptured or surface involvement
- Hysterectomy with bilateral salpingo-oophorectomy is the most cogent therapy for ovarian carcinoma.
- The role of adjuvant therapy in tumors of LMP has not yet been established.
- A GOG study reported no difference in survival for patients with stage Ic or II or poorly differentiated stages Ia and Ib cancer randomized to receive melphalan or intraperitoneal ^{32}P. The same report showed no advantage to adjuvant treatment with melphalan for patients with stage Ia or Ib, well-differentiated or moderately differentiated tumor.
- Disease-free survival and overall survival were similar in 347 patients with epithelial ovarian cancer without residual tumors following primary surgery and use of cisplatin or intraperitoneal ^{32}P.
- No difference in the overall survival could be detected in 92 patients with stage Ia or Ib grade 2 or 3 tumors who received six cycles of cisplatin or no treatment.
- Treatment of dysgerminoma is conservative surgery. Although the recurrence rate is 20% in stage I, the overall survival rate is 95% because of the exceptional response to radical radiation therapy or chemotherapy.
- Spill of tumor during surgery results in decreasing survival rate in some studies or no negative influence on the outcome for patients in others. Manipulation that provokes rupture during surgery probably does not have a negative influence on the outcome for patients. However, rupture occurring at some interval before surgery may lead to seeding of the peritoneal cavity. DiSaia and Creasman recommend a course of platinum-based chemotherapy followed by a "second-look" procedure. Lavage of the peritoneal cavity with sterile water is recommended to cause lysis of cells.
- In a national survey of 12,316 ovarian cancer cases, Averette and Nguyen found that 18.2% of patients reported previous hysterectomy with ovarian conservation.
- Prophylatic oophorectomy should be offered to all perimenopausal (40- to 50-year-old) patients undergoing pelvic surgery after being informed of advantages and possible adverse effects. It is estimated that at least 1000 cases of ovarian cancer could be prevented if prophylactic oophorectomy is diligently practiced after the age of 40.

QUESTIONS

Directions for Questions 1–32: Select the one best answer.

1. Anatomically the adnexa consists of the following structures *except:*
   A. fallopian tubes
   B. ovaries
   C. broad ligaments
   D. levator ani
2. What is the percentage of women in the United States who will undergo a surgical procedure for a suspected ovarian malignancy?
   A. 2%–5%
   B. 5%–10%
   C. 10%–15%
   D. 15%–20%
3. Management of an adnexal mass depends on a combination of many predictive factors; the most important is/are:
   A. age
   B. size of mass, ultrasonographic features, unilaterality vs. bilaterality
   C. menopausal status
   D. CA-125 level
4. In premenarchal patients, most neoplasms of ovary are:
   A. epithelial
   B. germ cell
   C. stromal
   D. metastatic
5. In postmenopausal women, the histogenesis of ovarian neoplasms is from:
   A. germ cell
   B. stroma
   C. surface epithelium
   D. all of the above

6. True statements concerning the diagnosis of an adnexal mass are the following *except:*
   A. diagnosis varies with age of the patient
   B. in patients in the reproductive age period, a cystic mass larger than 5 cm should be explored immediately
   C. in premenarchal patients, most neoplasms are germ cell in origin and require surgical exploration
   D. in postmenopausal women, enlargement of the ovary is abnormal and should be considered malignant until proven otherwise
7. Uterine masses included in the differential diagnosis of an adnexal mass are:
   A. pregnancy
   B. myomas and leiomyosarcomas
   C. adenomyosis and endometrial carcinoma
   D. all of the above
8. Theca lutein cysts are found in patients with the following *except:*
   A. hydatidiform mole
   B. fetal death syndrome
   C. choriocarcinoma
   D. induction of ovulation
9. The most common benign cystic neoplasms of the ovary are:
   A. serous cystadenomas
   B. mucinous cystadenomas
   C. cystic teratomas
   D. all of the above
10. The most common symptoms at initial presentation in children with adnexal mass are/is:
    A. menstrual irregularity
    B. amenorrhea, primary and secondary
    C. pain and abdominal mass
    D. increase in abdominal girth
11. Indications for surgery of an adnexal mass include:
    A. a solid ovarian lesion or a lesion with papillary vegetations on the cyst wall
    B. an adnexal mass with ascites or greater than 10 cm in diameter
    C. a palpable adnexal mass in a premenarchal or postmenarchal patient
    D. all of the above
12. Meigs' syndrome is often associated with which type of ovarian tumor?
    A. Brenner tumor
    B. serous cystadenocarcinoma
    C. fibroma
    D. teratoma
13. True statements concerning endometriosis are the following *except:*
    A. the most common sites are ovaries, ligaments of the uterus, peritoneal cul de sac, and bladder
    B. it is more common in white and nulliparous women
    C. the amount of endometriosis correlates with the intensity of pain
    D. nodularity of the uterosacral ligaments may be helpful in the differential diagnosis
14. The most common entity of the gastrointestinal tract that appears to be an adnexal mass is:
    A. diverticulitis
    B. fecal material
    C. regional ileitis
    D. periappendiceal abscess
15. "Hydrops tubal profluens," the colicky lower abdominal pain relieved by profuse vaginal serosanguineous discharge, is typical of:
    A. cervical carcinoma
    B. endometrial carcinoma
    C. tubal carcinoma
    D. ovarian carcinoma
16. Choose the *false* statement relative to the diagnostic evaluation of a woman with an adnexal mass:
    A. ultrasound examinations should be used in most patients with an adnexal mass
    B. bilaterality is an important finding that suggests malignancy
    C. one may initially presume that an ovarian mass during the reproductive years is a functional change of the ovary
    D. ovarian enlargement in the premenarchal or postmenopausal period necessitates surgical intervention
17. Choose the *false* statement regarding the adnexal mass:
    A. many malignant ovarian tumors are clinically indistinguishable from benign tumors
    B. malignant ovarian tumors develop from benign tumors
    C. clinically persistent adnexal enlargements should be considered malignant until proven otherwise
    D. pseudomyxoma peritonei may arise from benign or malignant ovarian tumors
18. Choose the *false* statement regarding the postmenopausal palpable ovary:
    A. ten percent of patients with postmenopausal palpable ovaries are found to have ovarian malignancy
    B. when laparotomy is performed, it should be similar to an ovarian cancer staging procedure
    C. diagnostic laparotomy is indicated for the patient with postmenopausal palpable ovary
    D. the volume of the postmenopausal ovary is increased in obese and multiparous women
19. The following is true for CA-125 *except:*
    A. in patients younger than 50 years, an elevated CA-125 level is associated with a malignant mass 25% of the time
    B. in patients older than 50 years, an elevated CA-125 level is associated with a malignant mass 80% of the time
    C. CA-125 level is sometimes elevated in patients with endometriosis
    D. in patients with stage I epithelial cancer of the ovary, CA-125 level is elevated 100% of the time
20. Choose the *false* statement regarding the adnexal mass:
    A. a high false-positive rate is expected from surgical exploration of pelvic masses initially detected by CT, MRI, or ultrasound
    B. treatment of pseudomyxoma is primarily surgical

C. failure of the ovarian mass to regress over a 4- to 6-week period mandates surgical intervention
D. intraperitoneal cisplatin should be considered for adjuvant use in the pseudomyxoma patient

21. Indicate the *false* statement concerning ultrasonographic examination of the pelvis:
A. transvaginal ultrasound is a reliable and consistent method for evaluation of the size and consistency of a pelvic mass
B. using strict criteria, physicians accurately predict benign masses in 95% of patients
C. functional cysts of ovary and dermoid cysts have characteristic appearances
D. laparoscopy should be used on all ovarian masses with suspicious ultrasound findings

22. Choose the one *true* statement in reference to adnexal masses occurring in women of reproductive age:
A. any mass larger than 6 cm should be excised
B. laparotomy and excision is the method of choice for removal of these masses
C. oral contraceptives are contraindicated during the "monitoring phase" of the adnexal mass
D. failure of the mass to regress during a 2- to 3-week period mandates excision

23. Histologic criteria for borderline serous epithelial tumors are the following *except:*
A. epithelial stratification, papillary projections
B. stromal invasion
C. epithelial pleomorphism, atypicality
D. mitotic activity

24. Five-year survival in patients with ovarian serous borderline tumors with peritoneal implants is approximately:
A. 60%–70%
B. 70%–80%
C. 80%–90%
D. 90%–95%

25. Management of borderline lesions (low malignant potential) consists of:
A. unilateral salpingo-oophorectomy (or ovarian cystectomy), evaluation of the other ovary, peritoneal washing, partial omentectomy if the disease is unilateral
B. total abdominal hysterectomy and bilateral salpingo-oophorectomy, peritoneal cytologic studies, partial omentectomy, and selective pelvic and periaortic lymphadenectomy if the disease is more advanced
C. surgical removal of the disease with postoperative pelvic irradiation or chemotherapy
D. A and B

26. The incidence of unsuspected metastases to the diaphragm in stages I and II ovarian carcinoma is:
A. 5%
B. 10%
C. 15%
D. 20%

27. The management of early ovarian cancer, except in nulliparous young women, consists of total abdominal hysterectomy and bilateral salpingo-oophorectomy for the following reasons *except:*
A. the opposite ovary is removed because of the frequency of bilateral tumors or the possibility of occult metastases
B. hysterectomy is indicated because the prevalence of synchronous endometrial carcinoma is relatively high
C. hysterectomy is indicated because the uterine serosa and endometrium are often sites of occult metastasis
D. childbearing after ovarian carcinoma is potentially dangerous and the fetus could be abnormal

28. Management of dysgerminoma of the ovary stage I is:
A. unilateral salpingo-oophorectomy
B. total abdominal hysterectomy and bilateral salpingo-oophorectomy and radiation therapy
C. unilateral salpingo-oophorectomy and radiation therapy
D. chemotherapy

29. Concerning the spill of tumor during surgery, the following are true *except:*
A. some studies report a lower survival in patients with intraoperative rupture (stage Ic rupture)
B. other studies report no difference in survival in patients whose tumors had intact capsules and in those in whom tumor ruptured during surgery
C. rupture of the tumor before surgery has a negative influence on the outcome of patients as a result of seeding in the peritoneal cavity
D. in case of intraoperative rupture of the tumor, whole abdomen irradiation with pelvic boost should be given

30. A key issue in patients treated conservatively for stage Ia epithelial tumor of the ovary is:
A. parity
B. age
C. histology
D. close follow-up

31. Concerning the spill of tumor during surgery, the following are true *except:*
A. results of retrospective studies are conflicting but the majority show a decrease in survival in ruptured neoplasms
B. a course of chemotherapy, then a "second-look" procedure, could be offered to these patients
C. intraperitoneal ^{32}P could also be offered
D. if rupture occurs, lavage of the peritoneal cavity should be done with saline

32. Prophylactic oophorectomy should be offered to all perimenopausal patients (40 to 50 years old) undergoing pelvic surgery for the following reasons:
A. good methods of adequate substitution for the loss of ovarian function are available
B. reoperation because of benign ovarian disorder is 3% to 4%
C. ovarian carcinoma can occur in 6% to 12% of preserved ovaries
D. all of the above

Directions for Questions 33–43: For each numbered item, select the letter of the most appropriate answer. Each letter may be used once, more than once, or not at all.

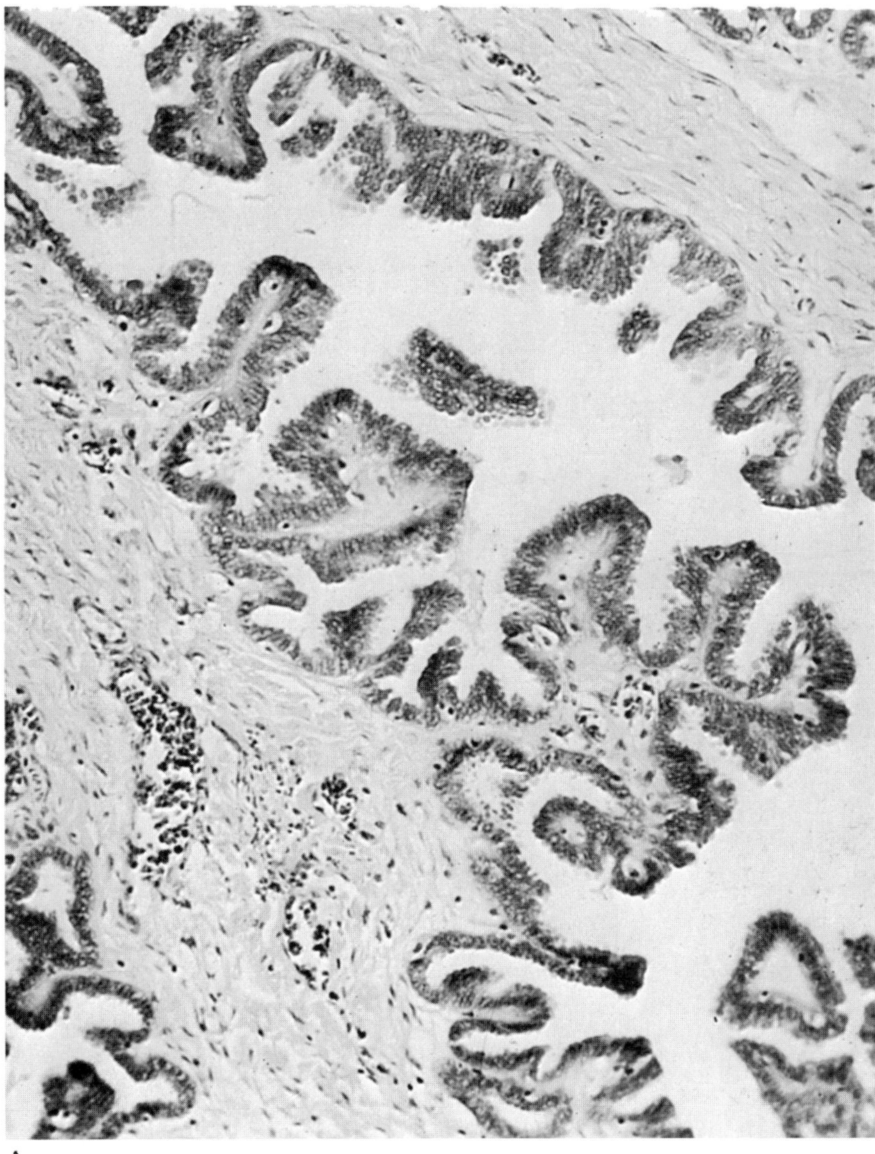

FIGURE 10–1. A

33–43. Match tumor characteristics to the appropriate benign tumor:
- A. serous cystadenoma
- B. Brenner tumor
- C. cystic teratoma
- D. fibroma

33. Nests of urothelial-like cells
34. Ectodermal, mesodermal, and endodermal tissues
35. Psammoma bodies
36. Hair, teeth, bone
37. Meigs' syndrome
38. Papillary projections
39. Longitudinal nuclear grooving

40–43. Match the histologic pictures in Figure 10–1 with the following ovarian tumors:

40. Brenner tumor of ovary
41. Fibroma of ovary
42. Mucinous adenoma of ovary
43. Borderline serous carcinoma of ovary

Answers

1. **D** page 259
   Levator ani are muscles of the pelvic floor; they are not part of the adnexa.
2. **B** page 259
   It is estimated that 5% to 10% of women in the United States will undergo a surgical operation for a suspected ovarian neoplasm. Thirteen to twenty-one percent of these women will be found to have an ovarian malignancy.
3. **A** page 259
   Among the predictive factors, age is probably the most important factor for determining the potential for malignancy of an adnexal mass.
4. **B** page 260
   Germ cell neoplasms constitute 40% of 42 malignant ovarian tumors in a study on 521 adnexal masses in childhood by Van Winter and colleagues. They need immediate surgical exploration.

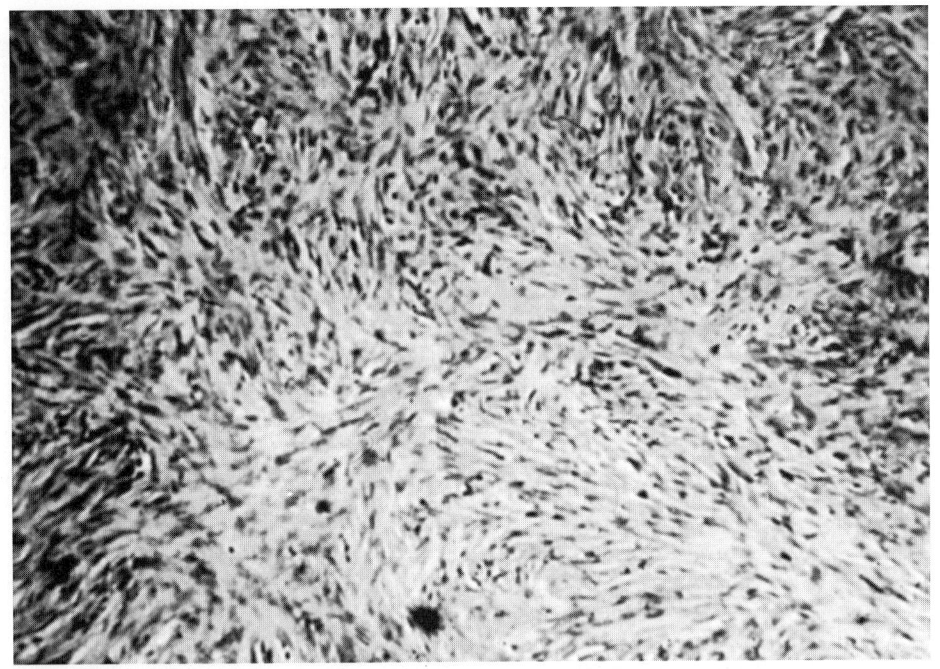

B

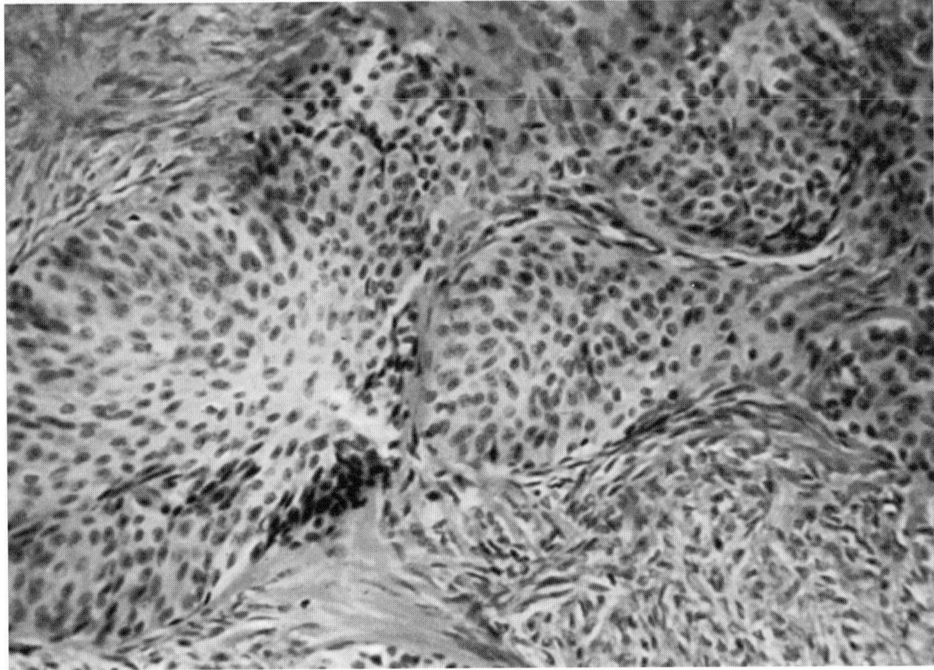

C

FIGURE 10–1. **B** and **C**

5. **D** page 260
Stromal, germ cell, and epithelial tumors all are seen in postmenopausal women.
6. **B** page 261
In patients in the reproductive age, cystic enlargement of the ovary is usually a functional cyst. These are the most common tumors of the ovary. They can reach 10 cm in diameter and can resolve spontaneously. Patients should be watched for 4 to 6 weeks before deciding on operative intervention.
7. **D** page 261
All choices of differing uterine conditions should be included in the differential diagnosis of an adnexal mass.
8. **B** page 262
Theca lutein cysts result from overstimulation of the ovary by human chorionic gonadotropin (hCG). Except for fetal death syndrome, the remaining entities account for a high serum hCG level. Theca lutein cysts may be found in twin pregnancies but are found rarely in single pregnancies.

FIGURE 10–1. D

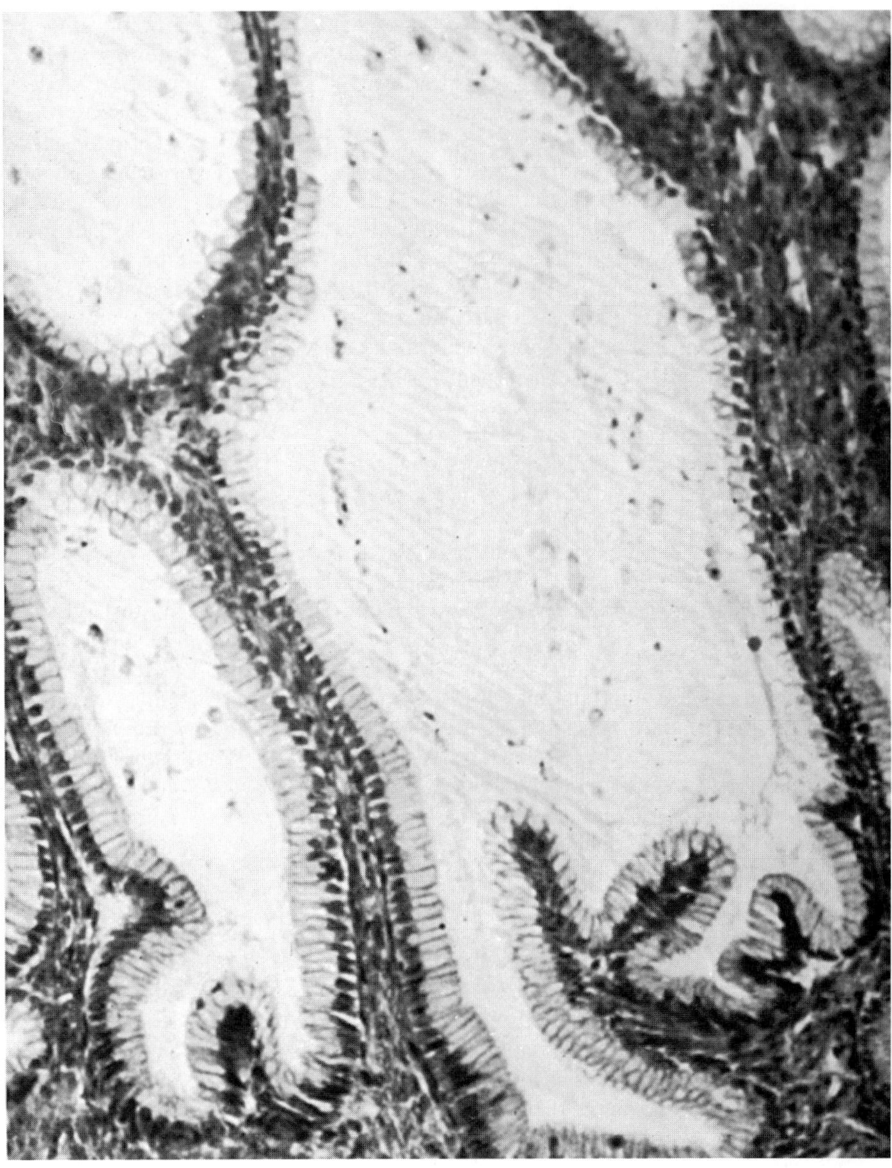

9. **D** page 262
   Serous and mucinous cystadenomas and cystic teratomas are the most common benign cystic true neoplasms of the ovary.
10. **C** page 271
    Pain and abdominal mass are the most frequent symptoms in children with adnexal mass.
11. **D** page 262
    The clinical situations enumerated above are indications for surgery to rule out malignancy.
12. **C** page 263
    Meigs' syndrome is an uncommon clinical entity that associates ascites and hydrothorax with a fibroma of the ovary.
13. **C** page 263
    The amount of endometriosis does not seem to correlate with the intensity of pain. In some patients, pain from small peritoneal implants is incapacitating.
14. **B** page 264
    All may appear as an adnexal mass, but the most frequent finding is fecal material in the sigmoid colon or cecum. The rectum and rectosigmoid should be empty when a pelvic examination is done.
15. **C** page 263
    Patients with carcinoma of the fallopian tube, a rare malignancy (less than 0.5% of all female genital tract malignancies), occasionally present with hydrops tubal profluens.
16. **A** page 265
    Ultrasound examination of all patients with a pelvic mass is discouraged for several reasons, the most important one being that the results of these tests do not influence management. Ultrasound is encouraged in a few specific situations: the pregnant patient, the obese patient, and the uncomfortable or uncooperative patient.

17. **B** page 266
It is not known whether malignant tumors arise de novo or develop from benign neoplasms. Both mechanisms of origin may exist.
18. **C** page 273
Only 10% to 15% of women with postmenopausal palpable ovaries have been found to have malignancy. In addition, serial ultrasound examinations in these patients has shown to be effective in determining the benign nature of the mass. CA-125 is very sensitive in the postmenopausal patient. This has led to the authors' revision of their previous recommendation for diagnostic laparotomy in all patients with postmenopausal palpable ovaries.
19. **D** page 275
Only 50% of patients with stage I epithelial cancer of the ovary have an elevated CA-125 level.
20. **D** page 269
Intraperitoneal alkylating agents after surgical evacuation of pseudomyxoma has shown some success. Cisplatin has been shown to be ineffective in these circumstances.
21. **D** page 267
If suspicious ultrasound findings are seen on an adnexal mass, laparotomy should be considered.
22. **B** page 268
The authors discourage use of the laparoscope for diagnosis or excision of the ovarian mass. Reasons are multiple but include the fact that a substantial proportion may be malignant and may be spread from the ovary by manipulation. In addition, a smooth, bland external appearance of the ovary does not reliably predict a benign state. Laparoscopy may be helpful, however, when the source of a pelvic mass is uncertain *and* nonsurgical therapy is contemplated. The authors recommend that any mass larger than 10 cm or any mass persistent beyond 4 to 6 weeks should be excised. They also note the propensity of many gynecologists to prescribe oral contraceptives in the presence of adnexal masses to accelerate involution.
23. **B** page 275
The presence of stromal invasion is diagnostic of serous adenocarcinoma. Borderline serous tumors have an increased incidence of bilaterality. The 5-year survival rate is very high, 90% to 95%, but these patients must be observed as closely as any patient with ovarian cancer because recurrent lesions may develop 20 to 50 years after the primary lesion. According to Julian and Woodruff, as many as 25% of the patients eventually succumbed to their tumors.
24. **D** page 278
Gershenson reported a 5-year survival of 95% in patients with ovarian serous borderline tumors with peritoneal implants. Kurman and Trimble reviewed 415 patients with stages II and III disease (excluding invasive peritoneal implants) and obtained a survival of 92%. On the other hand, Bell reported death from tumor was 4% at 5 years and 23% at 10 years.
25. **D** page 278
Appropriate treatment for stage I borderline tumors of the ovary, other than surgical resection, remains uncertain. Some authors suggest the use of intraperitoneal chromic phosphate as adjunctive therapy. Creasman reported on 55 patients with stage I borderline lesions of the ovary. Surgical removal of the disease was adequate therapy. The proper treatment of stage III disease also remains uncertain. Kurman and Trimble studied 415 patients with stages II and III. Excluding invasive peritoneal implants, survival after surgery was 92% with a mean follow-up of 7 years.
26. **C** page 280
The incidence of unsuspected metastases to the diaphragm with presumed stages I or II ovarian carcinoma was 15.7% (11.3% for stage I and 23.0% for stage II). Aortic node metastases were found in 10.3% of patients in stage I and 10.0% of patients in stage II. Omental metastasis was detected in 4.7% of patients. More than 29% of patients had malignant cytologic washings.
27. **D** page 279
There are no data demonstrating increased abnormality of pregnancy or of the product of conception after ovarian cancer. The normal-appearing opposite ovary could be the site of metastases 6% to 43% of the time, depending on the report and the stage of disease. For the young, nulliparous woman with a stage Ia tumor, the safety of more conservative operations to preserve childbearing is uncertain. Requirements for conservative management in stage Ia epithelial ovarian cancer should include the following: well-differentiated tumor, young woman of low parity, negative peritoneal washings, normal opposite ovary, negative omental biopsy result, and normal pelvic organs.
28. **A** page 282
Conservative surgery is performed in dysgerminoma stage I because of the exquisite radiosensitivity and chemosensitivity of this type of tumor. Although the recurrence rate is approximately 20% in stage I, the overall survival rate is 95%.
29. **D** page 282
Whole abdomen irradiation with pelvic boost should not be given because of numerous complications. DiSaia and Creasman recommend a course of platinum for six cycles, then a "second-look" procedure. Lavage of the peritoneal cavity with sterile water may be helpful.
30. **C** page 280
The key issue in patients treated conservatively for stage Ia epithelial tumors of the ovary is the histology. Close follow-up should be implemented for these patients. Mucinous and endometrioid lesions fare better than serous lesions, grade 1 and borderline lesions being the most easily treated conservatively. Serous lesions are said to be bilateral seven times more frequently than mucinous carcinomas.
31. **D** page 282
Lavage of the peritoneal cavity with sterile water has been recommended to cause lysis of the malignant cell. The peritoneal surfaces will absorb the water, so care should be taken to prevent delays in evacuating the fluid.

The use of platinum-based chemotherapy or intraperitoneal ^{32}P after spillage of the tumor during surgery are valid approaches, but at the present time there are no prospective studies comparing these two alternatives.

32. **D** page 284
The occurrence of ovarian carcinoma in patients who had previous pelvic surgery and in whom the ovaries could have been removed is certainly frustrating. Randall has shown that unilateral oophorectomy does not influence the subsequent incidence of ovarian carcinoma.
33. **B** page 270
The Brenner tumor is composed of nests of urothelial-like epithelial cells in a fibromatous stroma.
34. **C** page 271
The cystic teratoma is the only benign ovarian tumor commonly containing tissues from all three embryologic layers.
35. **A** page 268
Psammoma bodies may be found in any papillary tumor, including serous cystadenomas.
36. **C** page 271
Hair, teeth, or bone are found in cystic teratomas.
37. **D** page 272
Meigs' syndrome—the classic triad of ovarian neoplasm, ascites, and hydrothorax—was first described with fibroma.
38. **A** page 268
Papillary projections are usually found on the internal and/or external surfaces of the serous cystadenoma.
39. **B** page 270
The nuclei of cells in the Brenner tumor frequently exhibit longitudinal nuclear grooving, the so-called coffee bean nucleus. This phenomenon is also commonly seen in granulosa cell tumor.
40. **C** page 270
41. **B** page 272
42. **D** page 269
43. **A** page 276

chapter 11 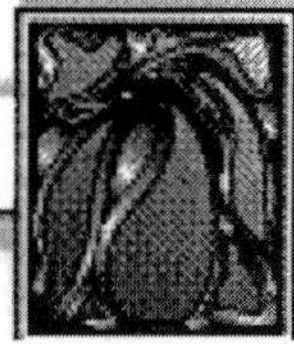

EPITHELIAL OVARIAN CANCER

Key Points to Remember

- Cancer of the ovary is the cause of more deaths than any other female genital tract cancer.
- About 25,400 new cases of malignant neoplasms of the ovary are diagnosed each year in the United States, and 14,500 deaths occur annually.
- Cancer of the ovary accounts for 5% of all cancers among women and 23% of gynecologic cancers. One in 58 women will develop this disease. Forty-seven percent of all deaths from cancer of the female genital tract occur in women with ovarian cancer.
- The majority (85% to 90%) of malignant ovarian tumors are epithelial (serous 42%, mucinous 12%, endometrioid 15%, undifferentiated 17%, and clear cell 6%).
- There is limited prognostic significance concerning the histology of ovarian cancer independent of clinical stage, extent of residual disease, and histologic grade. Histologic grade is an important independent prognostic factor in patients with epithelial tumors of the ovary.
- Malignant germ cell tumors are most commonly seen in women younger than 20 years of age, whereas epithelial cancers of the ovary are primarily seen in women older than 50 years. The largest number of ovarian cancer patients is found in the 60- to 64-year age group.
- Elderly women are more likely than younger women to be in advanced stages of ovarian cancer at initial diagnosis, and 5-year relative survival rates for elderly women are almost one half the rate observed in women younger than 65 years.
- The lifetime risk for ovarian cancer for a 35-year-old woman is approximately 1.6%; with one first-degree relative it is 5%, and with two or more first-degree relatives it rises to 7%.
- Three different hereditary syndromes of ovarian cancer have been identified: site-specific familial ovarian cancer syndrome, breast–ovarian cancer syndrome (associated with *BRCA1* or *BRCA2* gene), and Lynch's syndrome II (colorectal, endometrial, and ovarian cancer). They have a pattern of early onset cancer, and vertical transmission is consistent with autosomal dominant inheritance. Multiple family members are affected over several generations.
- A family history of breast or ovarian cancer, particularly before the age of 50 years in a first-order relative, and Ashkenazic Jewish ancestry are risk factors for *BRCA1* and *BRCA2* mutations. Experts recommend testing the family members who have cancer before testing the cancer-free members.
- Women with hereditary ovarian cancer syndrome should be maintained on oral contraceptive therapy (unless they desire childbearing), monitored closely before the age of 35 (ultrasonograpy, CA-125, pelvic examination), and encouraged to consider prophylactic oophorectomy at the age of 35 after completion of childbearing.
- Causative carcinogens of ovarian cancer (e.g., food, personal customs) are probably in the immediate environment.
- There is a reduction in incidence of ovarian cancer in women who use oral contraceptive agents (OCA). The trauma of ovulation may act as a promoting factor in epithelial ovarian cancer.
- Published data suggest that there is probably little relationship between fertility drug use and ovarian cancer. Women who use acetaminophen daily have a death rate from ovarian cancer 45% lower than that for women who do not use this agent.
- Early symptoms of ovarian cancer include vague abdominal discomfort, dyspepsia, and other mild digestive disturbances, especially for women between the ages of 40 and 69 years. Any persistent ovarian enlargement should be an immediate indication for exploratory laparotomy. The diagnosis rests with the pathologist.
- CA-125 and transvaginal ultrasonography cannot be used effectively for widespread screening.
- Routine pelvic examinations detect only 1 ovarian cancer in 10,000 asymptomatic women.
- Staging of ovarian cancer is surgical, based on the operative findings at the commencement of the procedure. Proper staging is the key to an accurate prognosis.
  - Stage I: growth limited to the ovaries.
    - Ia: one ovary, no ascites, to tumor on external surface, capsule intact
    - Ib: both ovaries, no ascites, to tumor on external surface, capsule intact
    - Ic: Ia or Ib with tumor on surface of one or both ovaries, or capsule ruptured, or with ascites or peritoneal washings positive for malignant cells
  - Stage II: growth involving one or both ovaries and with pelvic extension
    - IIa: extension to uterus or tubes
    - IIb: extension to other pelvic tissues
    - IIc: stage IIa or IIb with tumor on surface of one or both ovaries or with capsule ruptured or with ascites or peritoneal washings positive for malignant cells
  - Stage III: growth involving one or both ovaries and with peritoneal implants outside the pelvis

and/or positive retroperitoneal or inguinal nodes. Superficial liver metastasis

IIIa: microscopic seeding of peritoneal cavity, negative nodes

IIIb: abdominal implants smaller than 2 cm, negative nodes

IIIc: abdominal implants larger than 2 cm and/or positive retroperitoneal or inguinal nodes

Stage IV: growth involving one or both ovaries with distant metastases (pleural effusion positive for cancer, parenchymal liver metastasis)

- Epithelial borderline tumors (low malignant potential), which account for 15% of epithelial ovarian cancers, afflict a younger population, have a high 10-year survival rate (95%), and can recur as long as 20 years after therapy. The diagnosis must be based on examination of the original tumor. Standard surgical therapy is total abdominal hysterectomy and bilateral salpingo-oophorectomy (TAH-BSO). Treatment of stage III remains unsettled. Lymph node metastases occasionally develop, but hematogenous metastases and extension outside the peritoneal cavity are uncommon.
- All different histologic varieties of epithelial ovarian cancer (serous, mucinous, endometrial, and clear cell types) behave similarly, stage for stage and grade for grade. The most important variable influencing the prognosis in each case of ovarian cancer is the stage or extent of disease.
- Survival depends on stage of the lesion, grade of differentiation, gross findings at surgery, amount of postsurgery residual tumor, and additional treatment (5-year survival: stage Ia 84%, IIa 65%, IIIa 52%, IV 14%, overall 31%).
- Treatment of stages Ia, Ib, and Ic ovarian cancer consists of TAH and BSO with careful surgical staging. Pelvic and periaortic nodes should be evaluated because those nodes can be involved 10% to 20% of the time in apparent stage I disease. Omentectomy is also done in some institutions. Treatment of stages Ia and Ib grade 1 or 2: no chemotherapy; stage Ia grade 3: adjuvant chemotherapy; and stages Ib and Ic and undifferentiated histology: adjuvant chemotherapy (cisplatin, paclitaxel [Taxol]).
- In the young patient with stage Ia disease who is desirous of childbearing, unilateral salpingo-oophorectomy can be performed with minimal increased risk of recurrence, provided a careful staging procedure is performed and the grade of the tumor is evaluated.
- Treatment of stages IIa, IIb, and IIc: TAH-BSO, omentectomy, and instillation of ^{32}P. Other centers prefer a combination of pelvic irradiation and systemic chemotherapy, or chemotherapy alone with platinum-based combination therapy. Careful surgical planning is essential.
- Treatment of stage III: TAH-BSO, omentectomy, and removal of the bulk of the tumor. Survival rate is related to the residual tumor after surgery (< 2 cm). Multiple-agent platinum-based adjunctive chemotherapy is used for 6 to 12 months. Second-look procedure has had no impact on survival.
- Treatment of stage IV: removal of as much cancer as possible and follow-up with chemotherapy.
- The most important prognostic factors in stage III ovarian cancer are the histologic grade of the tumor and the size of the largest residual mass after surgery.
- Patients found to have small-volume disease survived longer than patients cytoreduced to small-volume disease at surgery.
- Unless the mass can be cytoreduced to less than 2 cm, residual diameter did not influence survival (4-year survival of microscopic disease 60%, < 2 cm 35%, > 2 cm 20%).
- Optimal debulking can be performed in stage IV ovarian cancer with beneficial effect. The percentage of patients with advanced ovarian cancer who can effectively undergo cytoreductive surgery ranges from 43% to 87%.
- DiSaia and Creasman routinely do pelvic and para-aortic lymphadenectomy if the patient's tumor can be optimally debulked. Benefits of lymphadenectomy remain questionable. Evaluation of ovarian cancer with laparoscopy is controversial, and several incidents of metastasis at the port site have been reported.
- Patients selected to have postoperative irradiation should receive treatment of the entire abdomen plus additional radiation to the pelvis (2500 to 3000 cGy to the abdomen with a 2000 to 3000 cGy pelvic boost). The effectiveness of abdominal and pelvic irradiation is independent of stage or histology. As a better understanding of the effects of chemotherapeutic agents in ovarian cancer has been gained, the role of radiation therapy in this disease has diminished in prominence. There are advocates for radiation therapy as a salvage treatment in patients with chemotherapy-resistant disease.
- ^{32}P (half-life 14.2 days) is the agent of choice for intraperitoneal therapy. It can be used in conjunction with pelvic radiotherapy: in one study the 5-year survival rate was 95% for stage Ia_1, 82% for stage Ia_2, 73% for Ib, 67% for stages IIa and IIb, and 50% for stage III with minimal or no residual tumor. Small bowel complications were high (24%) and were related to pelvic radiotherapy.
- Single-agent chemotherapy used in ovarian cancer consists of hexamethylmelamine, doxorubicin, cyclophosphamide, 5-fluorouracil, methotrexate, cisplatin, paclitaxel, Topotecan, **or** vinorelbine (Navelbine).
- Combination chemotherapy is more effective against ovarian cancer, but toxicity is greater than that with single-agent chemotherapy.
- All the successful combinations are cisplatin based. Cisplatin analogs such as carboplatin and iproplatin appear to have fewer marked side effects.
- Paclitaxel and cisplatin emerge as the gold standard for combination first-line chemotherapy for the treatment of ovarian cancer. Yet, clear evidence that the combination results in more long-term survivors than just platinum alone does not currently exist.
- Omura reported a sobering analysis of two large GOG studies involving 726 patients with stages III and IV disease and concluded that the impact of chemotherapy to date had been modest: less than 10% of patients were progression free at 5 years, and late failures continued to occur beyond 7 years. Results of studies did not support the concept that increased dose intensity will produce

greater therapeutic effect, even with a 3.3-fold increase of cisplatin doses.

- Studies by Stiff with high-dose chemotherapy and autologous bone marrow transplant in patients with recurrent epithelial carcinoma showed promise: 89% overall response rate, with 59% clinical complete responders, and a median survival of 29 months in 22 patients with large volume disease (>1 cm). Larger studies are needed. The toxicity of high-dose chemotherapy is a serious concern, as is the additional expense.
- The most important factor for long-term survival after high-dose chemotherapy is the completeness of the primary cytoreductive surgery.
- Immunochemotherapy using *Corynebacterium parvum* or BCG could improve the median survival of patients with advanced ovarian cancer, but more studies are needed for confirmation. Interferon alfa, biologic response modifiers, and cancer vaccines are under investigation.
- Patients with extraovarian peritoneal serous papillary carcinoma respond to therapy similar to patients with serous papillary carcinoma of the ovary.
- Small cell carcinoma of the ovary is very aggressive and should be treated with combination chemotherapy.
- Optimal follow-up strategy for the asymptomatic patient who has advanced ovarian cancer after initial treatment remains undecided. DiSaia and Creasman propose to monitor these patients with physical examination, serum CA-125, and liberal use of imaging every 2 months for 2 years, and every 6 months thereafter.
- In epithelial ovarian carcinoma, rising or falling levels of CA-125 correlate with disease progression or regression in 90% of patients. Virtually all patients with elevated serum CA-125 levels before second-look surgery have residual ovarian cancer at laparotomy or develop disease within the next 4 to 6 months. Patients in whom the CA-125 level reverts sharply to within the normal range by the third course of chemotherapy following surgery have a survival that is markedly and significantly improved over patients who have an elevation of CA-125 levels before their fourth course of chemotherapy. A 50% rise in the CA-125 level above normal ranges (35 units/mL) on two separate occasions is considered a likely indication of recurrence, especially if the value exceeds 100 units.
- Patients with stages I–II disease have a high correlation between a negative second-look operation and subsequent disease-free survival. Half of the patients with stage III–IV disease and negative second look after combination chemotherapy experience recurrences. Today the second-look procedure is used infrequently. However, second-look surgery remains valuable for providing information to select salvage therapy.
- Platinum sensitivity, which is defined by a response to first-line platinum-based therapy is found to predict response to subsequent retreatment with a platinum-based or nonplatinum-based salvage regimen (relapse within 6 months: platinum refractory; no relapse within 6 months: platinum sensitive). A response rate of 10% was observed for platinum-refractory patients, compared with a response rate up to 90% for platinum-sensitive patients treated with salvage therapy.
- There is limited evidence of sustained benefit from salvage therapy in patients with ovarian cancer (high-dose cisplatin, carboplatin, hexamethylmelamine, 5-fluorouracil, and intraperitoneal therapy). Only modest response rates with short durations of response have been reported.
- Intraperitoneal chemotherapy with cisplatin is an acceptable option of management with ovarian cancer in patients who have demonstrated response to intravenous therapy with persistence of minimal residual cancer (<0.5 cm). Other agents under trial are 5-FU, carboplatin, paclitaxel, interferon gamma, TNF, and interleukin-2.
- Paracentesis should not be done in patients whose findings are highly suggestive of ovarian cancer, except in cases of severe pain or respiratory embarrassment. Ascites and pleural effusion usually respond to systemic chemotherapy.
- Pleural effusion can be managed with obliteration of the pleural cavity by instillation of such agents as nitrogen mustard or tetracycline or bleomycin.
- The dose-limiting toxicity of cisplatin is neurotoxicity (nephrotoxicity can be eliminated by vigorous saline diuresis); that of carboplatin is myelosuppression.
- Drug resistance by malignant cells remains a barrier when treating micrometastasis.
- Terminal events for most patients with ovarian cancer are electrolyte imbalance and protein loss caused by gastrointestinal obstruction, malnutrition, and multiple paracenteses.

QUESTIONS

Directions for Questions 1–51: Select the one best answer.

1. The following are epithelial tumors of the ovary *except:*
   A. serous tumor
   B. mucinous tumor
   C. Brenner tumor
   D. endodermal sinus tumor
2. The following are germ cell tumors *except:*
   A. dysgerminoma
   B. Sertoli-Leydig tumor (arrhenoblastoma)
   C. teratoma
   D. gonadoblastoma
3. The following are neoplasms derived from specialized gonadal stroma *except:*
   A. granulosa theca cell tumors
   B. Sertoli-Leydig tumor
   C. mixed mesodermal tumor
   D. lipid cell tumor
4. The majority of malignant ovarian tumors are:
   A. epithelial tumors
   B. germ cell tumors
   C. gonadal stroma tumors
   D. metastatic tumors
5. Important prognostic factors in patients with epithelial carcinoma of the ovary include the following *except:*
   A. clinical stage
   B. extent of residual disease
   C. histologic type
   D. histologic grade

6. Patients with untreated or unsuccessfully treated ovarian cancer will usually die of:
   A. respiratory failure
   B. infection
   C. hemorrhage
   D. intestinal obstruction
7. Women younger than 20 years develop which type of ovarian cancer most commonly?
   A. epithelial
   B. germ cell
   C. gonadal stroma
   D. metastatic
8. The highest incidence rate of ovarian cancer patients is found in which age group?
   A. 1 to 25 years
   B. 25 to 45 years
   C. 45 to 65 years
   D. 65 to 85 years
9. A patient has a single, first-degree relative with ovarian cancer. Her risk of contracting the disease is increased to what percentage?
   A. 3%
   B. 5%
   C. 8%
   D. 10%
10. In families with site-specific ovarian cancer, the lifetime risk of ovarian cancer for each member is:
    A. 1 in 2
    B. 1 in 3
    C. 1 in 4
    D. 1 in 5
11. What is the pattern of inheritance in hereditary ovarian cancer syndromes?
    A. autosomal dominant
    B. autosomal recessive
    C. X-linked dominant
    D. multifactorial
12. The most frequent presenting symptom of ovarian cancer is:
    A. abdominal swelling
    B. abdominal pain
    C. dyspepsia and urinary frequency
    D. weight change
13. The following are true concerning the reduction in ovarian cancer incidence with the use of OCA *except:*
    A. the reduction of risk appears to persist as long as 10 years after use
    B. The "incessant ovulation" makes the epithelial lining of the ovary sensitive to constant trauma and acts as a promoting factor in the carcinogenic process
    C. five years of use by nulliparous women can reduce their ovarian cancer risk to the level of parous women who never used OCA
    D. there is no decrease in incidence of ovarian cancer in patients taking OCA who have a positive family history
14. The most important prognostic factor in ovarian cancer is the:
    A. histology
    B. grade
    C. stage or extent of disease
    D. presence of ascites
15. The following diagnostic techniques should be performed in patients suspected of having cancer of the ovary *except:*
    A. pelvic examination
    B. pelvic ultrasound examination or CT scan
    C. laparotomy
    D. paracentesis
16. Surgical therapy in ovarian cancer consists of:
    A. peritoneal cytologic examination
    B. determination of extent of disease and removal of all tumor possible
    C. TAH-BSO, node sampling, and partial omentectomy
    D. all of the above
17. Aortic lymph node metastases in stage I epithelial ovarian cancer occur in what percentage of cases?
    A. 2%
    B. 5%
    C. 7%
    D. 10%
18. Management of stage Ia grade 1 ovarian lesion after surgery consists of:
    A. no chemotherapy
    B. pelvic irradiation
    C. cisplatin-based chemotherapy
    D. monochemotherapy with hexamethylmelamine
19. The following can be said about ovarian tumors of low malignant potential (borderline malignancies) *except:*
    A. patients have a high survival rate
    B. lesions usually have an indolent course
    C. occasional spontaneous regression of peritoneal implants occurs
    D. the diagnosis should be based on extensive sectioning of the metastases
20. The standard surgical treatment of ovarian tumors of low malignant potential is:
    A. radical hysterectomy and pelvic node dissection
    B. total abdominal hysterectomy
    C. TAH-BSO
    D. unilateral salpingo-oophorectomy
21. Survival of patients with ovarian cancer depends on:
    A. stage and grade of the lesion
    B. gross findings at surgery and amount of residual tumor after surgery
    C. additional treatment after surgery
    D. all of the above
22. The overall 5-year survival rate for cancer of the ovary is approximately:
    A. 25%
    B. 35%
    C. 45%
    D. 55%
23. Survival in stage III ovarian cancer depends on cytoreductive surgery. A patient has a better survival chance when the diameter of a residual mass is:
    A. 3 cm
    B. 4 cm
    C. 5 cm
    D. no difference in survival

24. Rationale for omentectomy done in many institutions for stage I disease is the following *except:*
    A. omentectomy permits easier access to the ovaries and uterus
    B. the omentum may harbor microscopic disease
    C. radioactive substances (^{32}P) have a great affinity for the omentum
    D. removal of the omentum allows a greater amount of radioactive substance to be distributed over the peritoneal surfaces
25. Metastases to pelvic and periaortic nodes in stage I ovarian cancer occur in what approximate percentage of patients?
    A. 1%–10%
    B. 10%–20%
    C. 20%–30%
    D. 30%–40%
26. Successful therapy for ovarian carcinoma usually includes all *except:*
    A. TAH-BSO
    B. administration of platinum-based therapy
    C. second-look laparotomy
    D. omentectomy and maximal cytoreduction of all remaining tumor to 2 cm maximum diameter
27. Choose the true statement regarding surgery for epithelial ovarian carcinoma:
    A. new technology that increases efficacy and decreases the morbidity of debulking (ultrasound surgical aspiration, argon beam coagulator) increases survival
    B. successful debulking surgery is a valuable therapeutic maneuver and a significant prognostic indicator
    C. secondary cytoreduction is a clear benefit in the therapy for persistent ovarian carcinoma
    D. "optimal" debulking is associated with the increased negative second-look laparotomy rate and increased 5-year survival
28. The following concepts in reference to radiotherapy for epithelial carcinoma of the ovary are valid *except:*
    A. when given, radiation should be delivered to pelvis *and* abdomen
    B. expanded indications for use of radiotherapy in ovarian carcinoma have recently been described
    C. radioactive colloids and external beam therapy may be used together
    D. the most striking success seems to be with patients with low-stage or no residual disease
29. Which combination is considered to be the gold standard for the treatment of advanced ovarian carcinoma?
    A. Paclitaxel (Taxol) and cyclophosphamide
    B. cyclophosphamide and methotrexate
    C. cisplatin and paclitaxel
    D. cisplatin and hexamethylmelamine
30. Which is the dose-limiting toxicity of paclitaxel?
    A. nephrotoxicity
    B. myelosuppression
    C. cardiotoxicity
    D. pulmonary toxicity
31. Acute leukemia is most commonly seen following the use of which group of chemotherapy drugs?
    A. plant alkaloids
    B. antibiotics
    C. alkylating drugs
    D. the platinum drugs
32. The alkylating agent found to exhibit the highest success rate when used as a single agent in stages III and IV ovarian cancer is:
    A. melphalan
    B. cyclophosphamide
    C. thiotepa
    D. chlorambucil
33. Of nonalkylating drugs demonstrating significant activity when used as a single agent, the agent demonstrating highest activity against stages III and IV ovarian cancer is:
    A. cisplatin
    B. doxorubicin
    C. methotrexate
    D. hexamethylmelamine
34. The following statements relative to single versus combination chemotherapy are true *except:*
    A. long-term survival is significantly enhanced by the choice of combination over single-agent therapy
    B. response rates of up to 96% have been reported with combination therapy
    C. response rates of up to 60% have been reported with single-agent therapy
    D. the addition of progestins to the cytotoxic drug regimen is not clearly shown to be beneficial
35. The addition of nonspecific immunotherapy such as *Corynebacterium parvum* or BCG to cytotoxic chemotherapy is referred to as immunochemotherapy. Which of the following statements is true regarding immunochemotherapy?
    A. The addition of *C. parvum* to melphalan has not resulted in prolonged survival of patients with stage III ovarian cancer
    B. two recent phase III clinical trials demonstrate an improved response rate when BCG is added to combination chemotherapy
    C. BCG has modest, but definite, cytotoxic activity when used as a single agent
    D. *C. parvum* is derived from inactivated BCG
36. The following are true concerning high doses of chemotherapy and autologous bone marrow transplant *except:*
    A. High doses of cisplatin given to patients with stage III ovarian cancer result in a longer survival
    B. the most important factor for long-term survival after high-dose chemotherapy in advanced stage is the completeness of primary cytoreductive surgery
    C. autologous bone marrow transplant after high-dose chemotherapy with no prior chemotherapy after cytoreductive surgery results in an increase in 5-year survival
    D. autologous bone marrow transplant and high-dose chemotherapy on patients with recurrence of ovarian carcinoma who have failed first-line chemotherapy and have large-volume disease also results in an increase in survival

37. Which statement about biologic response modifiers (BRMs) is *not* correct?
    A. combining BRMs with standard chemotherapy is difficult because of unanticipated overlapping toxicities
    B. intraperitoneal alpha-interferon administration for patients with small residual ovarian cancer after surgery has resulted in complete pathologic responses at reassessment laparotomy
    C. IL-2 demonstrates significant utility when used as consolidation therapy after standard chemotherapy for patients with advanced ovarian cancer
    D. intraperitoneal IL-2 administration has demonstrated that lymphokines can cause egress of large numbers of leukocytes and macrophages into the peritoneal cavity
38. Features of extraovarian peritoneal serous papillary carcinoma include:
    A. serous tumor deposits confined to the omentum and ovaries
    B. serous tumor deposits found anywhere in the abdomen, including possible deposits on the surface of the ovaries
    C. serous tumor deposits metastatic to abdominal sites with a coexistent serous papillary neoplasm in the uterus, but not either ovary
    D. metastatic deposits of noninvasive (borderline) serous tumors from a histologically dissimilar neoplasm of the ovary
39. Small cell carcinoma of the ovary is:
    A. a variant of ovarian carcinoma occurring in older patients
    B. often associated with hypercalcemia
    C. sensitive to cisplatin-based chemotherapy
    D. associated with long-term survival rate after whole abdomen irradiation therapy
40. In patients *without* ovarian cancer, CA-125 is an antigenic determinant found in all the following tissues *except:*
    A. ovary
    B. pericardium
    C. pleura
    D. endometrium
41. In patients *with* advanced ovarian cancer:
    A. CA-125 will be detectable in the serum (>35 mIU/mL) in more than 95% of patients before therapy
    B. CA-125 will be detectable in the serum in more than 95% of patients immediately before a second-look operation where residual tumor is found
    C. CA-125 levels will be normal in almost all patients with a negative second-look operation
    D. the degree of elevation of CA-125 usually predicts the amount of residual disease or outcome
42. Serum CA-125 in a patient with advanced ovarian cancer in complete clinical remission:
    A. may be normal despite tumor deposits of up to 2 cm in size
    B. commonly rises because of cisplatin-associated nephrotoxicity
    C. is considered abnormal only when it rises to 100% over the lowest recorded level
    D. if demonstrating a sustained rise above normal levels, is sufficient indication to resume therapy
43. The following are accepted indications for second-look surgery (reassessment surgery) *except:*
    A. to restage a patient with potentially localized disease who has not had an optimal staging procedure
    B. to evaluate the effect of chemotherapy in patients receiving standard and investigational regimens
    C. to attempt "second-effort" tumor reduction for patients previously found to have unresectable disease
    D. to examine patients who are clinically free of disease after receiving what is considered a sufficient course of chemotherapy and who are eligible for discontinuation of therapy
44. Following a pathologically confirmed negative second-look operation, the likelihood of recurrence of ovarian cancer is:
    A. approximately 50%
    B. independent of stage at diagnosis
    C. the same regardless of the chemotherapy used before surgery
    D. less than 10%
45. Follow-up strategy for the asymptomatic patient who had advanced ovarian cancer after initial treatment consists of:
    A. laparoscopy every 6 months
    B. monitoring serum CA-125 level every 3 months
    C. computerized tomography every year
    D. physical examination, serum CA-125, liberal use of imaging on a quarterly basis for 2 years
46. Serum CA-125 has been used for monitoring the recurrence of ovarian cancer. The following are true for serum CA-125 *except:*
    A. patients on chemotherapy who have their serum CA-125 level reverted to normal after the third course have an improved survival rate
    B. patients who have their serum CA-125 still elevated after three courses of chemotherapy should be considered for alternative chemotherapy
    C. a 50% rise in CA-125 level above normal ranges on two separate occasions is considered a likely indication of recurrence
    D. histologic confirmation of recurrence is not necessary before any salvage therapy is offered
47. In patients who have not responded to first-line cisplatin chemotherapy:
    A. hexamethylmelamine is an active drug
    B. carboplatin is an active drug
    C. cisplatin dose escalation has been associated with an increased response rate
    D. doxorubicin is an active drug
48. Patients are defined as platinum sensitive when they respond to treatment and have a progression-free interval of greater than how many months off treatment?
    A. 3 months
    B. 6 months

C. 9 months
D. 12 months

49. A drug is likely to be suitable for intraperitoneal administration (IP) if:
A. it is rapidly cleared from the peritoneal cavity and has low plasma clearance
B. it is highly ionized, water soluble, and of high molecular weight
C. it is ideally administered in a small solute volume
D. it is a vesicant

50. For patients with ovarian cancer, the most ideal setting for intraperitoneal administration of cytotoxic drugs is:
A. in a patient following initial tumor reduction who has bulky residual tumor nodules in an unresectable location
B. in a patient who has failed to respond to platinum-based chemotherapy administered systemically
C. in a previously untreated patient with significant bone marrow compromise
D. in a patient with minimal residual ovarian cancer following systemically administered platinum-based chemotherapy

51. The following are reasons for not performing a paracentesis in patients whose findings are highly suggestive of ovarian malignancy *except:*
A. rapid fluid shifts following paracentesis commonly result in significant hypovolemia
B. cytologic examination of fluid may be negative even in the presence of malignancy, and laparotomy is still indicated
C. even if the cytologic examination is positive, it seldom provides sufficient clues to the origin of the tumor; laparotomy is still indicated
D. rupture of a cyst and seeding into the peritoneal cavity may occur, often long before the laparotomy

Directions for Questions 52–66: For each numbered item, select the letter of the most appropriate answer. Each letter may be used once, more than once, or not at all.

52–55. Match the stage with the ovarian tumor:
A. Stage Ic
B. Stage IIIa
C. Stage Ia
D. Stage IIb

52. A tumor involving one ovary with histologically confirmed microscopic metastases to the small bowel
53. Tumor involving both ovaries with no ascites but positive peritoneal washings
54. Tumor involving both ovaries with excrescences on one ovary, with no ascites, and with negative peritoneal washings
55. Tumor involving one ovary with extension to broad ligament, with no ascites, and with negative peritoneal washings

56–62. Match the surgical findings most applicable to either benign or malignant ovarian tumors.
A. benign
B. malignant

56. Surface papillae
57. Solid areas
58. Bilaterality
59. Ascites
60. Peritoneal implants
61. Capsule intact
62. Totally cystic

63–66. Match the treatment with the appropriate stage of epithelial ovarian cancer.
A. unilateral salpingo-oophorectomy
B. total abdominal hysterectomy (TAH) with bilateral salpingo-oophorectomy (BSO), omentectomy
C. TAH-BSO, omentectomy, intraperitoneal ^{32}P or platinum-based chemotherapy
D. TAH-BSO, omentectomy, debulking, platinum-based chemotherapy

63. Stage I, grade 3 tumor of ovary
64. Stage Ia or Ib with grade 1 or 2 disease
65. Stage Ia disease in a young woman desiring further childbearing
66. Stage III ovarian cancer

Answers

1. **D** page 290
Endodermal sinus tumor (or yolk sac tumor) is a neoplasm derived from germ cells.
2. **B** page 290
Arrhenoblastoma is a gonadal stromal tumor.
3. **C** page 290
Mixed mesodermal tumor of the ovary is an epithelial tumor.
4. **A** page 289
The majority (85%–90%) of malignant ovarian tumors in the United States are epithelial: serous 42%, mucinous 12%, endometrioid 15%, undifferentiated 17%, and clear cell 6%.
5. **C** page 290
Histologic type of the tumor is of limited prognostic significance in epithelial ovarian cancer as opposed to the significant importance of clinical stage, extent of residual disease, and histologic grade.
6. **D** page 290
As the tumor spreads over the surface of the bowel, the patient will have bouts of intestinal obstruction and develop inanition and malnutrition.
7. **B** page 291
Women younger than 20 years develop germ cell tumors of the ovary most commonly. Epithelial cancers of the ovary are primarily seen in women older than 50 years.
8. **D** page 291
The highest incidence of ovarian cancer occurs in the 66- to 85-year age group, within which the peak of 54 cases per 100,000 is found in the 75- to 79-year age group.
9. **B** page 292
A history of a single, first-order relative with ovarian cancer increases the individual's risk to approximately 5%, whereas the lifetime probability of ovarian cancer in a 35-year-old woman is 1.6% without a family history of ovarian cancer.

10. **A** page 293
The lifetime risk for ovarian cancer for first-degree relative is 1 in 2 in the 19 families with site-specific ovarian cancer according to a study of Houlston.
11. **A** page 292
All three syndromes of hereditary familial ovarian cancer have a pattern of early onset cancer and vertical transmission consistent with autosomal dominant inheritance. Women suspected of having hereditary ovarian cancer syndrome should be followed closely by a physician for determination of a family pedigree. They should be on oral contraceptives, followed by pelvic examination, ultrasonography, and serum CA-125 every 6 months. At the age of 35, they should be encouraged to consider prophylactic oophorectomy.
12. **A** page 296
All choices are presenting symptoms of ovarian cancer, but the most frequent symptom is abdominal swelling, marking the occurrence of ascites and extension of tumor to the abdomen. Physicians should not dismiss the possibility of early ovarian cancer in women between age 40 and 69 who have persistent gastrointestinal symptoms.
13. **D** page 295
Studies by Gross showed that 10 years of OCA use by women with a positive family history can reduce their risk to a level below that of women whose family history is negative and who never used OCAs. Patients with a family history of ovarian cancer should consider using OCAs.
14. **C** page 301
The stage represents the extent of disease and is the most important prognostic factor in epithelial ovarian cancer. Also important are the gross findings at surgery and the amount of tumor remaining after surgery. Five-year survival in stage Ia is 84%, IIa 65%, and IIIa 52%.
15. **D** page 301
Diagnostic paracentesis in a patient with ascites and a pelvic abdominal mass is unnecessary and dangerous. It can result in a spillage of malignant cells in the abdominal cavity. Laparotomy is necessary to remove the tumor, establish the diagnosis, and evaluate the extent of the disease. Confirmation of the diagnosis rests with histologic examination of the specimen.
16. **D** page 301
Surgical therapy should be extensive and complete because the prognosis and therapy rest on accurate surgical establishment of the extent of the disease. Any peritoneal fluid should be aspirated and submitted for cytologic examination. In the absence of peritoneal fluid, four washings should be taken: undersurface of diaphragm, peritoneal surfaces lateral to ascending and descending colons, and pelvic peritoneal surfaces. Proper staging is the key to an accurate prognosis and a correct treatment.
17. **C** page 301, Table 11–14
Among 141 patients with stage I ovarian cancer, 10 were found to have aortic lymph node metastases (7%). Aortic lymph node metastases occurred in 25% and 47% of patients with stages II and III ovarian carcinoma, respectively.
18. **A** page 304
In management of patients with low-grade lesions, DiSaia and Creasman advise against chemotherapy because the risks of adjuvant chemotherapy outweigh the possible benefits. However, they think that patients with stage I grade 3 ovarian cancer should receive chemotherapy.
19. **D** page 304
The diagnosis must be based on examination and extensive sectioning of the original ovarian tumor and not on implants or metastases. Therapy, however, may be based on extensive histologic study of the primary tumor and its metastatic implants.
20. **C** page 305
The standard surgical therapy for serous and mucinous tumors of low-grade malignancy is TAH-BSO. Unilateral salpingo-oophorectomy is reserved only for patients who have not completed their families and have early stage disease. Radical hysterectomy with pelvic node dissection is performed for cancer of the cervix.
21. **D** page 307
The survival of patients depends on all factors enumerated.
22. **B** page 304, Table 11–15
A recent FIGO determination of overall 5-year survival for cancer of the ovary was 39%; stage I was 78%, stage II 61%, stage III 23%, and stage IV 14%.
23. **D** page 313
Gynecologic Oncology Group (GOG) investigators found that cytoreduction to the largest residual mass smaller than 2 cm results in a significant survival benefit but that all patients with residual diameters larger than 2 cm have equivalent survival. Patients with microscopic disease have a 4-year survival rate of about 60%. Patients with gross disease smaller than 2 cm have a 4-year survival of 35%. Patients whose disease cannot be cytoreduced to smaller than 2 cm have a 4-year survival rate of less than 20%.
24. **A** page 311
Ovaries and uterus are easily accessible without omentectomy in stage I disease.
25. **B** page 310
Pelvic and periaortic nodes may be involved in 10% to 20% of patients with stage I disease. These nodes should be thoroughly evaluated to assess the true extent of the disease.
26. **C** page 316
Data from Munnell demonstrate threefold to sixfold improvement in survival in patients undergoing "maximal surgical effort," including (but not limited to) hysterectomy, BSO, and omentectomy. Aure has shown threefold increased survival in patients in whom no gross tumor remains after resection. Griffiths determined the "critical diameter" of residual tumor mass to be 1.6 cm. Multiple authors have demonstrated the value of combination chemotherapy: all of the most successful regimens are platinum-based. Second-look laparotomy is a

diagnostic tool, not a therapeutic measure, and does not appear to influence survival.

27. **D** page 309
Multiple studies demonstrate association of "optimal" debulking with negative second-look surgery (Table 11–20). A report by the MD Anderson Cancer Center of large numbers of patients with stages II and III disease demonstrates the association between optimal debulking and improved survival. New technology that decreases the morbidity of optimal debulking has not yet been shown to have a survival advantage. Whether successful debulking is therapeutic or prognostic, or both, is not clear. The literature on secondary cytoreductive surgery in the treatment of advanced ovarian carcinoma is fairly evenly divided between those who believe it is of benefit and those who do not.

28. **B** page 318
Radiotherapy is not effective in patients with bulky residual disease. Because of potential great toxicity, great effort has been undertaken to define subgroups of patients who may benefit from radiotherapy without excessive toxicity. Thus, indications for radiotherapy have become more refined and narrowed. It has not been conclusively shown to be superior to chemotherapy.

29. **C** page 324
A combination of paclitaxel (Taxol) and cisplatin should be considered the treatment of choice for advanced ovarian carcinoma.

30. **B** page 322
Myelosuppression manifested primarily as neutropenia was the dose-limiting toxicity in patients receiving paclitaxel. Cardiac problems are rare. Neuropathy is seen only in patients receiving large doses of paclitaxel (>200 mg/m^2).

31. **C** page 321
The alkylating agents are the most leukemogenic class of cytotoxic antitumor drugs. Reimer estimated that as many as 10% of 10-year survivors may develop leukemia.

32. **B** page 321
High-dose cyclophosphamide demonstrated the highest response (61%) when compared with other alkylating agents (Table 11–25).

33. **D** page 321
Hexamethylmelamine (altretamine) exhibited the highest average percent response of 42%.

34. **A** page 322
The most successful regimens are platinum based. There is no substantial proof that combination therapy, or the addition of any agent to a platinum-based drug, significantly increases long-term survival. The toxicity of combination therapy is clearly greater, however.

35. **A** page 327
There are no clinical trials in patients with gynecologic cancers demonstrating the usefulness of *Corynebacterium parvum* in increasing response or prolonging survival. The role of BCG is less clear. Alberts reported a phase III trial showing that the addition of BCG to doxorubicin and cyclophosphamide (AC BCG) resulted in improved response rates and prolonged survival when compared with those of patients receiving AC alone. A similar trial using cisplatin-based combinations with or without BCG (CAP vs. CAP BCG), performed by the Gynecologic Oncology Group, failed to show improved response or survival.

36. **A** page 325
There are no data to support the utility of dose intensity of cisplatin over a 3.3-fold range of doses. Studies by Mukarami and Stiff on autologous bone marrow transplant and high-dose chemotherapy on patients with no prior chemotherapy (42) or patients who failed first-line chemotherapy (30) showed some promise, but larger studies are needed before this becomes standard therapy.

37. **C** page 327
Attempts to use BRMs in the treatment of advanced ovarian cancer have stalled, awaiting the introduction of more effective BRMs. In addition, the toxicity of these agents seems to be additive to that of standard therapy. Despite these frustrations, BRMs have shown activity in a limited number of settings. Intraperitoneally administered IL-2 has been shown to initiate a series of events that results in more leukocytes and macrophages entering the peritoneal cavity. Alpha-interferon, given IP, has shown significant activity in phase II trials in patients with small-volume disease. Berek rendered 4 of 11 patients with small-volume residual disease after standard chemotherapy free of disease as assessed by repeat laparotomy.

38. **B** page 328
Extraovarian peritoneal serous papillary carcinoma is a term used to describe peritoneal carcinomatosis of serous papillary neoplasms with no apparent primary site in the ovaries. Tumor deposits may be found on the ovarian surface, but there is no evidence of in situ or primary ovarian cancer. In most reports, the metastatic implants are frankly invasive but a syndrome of metastatic "noninvasive implants" has been described. The natural history of the illness and the response rates to standard chemotherapy are similar to those of patients with ovarian cancer.

39. **B** page 329
Small cell carcinoma of the ovary is a newly described and rare neoplasm that affects children and young adults (ages 10 to 40). It is extremely aggressive, and few long-term survivors are reported. Hypercalcemia is commonly observed in these patients, suggesting a paracrine secretion.

40. **A** page 329
Traces of CA-125 are expressed in adult tissues derived from coelomic epithelium, including mesothelial cells lining the pleura, pericardium, and peritoneum, as well as the epithelial components of the fallopian tube, endometrium, and endocervix. CA-125 is not found in adult or fetal ovaries.

41. **C** page 330
CA-125 level is elevated in 80% of patients with ovarian cancer; it is usually not elevated in patients with mucinous carcinomas of the ovary. Virtually all

patients with elevated serum CA-125 levels before second-look surgery will have residual ovarian cancer. Normal serum CA-125 levels, before second-look surgery, are of limited value. Over 50% of patients with such findings (normal CA-125 and negative clinical examination results) will have persistent disease. The degree of elevation of CA-125 by itself does not predict the amount of residual disease or outcome.

42. **A** page 330
Although serum CA-125 levels may rise in patients with significant renal compromise, cisplatin toxicity is rarely the cause of an observed rise. The patient in complete clinical remission may have significant nodules, often up to 2 cm in size, and remain CA-125 negative. There is no universally recognized criteria for absolute evidence of recurrence, but most consider a 50% rise of CA-125 over normal range on two separate occasions to be evidence of recurrence. The authors, however, recommend histologic or cytologic confirmation of disease recurrence before consideration of additional therapy.

43. **C** page 331
"Second-effort" laparotomy does not increase survival and is no longer considered indicated. The remaining choices are the traditional indications for this procedure, although all three are under scrutiny. Response D, using second look as a prelude to discontinuing chemotherapy, is the most widely used indication, but even this indication is not universally accepted. That was the result of secondary cytoreductive surgery done at Memorial Sloan Kettering and MD Anderson Hospitals. However, a recent report from the European Oncology group in 1995 noticed an increase in progression-free and overall survival for patients who underwent secondary tumor reductive surgery.

44. **A** page 331
The likelihood of recurrence of patients with stages III and IV ovarian cancer treated with cisplatin-based chemotherapy is around 50%. The likelihood of recurrence is considerably smaller in patients with stage I or II disease. In addition, the rate is smaller for patients achieving a negative second look after treatment with single-agent alkylating therapy. This is difficult to explain, but many have rationalized that since a greater percentage of patients have a negative second look after combination therapy, the apparent difference is not real.

45. **D** page 330
The optimal follow-up after initial treatment remains undecided. DiSaia and Creasman advise monitoring patients following negative reassessment laparotomy with physical examination, serum CA-125, and liberal use of imaging every 3 months for 2 years, and every 6 months thereafter.

46. **D** page 330
Histologic confirmation is necessary before any salvage chemotherapy is offered. Instead of performing a full surgical exploration, one could consider an open diagnostic laparoscopy.

47. **C** page 333
Phase II trials have not demonstrated activity for doxorubicin, carboplatin, or hexamethylmelamine in patients who have previously progressed while taking cisplatin. With intense dose escalation Ozols reported a 32% response rate in patients who previously had progressed on lower doses of the drug. Unfortunately, the toxicity was severe, with neurotoxicity being the limiting factor.

48. **B** page 332
Platinum sensitivity, which is defined by a response to first-line platinum-based therapy, is found to predict the response to subsequent retreatment with a platinum-containing treatment used for salvage therapy. The response rates to salvage therapy are strikingly different in these two groups, who relapse within 6 months of therapy or who have a progression-free interval 6 months (10% in comparison to nearly 90% for patients with a progression-free interval of 21 months).

49. **B** page 334
An ideal drug for intraperitoneal use should have low peritoneal clearance and high systemic clearance. Determinants of clearance include molecular size and lipid solubility; a useful drug should be highly ionized and water soluble and have a high molecular weight. To ensure even distribution in the peritoneal cavity, there should be minimal adhesions causing the agent to loculate. Distribution can be improved by using a high volume of solution to distend the abdomen.

50. **D** page 335
Intraperitoneal (IP) platinum-based chemotherapy appears to be an efficacious salvage regimen for patients with persistent small volume disease after platinum-based intravenous chemotherapy. The use of IP therapy as initial therapy is investigational. The use of IP platinum-based therapy in the setting of bulky disease is disappointing.

51. **A** page 337
Although large fluid shifts may occur, hemodynamic instability is not as common in this setting as it is when used to treat a patient with hepatic dysfunction. Answers B and C are classic reasons paracentesis is not performed in this setting. An additional reason is that paracentesis may be associated with rupture of an abdominal viscus, bleeding, or infection. If the patient has significant respiratory embarrassment or severe pain, paracentesis may be indicated for symptom control.

52. **B** page 300
Stage IIIa refers to gross tumor limited to the true pelvis (one or both ovaries) with histologically or cytologically confirmed microscopic seeding of abdominal peritoneal surfaces.

53. **A** page 300
Stage Ic refers to tumor stage Ia or Ib but with tumor on the surface of one or both ovaries, or with capsule ruptured, or with ascites present containing malignant cells or with positive peritoneal washings.

54. **A** page 300
A tumor involving one or both ovaries (stage Ia or Ib) with tumor on the surface of one or both ovaries is classified as stage Ic.

55. **D** page 300
Stage II refers to growth involving one or both ovaries with pelvic extension; IIa extension to uterus and tubes, IIb extension to other pelvic tissues.
56. **B** page 298, Table 11–8
Surface papillae are rare in benign tumors and very common in malignant tumors of the ovary.
57. **B** page 298, Table 11–8
Solid areas of the tumor are very common in malignant ovarian tumors.
58. **B** page 298, Table 11–8
Bilaterality is rare in benign ovarian tumors and common in malignant tumors.
59. **B** page 298, Table 11–8
Ascites of more than 100 mL is rare in benign ovarian tumors (except in Meigs' syndrome with ovarian fibroma) but common in ovarian cancer.
60. **B** page 298, Table 11–8
Peritoneal implants are common in ovarian cancer.
61. **A** page 298, Table 11–8
In benign ovarian tumors, an intact capsule is commonly found; the reverse is true in advanced malignant tumors.
62. **A** page 298, Table 11–8
Malignant ovarian tumors are rarely totally cystic; they often have solid areas with necrosis. The reverse is true for benign ovarian tumors.
63. **C** page 307
According to DiSaia and Creasman, patients with stage I grade 3 lesions present a difficult problem. The recurrence rate in this group of patients is nearly 50%. They constitute a group of youthful patients who are better able to tolerate vigorous adjuvant therapy than are older patients. DiSaia and Creasman favor a platinum-based multiagent therapy.
64. **B** page 309
A study by the Gynecologic Oncology Group and the Ovarian Cancer Study Group randomized patients with stages Ia and Ib grade 1 or 2 disease between those who received melphalan for 12 cycles and those who received no further therapy. The 5-year survival in both was excellent (90%).
65. **A** page 308
Unilateral salpingo-oophorectomy could be performed in a young patient with stage Ia disease who desires further fertility. There is minimal increased risk of recurrence provided a careful staging procedure has been performed. Consideration should be given to hysterectomy and salpingo-oophorectomy when childbearing is completed.
66. **D** page 311
In stage III disease, surgery consists of removal of the uterus, both adnexae, and the bulk of the tumor, including large omental metastases. The survival rate is related to amount of residual tumor after surgery. Multiple-agent platinum-based chemotherapy is used postoperatively. Abdominal and pelvic irradiation has found less and less favor in recent years because of the long-term morbidity of radiation and its limited efficacy.

chapter 12 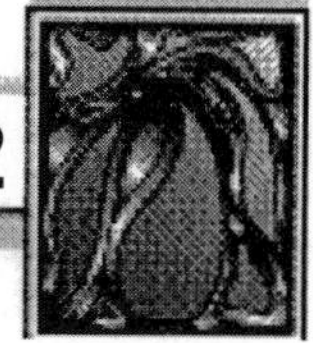

GERM CELL, STROMAL, and OTHER OVARIAN TUMORS

KEY POINTS TO REMEMBER

- Germ cell tumors are derived from the primitive germ cells of the embryonic gonad.
- Germ cell tumors represent 20% of all ovarian tumors and occur mostly in young women in the second and third decades of life.
- Symptoms are palpable abdominal mass, pain, or, rarely, hemoperitoneum (due to rupture of a dysgerminoma).
- Dysgerminoma, accounting for 3% to 5% of ovarian malignancies, is composed of germ cells that have not differentiated to form embryonic or extraembryonic structures. Histologically, it is composed of germ cells, a stroma infiltrated with lymphocytes, and occasionally syncytiotrophoblastic cells producing hCG. An elevated LDH or hCG level may be present in these patients.
- Dysgerminoma is one of the two most common ovarian neoplasms observed in pregnancy (the other is serous cystadenocarcinoma of low malignant potential [LMP]). It can be discovered incidentally in patients with gonadal dysgenesis and gonadoblastoma. It is the only germ cell tumor in which the opposite ovary may be involved with the tumor process (10% to 15%). Dysgerminoma may occur at any age.
- Dysgerminomas are notable for their predilection for lymphatic spread and their sensitivity to irradiation and chemotherapy. Conservative surgery (unilateral salpingo-oophorectomy) is indicated in the young woman who has a unilateral encapsulated dysgerminoma and who desires future childbearing. Patients should be followed closely because 90% of recurrences appear in the first 2 years after initial therapy. Recurrences can be treated successfully with irradiation or chemotherapy.
- Chemotherapy appears to be the treatment of choice for dysgerminoma after surgery: doxorubicin and cyclophosphamide, or cisplatin, vinblastine, and bleomycin (BVP), or etoposide. Complete responses in the 80% to 100% range have been reported with stages II–IV disease.
- It may be prudent to conserve the uterus, even in cases of bilateral oophorectomy (future in vivo fertilization).
- Prognosis of and therapy for dysgerminoma mixed with other malignant germ cell components are determined by the latter.
- Endodermal sinus tumor is the second most common form of malignant germ cell tumor of the ovary, accounting for 22% of germ cell lesions. Median age is 19 years. It is characterized by extensive rapid growth and intra-abdominal spread.
- The biochemical hallmark of endodermal sinus tumor is the elevation of alpha-fetoprotein (AFP), and its anatomic characteristic is the Schiller-Duval body. Serum AFP is an ideal tumor marker.
- Treatment consists of surgery and multiple chemotherapy: VAC (vincristine, dactinomycin, cyclophosphamide) or MAC (methotrexate, dactinomycin, chlorambucil), BEP (bleomycin, etoposide, cisplatin), or VBP (vincristine, bleomycin, cisplatin).
- The 4-year disease-free survival rate was 73% according to a GOG study of 48 patients who had stages I–III completely resected endodermal sinus tumor (EST); no patient with stage I disease treated with unilateral oophorectomy and VAC (or PBV) died, according to a study of 21 patients in Japan.
- Embryonal carcinoma, one of the most malignant ovarian cancers, is rare (4% of malignant germ cells) and consists of syncytiotrophoblast cells and large primitive cells with secretion of hCG and AFP. Half of the patients have hormonal abnormalities (precocious puberty, hirsutism, irregular bleeding). Treatment is with VAC or VBP and surgery. Actuarial survival for all stages is 30%.
- Polyembryoma is rare, highly malignant, and not sensitive to radiotherapy. Response to chemotherapy is unknown.
- Choriocarcinoma secretes hCG and is often mixed with other neoplastic germ cell elements. It occurs in children and young adults and is treated with MAC combination chemotherapy.
- Mixed germ cell tumor contains at least two malignant germ cell elements; dysgerminoma is the most common element. Treatment is with surgery and MAC. Survival was 79% in patients with stage I tumor.
- Mature cystic teratoma is the most common ovarian tumor in the second and third decades of life. It contains mature tissue of ectodermal, mesodermal, and endodermal origin. Complications include torsion, rupture, and infection (coliform, *Salmonella*). Mature solid teratoma is considered benign.
- Immature teratoma occurs in the first two decades of life. It is uncommon (less than 1% of teratomas), never bilateral, and contains immature neural elements. The quantity of immature neural tissue determines the grade (grade 0: all tissue mature; grade 1: neuroepithelium limited to 1 low-power field [LPF] in any one slide; grade 2: neuroepithelium does not exceed 3 LPF; grade 3: neuroepithelium occupies 4 or more LPF in any slide). Prognosis is closely related to the histologic grade of the tumor and the implants (survival rates: 82%

with grade 1, 63% with grade 2, and 30% with grade 3). A VAC regimen has proved to be effective. Chemotherapeutic retroconversion of immature teratoma, by which peritoneal implants contain exclusively mature elements, can occur and harbor a good prognosis. Conservative surgery (unilateral oophorectomy) followed by chemotherapy gives excellent results. Stage Ia grade 1 immature teratoma is treated with unilateral oophorectomy alone.

- Struma ovarii is usually benign and is treated by simple resection.
- Primary carcinoid tumor of the ovary is uncommon and is treated with excision. One third of the reported cases have typical carcinoid syndrome, despite the absence of metastasis.
- Gonadoblastoma occurs in patients with dysgenetic gonads (45,X or 45,X/46,XY). The prognosis is excellent if the tumor and the contralateral gonad are excised. The uterus should be retained. Sixty percent are virilized. It is associated with dysgerminoma in 50% of cases.
- Second-look laparotomy (SLL) in germ cell tumor is not well defined. The MD Anderson group used SLL for surgical debulking in the management of recurrences and obtained a rate of 29% of patients who were disease free using different chemotherapeutic regimens.
- Granulosa theca cell tumors produce estrogen. Granulosa cell occurs in two subtypes: adult (95%) and juvenile (5%). Adult granulosa cell occurs commonly in postmenopausal women. Histologic characteristics are the coffee bean–grooved cells, mature follicles, and Call-Exner bodies. Hyperplasia of the endometrium is not uncommon (55%). Juvenile granulosa cell occurs in young adults or children with sexual precocity. Histologically, the tumor has cell pleomorphism and numerous mitoses.
- Granulosa cell tumors are low-grade malignancies. The prognosis is excellent with surgery: long-term survival from 75% to 90% has been reported. Recurrences can occur more than 5 years after initial therapy (5% to 10% of stage I).
- Good prognostic factors include low-stage, mitotic activity less than 4/10 HPF and euploidy. Inhibin has been suggested as a tumor marker for granulosa cell tumor. Recurrent granulosa cell tumor is treated with systemic chemotherapy (Adriamycin, bleomycin, cisplatin, and vinblastine). Serum inhibin is used as a marker for monitoring treatment and recurrence.
- Theca cell tumor, or thecoma, is composed of benign theca cells, always unilateral, and never malignant. Unilateral oophorectomy may be done in young patients.
- Sertoli-Leydig cell, or androblastoma, which represents 0.5% of all ovarian tumors, occurs in all age groups but most often in young women who become masculinized. Prognosis depends on degree of differentiation of tumor. Considered to be a low-grade malignancy, the 5-year survival of these patients is 70% to 90%. Advanced or recurrent lesions are treated with chemotherapy (VAC or BEP).
- Lipid cell tumors are a heterologous group of tumors that have in common a parenchyma composed of polygonal cells containing lipids. They could be benign or malignant. Neoplasms less than 8 cm in diameter are benign.
- Mixed mesodermal sarcoma of the ovary is rare and is invariably fatal.
- Malignant lymphoma of the ovary is rare and of non-Hodgkin's type. Treatment is unilateral surgical resection and chemotherapy.
- Ten percent of ovarian cancers are metastases, mostly from carcinoma of the breast (second most frequent) and adenocarcinomas of the large intestine (most frequent) and endometrium.
- Krukenberg tumor is restricted to metastases that contain signet ring cells in a cellular stroma and arise from stomach, breast, and intestine.
- Ovarian endometrioid carcinoma is associated with endometrial carcinoma in one third of cases and probably represents two primaries.
- Most ovarian cancers in children are of germ cell origin (immature teratoma, endodermal sinus tumor).
- Granulosa theca cell tumors are the most common ovarian neoplasms found in children with isosexual precocity and adnexal enlargement. Fortunately, the most common germ cell neoplasm is the benign teratoma. Patients are treated in a manner similar to that of the adolescent.

QUESTIONS

Directions for Questions 1–22: Select the one best answer.

1. Characteristics of germ cell tumors include the following *except:*
   A. they can be found in extragonadal locations along the line of migration of primitive germ cells
   B. there is remarkable homology between various tumor types in men and women
   C. they represent about 15% to 20% of all ovarian tumors
   D. most of these neoplasms occur in older women
2. The two most common ovarian neoplasms observed in pregnancy are:
   A. dysgerminoma and serous cystadenocarcinoma of LMP
   B. dysgerminoma and teratoma
   C. teratoma and gonadoblastoma
   D. mucinous cystadenoma and teratoma
3. Findings in germ cell tumors include:
   A. rapidly enlarging abdominal mass
   B. hemoperitoneum
   C. palpable abdominal mass and pain
   D. all of the above
4. Which malignancy often develops from a gonadoblastoma?
   A. squamous cell carcinoma
   B. adenocarcinoma
   C. dysgerminoma
   D. choriocarcinoma
5. The following are true concerning the treatment of dysgerminomas *except:*
   A. in the young woman with a unilateral encapsulated dysgerminoma who desires future childbearing, conservative management is indicated
   B. it is routine to bivalve or wedge the opposite ovary even if it is normal size, shape, and consistency

C. the majority of recurrences can be successfully eradicated by radiation therapy or chemotherapy
D. multiagent chemotherapy consists of doxorubicin and cyclophosphamide or cisplatin, vinblastine, and bleomycin

6. The biochemical marker for endodermal sinus tumor is:
A. hCG
B. CEA
C. alpha-fetoprotein (AFP)
D. estradiol

7. The best treatment for endodermal sinus tumor is:
A. surgery
B. surgery and radiation
C. surgery and chemotherapy
D. all of the above

8. Treatment of endodermal sinus tumor of the ovary stage I consists of:
A. unilateral oophorectomy
B. total abdominal hysterectomy, bilateral salpingo-oophorectomy, and pelvic node dissection
C. chemotherapy with VAC (vincristine, actinomycin, cyclophosphamide) or PBV (cisplatin, bleomycin, vincristine)
D. unilateral oophorectomy and postoperative VAC or BEP

9. The most common complication of mature cystic teratoma is:
A. rupture
B. torsion
C. chemical peritonitis
D. infection

10. The following statements regarding germ cell tumors are true *except:*
A. the presence of AFP may help to differentiate an endodermal sinus tumor from an embryonal carcinoma
B. combination chemotherapy is warranted in most cases of malignant germ cell tumors
C. dysgerminoma is the most frequent component of mixed germ cell tumors
D. teratomas account for 15% of ovarian tumors

11. Choose the germ cell tumor *least* likely to be associated with menstrual irregularity:
A. choriocarcinoma
B. embryonal carcinoma
C. mature teratoma
D. gonadoblastoma

12. The following are adequate treatment of immature teratoma of the ovary stages I and II *except:*
A. unilateral oophorectomy
B. chemotherapy should be given in all cases
C. chemotherapy should be given after surgery only in stages I and II grade 3 tumors or in stage III
D. chemotherapy used is a cisplatin-based regimen

13. The histology of the endometrium in granulosa cell tumor of the ovary is most often:
A. proliferative endometrium
B. atrophic endometrium
C. hyperplastic endometrium
D. adenocarcinoma

14. The following are prognostic factors in granulosa cell of the ovary *except:*
A. stage
B. mitotic activity
C. ploidy
D. S-phase fraction

15. Which substance can be used as a tumor marker for granulosa cell tumor?
A. inhibin
B. CA-125
C. CEA
D. alpha-fetoprotein

16. Treatment of granulosa cell tumor in the perimenopausal patient should be:
A. total abdominal hysterectomy and bilateral salpingo-oophorectomy (TAH-BSO)
B. radical hysterectomy with bilateral salpingo-oophorectomy
C. unilateral salpingo-oophorectomy
D. bilateral salpingo-oophorectomy

17. The following are true concerning thecoma of the ovary *except:*
A. it is of ovarian stromal origin
B. it is virtually never malignant
C. it is often bilateral
D. treatment consists of unilateral oophorectomy or TAH-BSO, depending on age of the patient

18. Treatment recommendations by DiSaia and Creasman for stages II and III or recurrent granulosa cell tumor are:
A. radiotherapy
B. chemotherapy
C. radical hysterectomy and bilateral pelvic lymphadenectomy
D. pelvic exenteration

19. The prognosis of Sertoli-Leydig cell tumor depends on its:
A. presence of heterologous elements
B. histologic differentiation
C. quantity of Leydig cells
D. degree of clinical masculinization

20. Which is the most common primary carcinoma metastatic to the ovary?
A. breast
B. large intestine
C. endometrium
D. cervix

21. The most common pathway of metastatic spread to the ovary is:
A. direct continuity
B. surface implantation
C. lymphatic metastasis
D. hematogenous spread

22. Most ovarian cancers in children are of which origin?
A. epithelial
B. germ cell
C. stromal
D. metastatic

Directions for Questions 23–51: For each numbered item, select the letter of the most appropriate answer.

Each letter may be used once, more than once, or not at all.

23–27. Match the characteristics of endodermal sinus tumor and dysgerminoma.
- A. endodermal sinus tumor
- B. dysgerminoma
- C. both
- D. neither

23. Sensitivity to radiation
24. Chemotherapy
25. Progestins
26. Germ cells and lymphocytes
27. Schiller-Duval body

28–33. Match the germ cell tumors to their appropriate therapy.
- A. unilateral oophorectomy or salpingo-oophorectomy
- B. combination chemotherapy
- C. oophorocystectomy
- D. A plus B
- E. none of the above

28. Choriocarcinoma
29. Embryonal carcinoma
30. Mature teratoma
31. Immature teratoma
32. Primary ovarian carcinoid
33. Gonadoblastoma

34–41. Match the tumors with their characteristics.
- A. polyembryoma
- B. struma ovarii
- C. embryonal carcinoma
- D. dysgerminoma
- E. gonadoblastoma
- F. immature teratoma
- G. primary ovarian choriocarcinoma

34. Lack of second X chromosome
35. Metastases are better differentiated than is the primary tumor
36. AFP negative, hCG positive
37. Usually has widespread metastases
38. Thyroid parenchyma
39. Tumor grading system includes amount of neural tissue
40. AFP positive, hCG positive
41. Most common component of mixed germ cell tumor

42–46. Match the histologic formations with the most appropriate type of ovarian tumor.
- A. granulosa cell tumor
- B. Krukenberg tumor
- C. Leydig cell tumor
- D. immature teratoma

42. Call-Exner bodies
43. Coffee bean nucleus
44. Immature neural tissue
45. Signet ring cells
46. Reinke crystals

47–51. Match the figures representing germ cell tumors in Figure 12-1 with their characteristics:

47. Call-Exner bodies
48. Sensitive to radiation and chemotherapy
49. Alpha-fetoprotein
50. Schiller-Duval bodies
51. Immature neural tissue

Answers

1. **D** page 351
   Since most germ cell neoplasms occur in young women, treatment of the disease involves decisions concerning childbearing and probabilities of recurrence.
2. **A** page 352
   Dysgerminoma and serous cystadenocarcinoma of LMP are the two most common ovarian neoplasms observed in pregnancy. The finding of dysgerminoma in pregnant patients is nonspecific and is related to age of the patient rather than to the pregnancy state.
3. **D** page 352
   Most germ cell tumors are found in the second and third decades of life. They are frequently diagnosed by finding a palpable abdominal mass, often associated with pain. Rapid enlargement, rupture, or torsion of the tumor causes considerable pain. Dysgerminoma can rupture and cause hemoperitoneum.
4. **C** page 355
   Gonadoblastoma, a benign mixed tumor composed of germ cell and gonadal stromal elements, is found in patients with abnormal sex chromosomes 45,X or 45,X/46,XY. Dysgerminoma may develop from germ cells in a gonadoblastoma.
5. **B** page 355
   Although the opposite ovary may be involved with dysgerminoma in 10% to 15% of cases, DiSaia and Creasman advise not to wedge or bivalve the opposite ovary if it is of normal size, shape, and consistency to maximize fertility.
6. **C** page 355
   Alpha-fetoprotein (AFP) levels are elevated in endodermal sinus tumors. AFP determination can be used to monitor the result of treatment and to detect recurrences.
7. **C** page 357
   Surgery alone is unsuccessful in curing this disease. The tumor is not sensitive to radiation. Conservative surgery plus chemotherapy results in an appreciable number of successful pregnancies after treatment. Chemotherapy often consists of vincristine, dactinomycin, and cyclophosphamide (VAC). VBP (vincristine, bleomycin, and cisplatin) induces a substantial number of durable complete responses even in patients with prior chemotherapy. BEP (bleomycin, etoposide, cisplatin) is more effective and has less neuromuscular toxicity than VBP.
8. **D** page 355
   Fujita treated 21 patients with unilateral oophorectomy followed by postoperative VAC or PBV. None of the stage I patients died. More aggressive surgery did not improve survival.
9. **B** page 361
   Up to 16% of patients are reported to have torsion, which is more common in pregnancy. Rupture and infection occur in about 1% of cases. Chemical peritonitis may follow rupture.
10. **A** page 357
    Endodermal sinus tumor and embryonal carcinoma contain AFP. The other criteria used to differentiate one from the other are histopathology and the

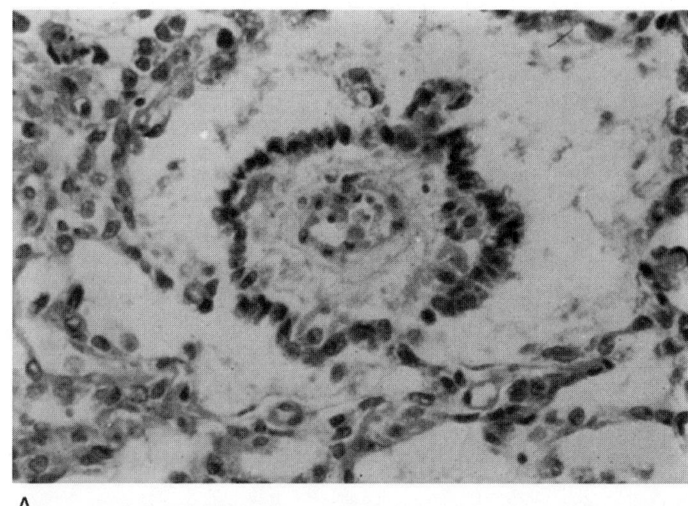
A

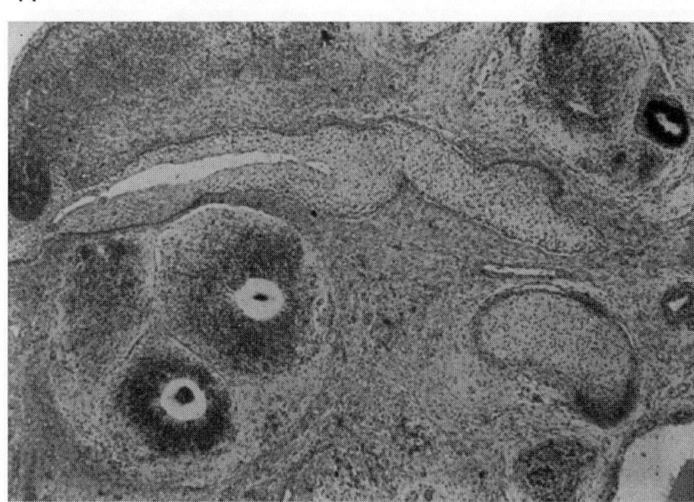
B

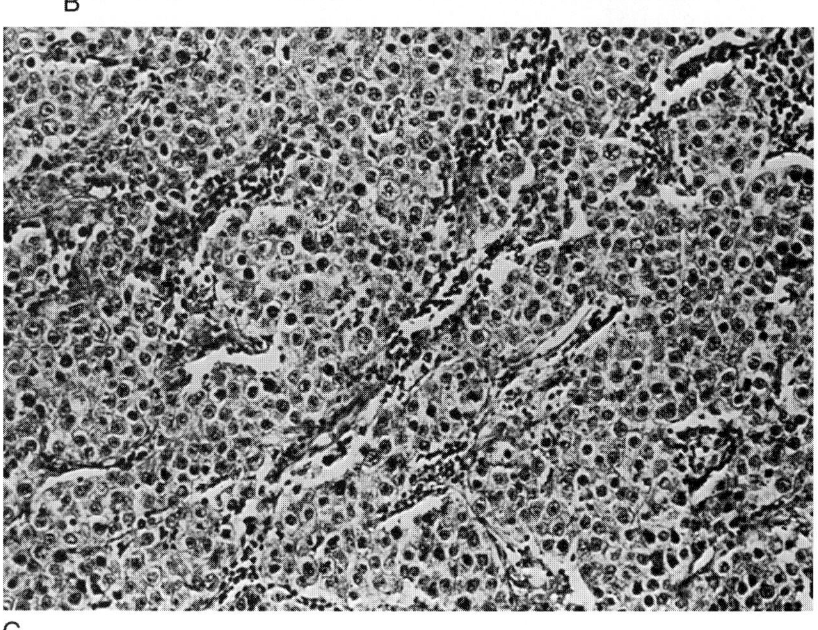
C

FIGURE 12–1. A, B, and C

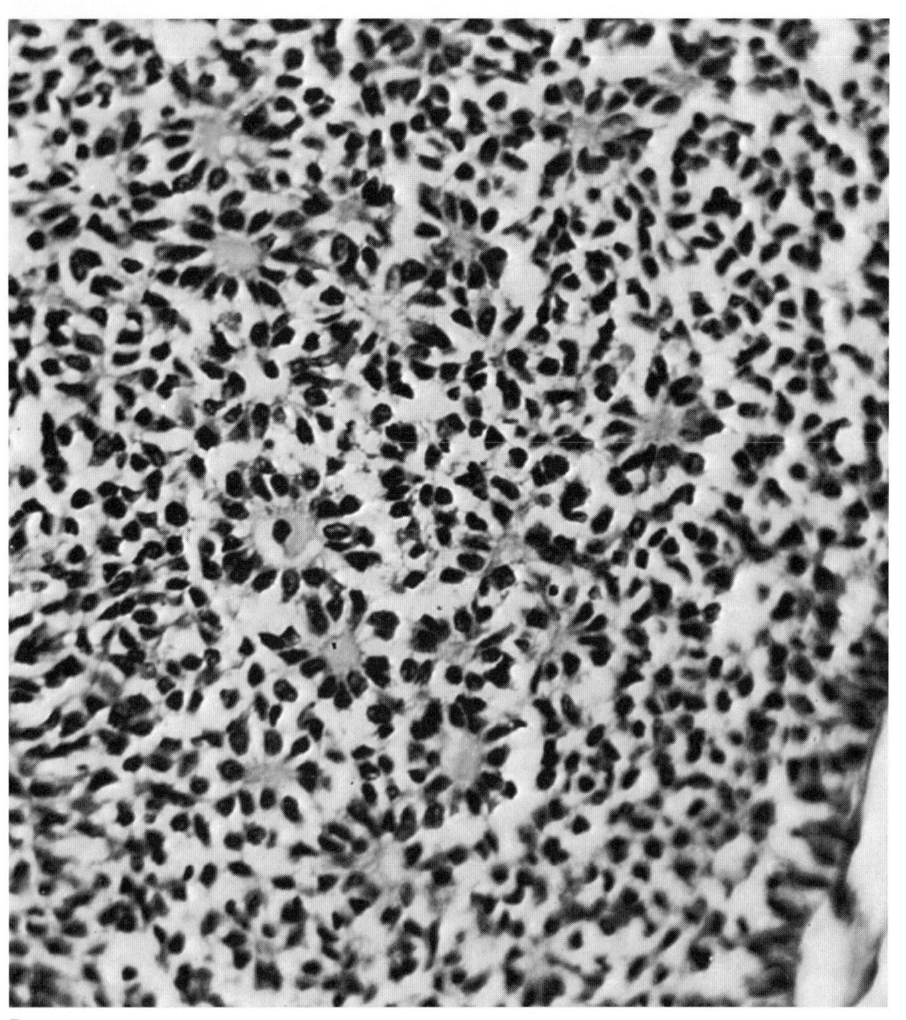
D

FIGURE 12–1. D

presence of hCG in embryonal carcinoma and its absence in EST.

Most malignant germ cell tumors are treated by simple excision plus combination chemotherapy. VAC, VBP, and MAC are favored regimens. The only exception seems to be stage Ia grade 1 immature teratoma, which can be treated by simple excision only.

11. **C** page 360
Embryonal carcinoma and choriocarcinoma secrete hCG, which interferes with menstrual function.
Patients with gonodoblastoma are usually found to have primary amenorrhea, virilization, or developmental genital abnormalities.
12. **B** page 363
Chemotherapy is not given by Bonazzi and colleagues with stages I and II and grades 1 and 2. They used fertility-sparing surgery in 30 patients. All patients were alive and disease free at a median of 47 months. Seven pregnancies occurred with delivery of seven normal infants.
13. **C** page 365, Table 12–9
Based on data from Evans, hyperplastic endometrium is found in 55% of endometria of patients with granulosa cell tumor. Proliferative endometrium is found in 25% and adenocarcinoma in 13%.
14. **D** page 367
In a study of 54 patients from Sweden, in patients with a mitotic rate of less than 4 MF/10 HPF there was no death. Those with more than 10 MF/10 HPF died—the longest survival was 4 years. Patients with mitotic rate of 4–10 MF/10 HPF had a median survival of 9 years. Patients with aneuploidy tumors died of disease. S-phase fraction was not correlated with any clinical or histologic parameter.
15. **A** page 367
Inhibin is a glycoprotein secreted by granulosa cells of the ovary during the menstrual cycle and during pregnancy. It is not secreted in postmenopausal women. The relationship of tumor to the level of inhibin appears to be very good.
16. **A** page 367
Granulosa cell tumors are low-grade malignancies that recur very late (75%–90% long-term survival for all stages). Twenty-three percent of recurrences are more than 13 years after initial therapy. Most recurrences occur in preserved genital tract structures. The authors recommend the preserved internal genitalia be removed in the perimenopausal patient. Preservation of internal genitalia may be appropriate during the childbearing period.

17. **C** page 368
Whereas granulosa cell tumors are found to be bilateral in 2% to 5% of patients, thecomas are almost always confined to one ovary. In cases in which preservation of fertility is important, a thecoma may be treated adequately by unilateral oophorectomy. TAH-BSO is recommended in postmenopausal and perimenopausal women.
18. **B** page 368
The authors recommend no further therapy in stage I lesions. Stages II and III or recurrent granulosa cell tumors are best treated with systemic chemotherapy. The optimal chemotherapeutic regimen has not yet been determined. Adriamycin, bleomycin, cisplatin, and vinblastine used singly or in combination (VBP, BEP) appear to be effective. If not yet done, a total hysterectomy and salpingo-oophorectomy should be performed.
19. **B** page 368
The degree of differentiation of the tumor is probably of greatest importance in determining the prognosis of Sertoli-Leydig cell tumors. In a report by Young and Scully, none of the 27 well-differentiated tumors and only 4 of 100 tumors of intermediate differentiation were known to be clinically malignant. Sertoli-Leydig tumors are considered to have low malignant potential, like granulosa cell tumors. The overall 5-year survival rate has been reported as 70% to 90%. Recurrences are treated often with the VAC or BEP chemotherapy regimen.
20. **B** page 370
Approximately 10% of ovarian tumors are not primary in origin. The most frequent metastasis comes from adenocarcinoma of colon, followed by breast cancer.
21. **C** page 370
Lymphatic metastasis is undoubtedly the most common pathway of spread to the ovary.
22. **B** page 370
Most ovarian cancers in children are of germ cell origin. Pain is the most frequently reported symptom. A palpable abdominal mass is found in half of the patients. Approximately 10% have isosexual precocity. In a study by Cangir on 21 girls, 8 had malignant teratomas, 6 had mixed germ cell tumors, 6 had endodermal sinus tumors, and 1 had a Sertoli-Leydig type stromal cell tumor.
23. **B** page 352
24. **C** page 356
25. **D** page 356
26. **B** page 352
27. **A** page 355
Dysgerminoma is notable for its sensitivity to radiation and its propensity for early lymphatic spread. Chemotherapy with multiple agents can be used for both diseases. Progestins have no effect on these tumors. The histologic features of dysgerminoma consist of nests of germ cells separated by bands of stroma peppered with lymphocytes. The histologic hallmark of endodermal sinus tumor is the Schiller-Duval body, a characteristic invaginated papillary structure with a central blood vessel reminiscent of glomeruli. There are also intracellular and extracellular hyaline globules, which contain alpha-fetoprotein.
28. **D** page 359
29. **D** page 359
30. **C** page 360
31. **D** page 362
32. **A** page 363
33. **E** page 364
Proper therapy for most malignant germ cell tumors (which usually appear as stage I or II) is unilateral oophorectomy or salpingo-oophorectomy followed by combination chemotherapy. Mature teratoma, the most common form of teratoma, is benign and is cured with conservative excision. Monodermal teratomas, such as struma ovarii or carcinoid, are best treated by excision alone. Gonadoblastoma, though benign, should be considered premalignant and should be excised by oophorectomy. In view of the very high association with a contralateral nonfunctional ovary or contralateral gonadoblastoma, the opposite ovary should also be excised.
34. **E** page 364
Gonadoblastoma is usually associated with 45,X or 45,X/46,XY mosaic genotypes. Eighty percent of patients with gonadoblastoma have female phenotypes.
35. **F** page 361
In the majority of cases of immature teratoma, the implants are more well-differentiated than the primary tumor.
36. **G** page 359
Choriocarcinoma is hCG positive and AFP negative.
37. **A** page 359
Although only a handful of polyembryomas have been reported, patients usually have extensive pelvic and abdominal disease. This is in contrast to the remainder of germ cell tumors, which are usually localized at the time of diagnosis.
38. **B** page 363
Struma ovarii is a teratoma composed predominantly of thyroid tissue. Twenty-five to thirty-five percent of patients will be clinically hyperthyroid.
39. **F** page 362
The grading system of immature teratoma by Norris includes the amount of neural tissue present, as well as traditional grading criteria such as atypia and mitoses (Table 12–6).
40. **C** page 352
Embryonal carcinoma is AFP and hCG positive.
41. **D** page 359
Dysgerminoma is the most common component of mixed germ cell tumors.
42. **A** page 367
Call-Exner bodies are cavities surrounded by granulosa cells, found in granulosa cell tumors.
43. **A** page 367
Oval or angular grooved nuclei (coffee bean appearance) are typical of granulosa cell tumor.
44. **D** page 361
Immature neural tissue is the hallmark of immature teratoma.

45. **B** page 370
Signet ring cells are found in Krukenberg tumors, which are metastases from the stomach, breast, or intestine.
46. **C** page 369
Reinke crystals, normally occurring in mature Leydig cells of the testes, are found in Leydig cell tumors of the ovary.
47. **D** page 367
Call-Exner bodies are found in granulosa cell tumor, especially in the microfollicular histologic type.
48. **C** page 354
Dysgerminomas are notable by their predilection for lymphatic spread and their acute sensitivity to irradiation. More recently, the use of multiple-agent chemotherapy is advocated and produces good results.
49. **A** page 355
Alpha-fetoprotein is the biochemical hallmark of EST.
50. **A** page 355
The Schiller-Duval body, a characteristic invaginated papillary structure with a central blood vessel, is the histologic hallmark of EST.
51. **B** page 361
Immature teratoma contains, by definition, immature neural tissue. The quantity of immature neural tissue determines grade of the tumor (Norris).

chapter 13 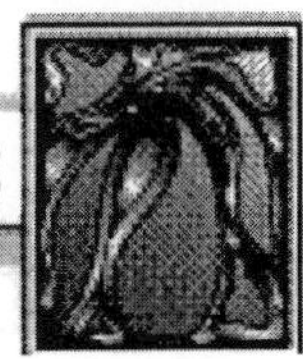

FALLOPIAN TUBE CANCER

KEY POINTS TO REMEMBER

- Adenocarcinoma of the fallopian tube is one of the rarest malignancies of the female genital tract: 1% or less of all gynecologic cancers, with an annual incidence of 3.6 in 1 million women. Primary infertility in 70% of patients has been reported in some series.
- Bilateral occurrence of tubal cancer (10% to 25%) is seen more frequently in infertile patients. One half of patients are nulliparous, with an average age of 50 years.
- Treatment of carcinoma in situ (CIS) of the tube involves the removal of the tube or tubes.
- Vaginal bleeding is the most common symptom of tubal carcinoma. Pain that is relieved with blood or watery discharges is referred to as *hydrops tubae profluens*. Ascites can occur with an adnexal mass interpreted as ovarian neoplasia or pedunculated fibroid. Delay of symptoms appears to be common (average 48 months).
- Positive cervical cytology, sometimes with psammoma bodies, is found in 23% of patients. More than 80% of patients have a pelvic or abdominal mass before surgery. CA-125 levels can be elevated in 20% of patients.
- Immunohistochemical staining for CA-125 is positive in 87% of tumors. The use of serum CA-125 levels becomes a valuable tool in monitoring patients during and after therapy.
- Diagnosis with abdominal and vaginal ultrasound is reported to be very accurate.
- More than 50% of patients have stage I or II at diagnosis (contrary to two thirds of ovarian cancers, which have stages III and IV disease).
- In tubal carcinoma, there is usually intraperitoneal involvement before ovarian involvement, and peritoneal cytology is extremely important.
- There is also high propensity for lymph node metastasis, as there is in ovarian cancer. Metastasis to retroperitoneal lymph nodes has been noted in one third of patients.
- Nearly all carcinomas of the tube are adenocarcinomas.
- Therapy should be essentially the same as that for ovarian carcinoma: total abdominal hysterectomy and bilateral salpingo-oophorectomy (TAH-BSO) and omentectomy are the minimal therapy for stage I lesions. Debulking to 1 cm lesions should be performed in patients with stage II and higher disease. Patients with negative cytologic findings had a 5-year survival of 67% vs. 20% for those with positive cytologic findings.
- FIGO staging (1991):
  - Stage 0: CIS
  - Stage I: fallopian tubes
    - Ia: one tube, extension into submucosa or muscularis, no ascites
    - Ib: both tubes, extension into submucosa or muscularis, no ascites
    - Ic: one or both tubes with extension to serosa, or ascites containing malignant cells, or positive peritoneal washings
  - Stage II: pelvic extension
    - IIa: extension to uterus and ovaries
    - IIb: extension to pelvis
    - IIc: stage IIa or IIb with ascites containing malignant cells
  - Stage III: peritoneal implant outside the pelvis or positive peritoneal or inguinal nodes; superficial liver metastasis
    - IIIa: microscopic seeding of abdominal peritoneal surfaces
    - IIIb: implants smaller than 2 cm
    - IIIc: implants larger than 2 cm or positive nodes
  - Stage IV: distant metastases, parenchymal liver metastases
- Optimal debulking appears to enhance survival, as it does in ovarian cancer: absence of gross residual disease after primary surgery was the best predictor of disease-free status at second-look laparotomy (SLL).
- Intraperitoneal ^{32}P or short-time cisplatin regimens can be used in patients who have positive cytologic findings.
- Adjuvant therapy in early stages of disease (stages I and II) has not shown a benefit in survival. Cisplatin-based chemotherapy does improve long-term survival of patients with advanced disease (overall 5-year survival 51%; stages II–IV with completely resected tumor 83% vs. 28% with gross disease remaining at primary laparotomy).
- Patients with negative disease at SLL had only 19% recurrence. Thirty percent of those found to have persistent disease at SLL were alive at 5 years.
- Stage, tumor grade, and amount of residual tumor are important prognostic factors. In stage I, the only statistically significant variable was depth of invasion within the tubal wall (80% 5-year survival with no invasion of the muscularis; 20% with invasion of more than half of the tubal muscularis). Recurrences appear to a lesser degree than in those with ovarian cancer.
- Five-year overall survival for all stages is 56% (FIGO 1998).
- Mixed mesodermal tumors of the tube are rare and are treated with surgery and chemotherapy. Prognosis is guarded. Mean survival is 16 months.

QUESTIONS

Directions for Questions 1–17: Select the one best answer.

1. In relationship to all gynecologic cancers, the frequency of carcinoma of the fallopian tube is:
   A. 1% or less
   B. 2% or less
   C. 3% or less
   D. 5% or less
2. Which is the most common symptom of tubal carcinoma?
   A. pain
   B. vaginal bleeding
   C. watery vaginal discharge
   D. ascites
3. What is the percentage of positive cervical cytologic findings in tubal carcinoma?
   A. 10%
   B. 25%
   C. 50%
   D. 60%
4. The diagnosis of tubal carcinoma is rarely made preoperatively. Which of the following are signs of this disease?
   A. abdominal mass
   B. pelvic mass
   C. abnormal cervical cytologic findings
   D. all of the above
5. The most frequent histologic type of tubal carcinoma is:
   A. squamous carcinoma
   B. endometrioid carcinoma
   C. adenocarcinoma
   D. adenosquamous carcinoma
6. Therapeutic guidelines for the surgical treatment of tubal carcinoma include the following *except:*
   A. total abdominal hysterectomy and bilateral salpingo-oophorectomy (TAH-BSO)
   B. peritoneal cytologic samplings
   C. debulking and partial omentectomy
   D. complete pelvic lymphadenectomy
7. Postoperative treatment of tubal carcinoma consists of:
   A. no further therapy in the case of disease limited to tubal mucosa and with limited muscle invasion
   B. intraperitoneal ^{32}P in the case of positive cytologic findings
   C. cisplatin-containing regimen in the case of bulk residual disease or positive nodes; and whole pelvic radiation with cisplatin-based chemotherapy in the case of residual disease only in pelvis
   D. all of the above
8. Negative second-look laparotomy (SLL) in tubal carcinoma is often found in patients with:
   A. negative-pattern peritoneal cytologic findings
   B. completely resected tumor followed with cisplatin-based chemotherapy
   C. gross disease remaining after primary laparotomy
   D. high doses and multiple cycles of cisplatin associated with paclitaxel (Taxol)
9. Prognostic factors in tubal carcinoma include:
   A. stage of the disease
   B. invasion of tubal muscularis in stage I disease
   C. positive peritoneal washings and amount of gross residual disease after surgery
   D. all of the above
10. What are the diagnostic criteria suggested by Hu for the histologic diagnosis of tubal cancer?
    A. papillary pattern of involved tubal mucosa
    B. transition between benign and malignant tubal epithelium
    C. main tumor in the tube
    D. all of the above
11. Important prognostic factors in tubal cancer are the following *except:*
    A. stage of disease
    B. grade of tumor
    C. lymphovascular invasion
    D. residual disease after primary laparotomy
12. The largest number of sarcomas of the fallopian tube are:
    A. leiomyosarcoma
    B. angiosarcoma
    C. mixed mesodermal tumor
    D. liposarcoma
13. Concerning fallopian tube cancer, the majority are in which stage?
    A. I
    B. II
    C. I or II
    D. III
14. Regardless of stage, the 5-year survival rate for all cases of carcinoma of the tube is around:
    A. 20%
    B. 40%
    C. 50%
    D. 60%

Directions for Questions 15–20: For each numbered item, select the letter of the most appropriate answer. Each letter may be used once, more than once, or not at all.

15–20. Match the stage of disease with the tumor:
   A. Ia
   B. Ic
   C. IIa
   D. IIb

15. A growth limited to one tube with extension into the muscularis and with ascites containing malignant cells
16. A growth limited to one tube with extension to the serosa, no ascites
17. A tumor of the fallopian tube extending to the right pelvic wall; negative pelvic washings
18. A growth limited to one tube with extension to the muscularis
19. A growth in both tubes extending to the uterus
20. A growth in one tube extending to both ovaries

ANSWERS

1. **A** page 377
   Adenocarcinoma of the fallopian tube is a rare malignancy, and its frequency is 1% or less of all gynecologic cancers. The recent average annual incidence of fallopian tube neoplasms was 3.6/1 million women.

2. **B** page 378
Vaginal bleeding is the most common symptom of tubal carcinoma and is present in more than 50% of patients. Pain with bloody vaginal discharge is a common finding. Pain with a profuse, watery vaginal discharge is referred to as *hydrops tubae profluens*. Ascites with positive peritoneal cytologic findings is being reported at an increasing frequency, although it is not yet the most frequently seen initial symptom.
3. **B** page 379
In a study of 115 patients, Peters found that 23% had positive cervical cytologic findings. A clinical smear with psammoma bodies increases the suspicion of tubal or ovarian cancer.
4. **D** page 379
More than 80% of patients have a pelvic or abdominal mass noted before surgery and 10% to 25% have abnormal cervical cytologic findings suggestive of adenocarcinoma. Uterine and ovarian pathologic conditions are often diagnosed before laparotomy. Preoperative diagnosis of tubal carcinoma is unusual. Ultrasound (abdominal and vaginal) has recently improved the preoperative diagnosis.
5. **C** page 380
Nearly all carcinomas of the tube are adenocarcinomas that can have papillary, alveolar, and medullary patterns. The other histologic types are rare.
6. **D** page 380
Surgical treatment of tubal carcinoma should follow the guidelines of ovarian carcinoma, which consists of TAH-BSO; peritoneal cytologic samplings from the pelvis, lateral paracolonic gutters, and subdiaphragmatic areas; debulking; and partial omentectomy. Complete pelvic lymphadenectomy is not performed. The lymphatic spread of tubal carcinoma is mainly to the periaortic nodes, and this area should be examined also. Selective pelvic and periaortic lymphadenectomy can be performed in stages I to IV.
7. **D** page 381
After surgical treatment of tubal carcinoma, DiSaia and Creasman suggest the use of intraperitoneal ^{32}P in the case of positive peritoneal cytologic findings and cisplatin-based chemotherapy and progestin chemotherapy in the case of residual disease or positive nodes. Whole pelvic irradiation is added to chemotherapy when the residual disease is localized to the pelvis only.
8. **B** page 382
Absence of gross disease at the completion of primary surgery was the best predictor of disease-free status at SLL. Low recurrence rate occurs in patients with negative SLL (19%). About 30% of those found to have persistent disease at SLL were alive at 5 years.
9. **D** page 382
All of the factors listed are significant prognostic factors in the 5-year survival of patients with tubal carcinoma.
10. **D** page 379
They are the diagnostic criteria suggested by Hu. This distinction between ovarian and tubal cancer in early stage is easily accomplished but in advanced disease is very difficult to recognize.
11. **C** page 382
Lymphovascular invasion is not a prognostic factor for survival; the other three factors are. In the Hellstrom study, patients receiving cisplatin chemotherapy had a superior survival rate (P = 0.006) compared with those not receiving chemotherapy.
12. **C** page 382
Mixed mesodermal tumor of the fallopian tube represents the largest number of sarcomas, yet fewer than 30 have been reported.
13. **C** page 379
More than 50% of patients have stage I or II disease. This is a more favorable situation than ovarian cancer.
14. **C** page 382
According to Sedlis, the 5-year survival rate for all cases of tubal carcinoma was 38%, regardless of stage. Barakat treated 38 patients with cisplatin-based chemotherapy. The overall survival was 51% at 5 years. It appears that cisplatin improved long-term survival in patients with advanced disease. Peters, in his review of 115 patients, found that in stage I disease, the only statistically significant variable was the depth of invasion within the tubal wall. The long-term survival of patients with no muscle involvement, less than 50%, and more than 50% muscle invasion is 80%, 60%, and 20%, respectively. In 1998, FIGO reported an overall survival of 56%
15. **B** page 380
16. **B** page 380
Note that staging of tubal carcinoma is surgical. The presence of ascites containing malignant cells or the extension of the tumor to the serosa of the tube when the tumor is limited to the tube classifies the tumor in stage Ic.
17. **D** page 378
Extension of the tumor to the pelvic wall puts the tumor in stage IIb. If pelvic washings are positive, the tumor is at stage IIc.
18. **A** page 380
19. **C** page 380
20. **C** page 380

chapter 14 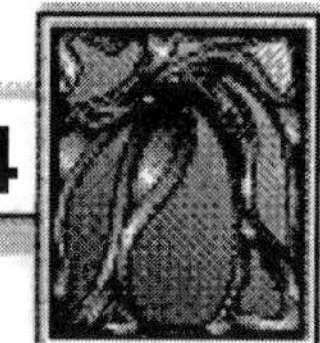

BREAST DISEASES

KEY POINTS TO REMEMBER

- Breast cancer is the most common neoplasm in women. One of every nine women, or about 11%, will develop breast cancer. The incidence rate is 110 per 100,000 per year. In 2000, 184,200 new invasive cancers were diagnosed.
- Breast cancer is the leading cause of cancer death in women after lung cancer, as well as the leading cause of death from all causes in women 40 to 44 years old. Death due to breast cancer occurs at the rate of one every 15 minutes. During 1999, 44,000 deaths in the United States were attributed to breast cancer.
- The cause of breast cancer is multifactorial (e.g., genetic predisposition, loss of immunologic defense mechanism, viruses, carcinogens). The most important aspect in combating the disease is diagnosis at an early state when the prognosis for cure is excellent.
- The 5-year survival rate for localized breast cancer has risen to 94%.
- The principal blood supply to the breast is from the internal mammary (60% of breast) and the lateral thoracic arteries (30%).
- Ninety-seven percent of lymph from the breast flows to the axillary nodes. Three percent flows to the internal mammary nodes.
- A method of delineating metastatic spread is to divide the axillary lymph nodes into three levels according to their relationship with the pectoralis minor muscle: levels I, II, and III lateral to the lateral border and behind and medial to the medial border of the pectoralis minor, respectively.
- Comparison of screening by clinical breast examination and mammography with no screening demonstrated a statistically significant decreased breast cancer mortality rate (20% and 71%, respectively).
- Fibrocystic changes are found in 58% of breasts. Atypical epithelial proliferation is the most important pathologic risk factor for progression to carcinoma. Moderate or florid hyperplasia without atypia was associated with slightly increased risk (1.5 to 2 times) for invasive carcinoma. Atypical hyperplasia is associated with a high risk for developing invasive carcinoma (8 to 10 times). Mild hyperplasia, adenosis, and apocrine and squamous metaplasias pose no increased risk for breast cancer.
- Fibroadenoma is the most common benign tumor of the breast found in many young women. Fibroadenomas are multiple and bilateral in about 14% to 25% of patients. Carcinoma rarely occurs in association with fibroadenoma. The most common carcinoma is lobular carcinoma in situ.
- Phyllodes tumor, an uncommon, slow-growing lesion, is most common in premenopausal patients. The increased cellularity with pleomorphism and mitotic activity of the connective tissue is characteristic of the tumor. It should be treated by a local excision with a wide margin of healthy tissue.
- Intraductal papilloma manifests as a serous, serosanguineous, or watery nipple discharge. It rarely undergoes malignant transformation and should be treated by surgery.
- Ductal ectasia manifests as a multicolored, sticky bilateral discharge from multiple ducts; it may simulate advanced breast carcinoma. Treatment consists of local excision of the inflamed area of breast tissue.
- Tubular and lactating adenomas are freely movable masses in young women.
- Sclerosing lesions of the breast can simulate breast carcinoma on mammographic, gross, and microscopic examinations. Local excision is the treatment of choice.
- A person with a breast mass during pregnancy should undergo biopsy, with meticulous hemostasis.
- Major risks for breast cancer:
  a. Age: most breast cancers occur during the postmenopausal years.
  b. Family history of breast cancer: if breast cancer is present in a mother or sister, there is approximately a twofold risk.
  c. Endogenous endocrine and reproductive factors: the younger a woman's age at menarche, the higher her risk for breast cancer. The later a woman's menopause occurs, the higher her risk of breast cancer.
  d. History of benign breast disease with atypical hyperplasia.
  e. Rate of exogenous hormones: there is a small increase in the risk of having breast cancer while on oral contraceptive agents (OCAs) and in the 10 years after stopping them. Six meta-analyses show no statistically significant increase risk of breast cancer with estrogen replacement therapy (ERT).
- Recommendations from ACS, NCI, and ACOG: monthly breast self-examinations by patients, yearly clinical breast examination by physicians, mammography every 1 to 2 years for women 40 to 49 years of age, and annually for women older than 50 years of age. ACOG also recommends regular screening beginning at age 35 years for women with a family history of premenopausal breast cancer in a first-degree relative.

- Mammography is the most accurate technique for the detection of early stage breast cancers, but a false-negative rate of 5% to 15% has been reported for clinically palpable masses. A fine-needle aspiration (FNA) or open biopsy should be performed on any clinically suspicious mass. Stereotactically guided core needle biopsy is more advantageous than FNA.
- The 5-year survival rate for localized breast cancer is 91%, with regional metastases 69%, and with distant metastasis 18%.
- Clinical staging correlates well with 5- to 10-year survival rate and is the basis for selection of therapy in many cases.
- One-fourth of patients with enlarged axillary nodes (clinical stage II) are without nodal metastasis; about 40% without palpable nodes (stage I) have nodal metastasis. The number of positive axillary nodes affects survival (10-year, disease-free survival 38% for one to three positive nodes and 13% for four or more positive nodes).
- Useful tests for detecting metastasis are bone scans and x-ray films of bones with abnormal uptake on the scan, as well as films of the chest and contralateral breast. Roberts and coworkers reported that 18% of new breast cancer patients with normal bone radiographic results had scans with evidence of bone metastasis.
- Standard radical mastectomy, modified radical mastectomy, and local excision plus irradiation give similar survival figures for treatment of invasive breast cancer.
- The modified radical mastectomy with partial axillary dissection (sparing of the pectoralis major and minor muscles) was accepted in 1979 by the NCI consensus conference.
- Tamoxifen, the first selective estrogen receptor modulator, appears to be advantageous to all women, irrespective of menopausal and lymph node status as long as the cancer was estrogen receptor positive. The current recommendation is for 5 years of use.
- The National Surgical Adjuvant Breast Project (NSABP) trial on 13,000 high-risk women reported a 49% reduction in the overall risk with invasive cancer and a 50% reduction for noninvasive cancer with the use of tamoxifen. There was a 2.5 times greater risk for development of endometrial cancer. High risk was determined by the Gail model, which includes age, number of affected first-degree relatives, age at menarche, age at first live birth, number of previous breast biopsies, and presence of atypical hyperplasia in biopsy specimen. Tamoxifen reduced the recurrence of estrogen receptor–positive tumors by 69%, but there was no difference in recurrence of estrogen receptor–negative tumors.
- The risk of invasive breast cancer was also 76% lower in the raloxifene group than in the placebo group.
- The increased use of screening mammography has led to a marked increase in the number of patients with a diagnosis of DCIS (ductal carcinoma in situ or intraductal carcinoma). Eighty-five percent of all DCIS is detected solely on mammography (one DCIS for two or three invasive breast cancers). Treatment is wide excision with negative margins (lumpectomy) followed by breast irradiation. Patients also benefit from the use of tamoxifen. DCIS recurs in the vicinity of the original surgery in the form of DCIS (50%) or invasive ductal carcinoma (50%).
- Lobular carcinoma in situ (LCIS) recurs in the opposite breast or in the ipsilateral breast in the form of DCIS, invasive ductal carcinoma, or lobular carcinoma. Tamoxifen also lowered rates of invasive tumors in women with a history of LCIS and atypical hyperplasia.
- Staging of breast cancer is based on size of primary tumor, regional lymph nodes, and distant metastasis.
  - Stage 0: CIS
  - Stage I: tumor smaller than 2 cm without node
  - Stage IIa: no evidence of primary tumor, movable ipsilateral axillary node(s), or tumor smaller than 2 cm with movable ipsilateral axillary node, or tumor larger than 2 cm but smaller than 5 cm, without node
  - Stage IIb: tumor smaller than 5 cm with movable ipsilateral axillary node, or tumor larger than 5 cm without node
  - Stage IIIa: no evidence of primary tumor with ipsilateral axillary nodes fixed to one another or to other structures, or tumor smaller than 2 cm with fixed axillary nodes, or tumor smaller than 5 cm with fixed axillary nodes, or tumor larger than 5 cm with movable or fixed axillary nodes
  - Stage IIIb: tumor of any size with extension to the chest wall and with or without axillary node, or any tumor with metastasis to the ipsilateral internal mammary node
  - Stage IV: any tumor with any axillary node and distant metastasis
- Six prospective randomized trials on 4114 patients comparing mastectomy with conservative surgery plus irradiation for stages I and II breast cancer showed no difference in survival or disease-free survival between the two treatments at a follow-up of up to 18 years.
- In a comparison of conservative surgery alone with conservative surgery and irradiation, there was a reduction rate of recurrence of 84% in the irradiated breast.
- The clinician can recommend lumpectomy plus irradiation to patients instead of mastectomy.
- There were no significant differences between two groups of patients who had clinically positive nodes treated by radical mastectomy or by total mastectomy without axillary dissection but with regional irradiation. Survival at 10 years was about 38% in both groups (Fisher, 1985). The use of sentinel node is under study.
- Disease-free survival after segmental mastectomy plus irradiation was better than disease-free survival after total mastectomy and overall survival after total mastectomy. Breast irradiation has value for reducing the incidence of tumor in the ipsilateral breast after segmental mastectomy.
- The concept of Halsted that cancer of the breast spreads in an orderly fashion is untenable because it may metastasize to a distant site before, during, or after it spreads to the lymph nodes. Breast cancer is often a systemic disease, even in its early stages.
- Up to 5 years of tamoxifen use reduces recurrence (50%) and mortality (36%) in women with estrogen receptor–positive tumors, irrespective of age and menopausal status and whether the lymph nodes are positive or negative, even if cytotoxic chemotherapy has been given. There

is no clear evidence of benefit in women with estrogen-poor tumors. An adverse effect is a significant increase in endometrial cancer.

- High-risk factors for recurrence in patients with node-negative breast cancer include tumor size larger than 2 cm, high histologic and nuclear grade, estrogen receptor negative, and lymphatic and vascular invasion.
- Node-negative premenopausal and postmenopausal patients who are at low risk for recurrence can be advised not to have adjuvant systemic therapy. For those women who are at intermediate risk and are estrogen receptor positive, tamoxifen for 5 years should be the first treatment. Women who are at high risk should have systemic therapy as should women who have estrogen receptor–negative tumors.
- Chemotherapy consists of CMF (cyclophosphamide, methotrexate, 5-fluorouracil) or AC (doxorubicin, cyclophosphamide). Women older than 70 years and at high risk should take only tamoxifen.
- For node-positive breast cancer patients, the Canadian Consensus states that polychemotherapy (CMF or AC) should be offered to all premenopausal women with stage II breast cancer. Postmenopausal women with stage II estrogen receptor–positive tumors should be offered tamoxifen.
- Paclitaxel (Taxol) and trastuzumab (Herceptin) are used in clinical trials and have shown promising antitumor activity.

QUESTIONS

Directions for Questions 1–33: Select the one best answer.

1. The following are true for breast cancer *except:*
   A. breast cancer is the leading cause of cancer death in women as well as the leading cause of death from all causes in women 40 to 44 years old
   B. its cause seems to be multifactorial
   C. its incidence has increased about 3% a year since 1980
   D. it is the most common neoplasm in women: one of every 11 women will develop breast cancer
2. Blood supply of and lymphatic flow from the breast are the following *except:*
   A. 60% of the breast is supplied by the internal mammary artery
   B. 30% of the breast is supplied by the lateral thoracic artery
   C. 97% of the lymph from the breast flows to the internal mammary chain, and 3% flows to the axillary nodes
   D. the lymph flow is unidirectional and centrifugal from the deep subcutaneous and intramammary lymphatic vessels toward the axillary and internal mammary lymph nodes
3. Malignant lesions of the breast most often occur in:
   A. upper outer quadrant
   B. lower outer quadrant
   C. upper inner quadrant
   D. lower inner quadrant
4. Treatment of fibrocystic disease of the breast consists of the following *except:*
   A. avoidance of dimethylxanthines and nicotine
   B. vitamins A and D
   C. vitamin E
   D. norethynodrel, danazol, tamoxifen, and bromocriptine
5. Concerning risk of developing cancer from fibrocystic disease of the breast, the following are *not* true *except:*
   A. there is a greater incidence of microscopic fibrocystic disease in cancerous breasts than in noncancerous breasts studied at autopsy
   B. epithelial hyperplasia is more common in the cancerous breast
   C. the percentage of previous biopsies in patients with cancer is higher than in patients with benign disease
   D. the degree and nature (typical or atypical) of epithelial proliferation are the most important pathologic risk factors for the subsequent development of carcinoma
6. The patient with the highest risk for breast cancer has the following pathologic characteristics and/or family history:
   A. proliferative, no atypia
   B. atypical hyperplasia
   C. atypical hyperplasia and positive family history of breast cancer
   D. cysts and family history of breast cancer
7. The most common benign tumor of the breast is:
   A. fibroadenoma
   B. intraductal papilloma
   C. ductal ectasia
   D. phyllodes tumor
8. The most common carcinoma involving fibroadenomas is:
   A. intraductal carcinoma
   B. infiltrating ductal carcinoma
   C. lobular carcinoma in situ
   D. infiltrating lobular carcinoma
9. Concerning phyllodes tumor of the breast, the following are true *except:*
   A. it is a fibroepithelial tumor
   B. the connective tissue is hypercellular and pleomorphic and has high mitotic activity
   C. its clinical course is variable and often unpredictable
   D. the preferred treatment is radical mastectomy
10. Patients with the following entities have a nipple discharge *except:*
    A. tubular adenoma
    B. ductal ectasia
    C. intraductal papilloma
    D. patients taking phenothiazines
11. Characteristics of a nipple discharge due to ductal carcinoma are:
    A. milky
    B. green, yellow, sticky
    C. clear, watery
    D. pink, serosanguineous

12. Which is the best diagnostic tool for a breast mass found during pregnancy or lactation?
    A. mammogram
    B. follow-up breast examination
    C. fine needle aspiration with cytology
    D. excisional biopsy
13. Major risk factors for breast cancer include the following *except:*
    A. age
    B. family history of breast cancer
    C. atypical hyperplasia in benign breast disease
    D. multiparity
14. Guidelines for early detection of breast cancer consist of:
    A. breast self-examination every month
    B. clinical breast examination on all patients during a periodic examination by a physician
    C. mammogram every 1 to 2 years for patients between 40 and 50 years of age and annually for women older than 50 years of age
    D. all of the above
15. The following are true concerning estrogen therapy and breast cancer *except:*
    A. there is no evidence that estrogen replacement therapy for menopausal women increases the risk of breast cancer
    B. for patients who developed breast cancer during estrogen replacement therapy, the relative survival rate was 10% higher than those who did not have estrogen
    C. there is a significantly improved survival rate in breast cancer patients who use oral contraceptives
    D. an early surgically induced menopause was found to be a risk factor for development of breast cancer
16. True statements concerning breast cancer and oral contraceptives (OC) are the following *except:*
    A. there is a small increased risk of developing breast cancer for OC users
    B. OCs protect from endometrial and ovarian cancers
    C. cancer of the breast in OC users is always in an advanced stage
    D. the evidence available at this time does not warrant any change in prescribing patterns for OCs.
17. Breast cancer nonfamilial risk factors include:
    A. woman older than 40 years
    B. proliferative fibrocystic changes with or without atypia
    C. nulliparous or late parity (first birth after age 34)
    D. all of the above
18. Pathologic evaluation of a specimen resected for ductal carcinoma in situ of the breast (DCIS) should include:
    A. nuclear grade, architectural subtype
    B. extent of the disease
    C. distance between DCIS and resection margins
    D. all of the above
19. Mammography has a false-negative rate for clinically palpable masses. It is:
    A. 5–15%
    B. 15–20%
    C. 20–25%
    D. 25–30%
20. The positive predictive value of excisional biopsies has been reported in the range of:
    A. 15–20%
    B. 10–40%
    C. 10–20%
    D. 20–30%
21. Baseline mammogram should be considered in women:
    A. age 25 to 30
    B. age 30 to 35
    C. age 35 to 40
    D. age 40 to 45
22. A 2-cm-diameter breast tumor without axillary and internal mammary nodes and no distant metastases is classified as stage:
    A. I
    B. II
    C. III
    D. IV
23. A 2-cm breast tumor with movable ipsilateral axillary nodes and no distant metastases is classified as stage:
    A. I
    B. IIa
    C. IIb
    D. IIIa
24. With the use of mammography, one can reduce mortality from breast cancer from 50% to 30%. What is its false-negative rate for clinically palpable masses?
    A. 2%–5%
    B. 5%–15%
    C. 15%–20%
    D. 20%–25%
25. The following are true concerning survival in breast cancer *except:*
    A. the 5-year survival rate for localized breast cancer has risen from 78% in the 1940s to 91% today
    B. the number of positive axillary nodes definitely affects survival
    C. staging is very important because survival is related to stage
    D. large clinical series indicate at the time of presentation a frequency of 1% to 2% of clinical stage IV disease, which has a poor survival rate
26. Survival figures are highest following which type of treatment for cancer of the breast?
    A. standard radical mastectomy
    B. modified radical mastectomy
    C. local excision and radiation
    D. no difference in survival
27. The following are true concerning estrogen receptors and breast cancer *except:*
    A. estrogen receptors are proteins found in hormonally dependent malignant and nonmalignant tissues
    B. the amount of estrogen receptors present in the cancer specimen is predictive of the success or failure of endocrine therapy
    C. patients with estrogen receptor–poor and progesterone receptor–positive tumors have no reduction in recurrence and mortality

D. not all patients with significant estrogen receptor content respond to hormone treatment

28. The following are true concerning oophorectomy *except:*
    A. women younger than 50 years with one to three axillary nodes involved by carcinoma benefit from prophylactic oophorectomy
    B. women who had cancer confined to the breast show no benefit from prophylactic oophorectomy
    C. patients 50 years of age or older benefit from oophorectomy
    D. bilateral oophorectomy appears to be the most useful treatment for a premenopausal patient with an estrogen receptor–containing tumor when the disease is metastatic or locally recurrent
29. Combination therapy yields clinical results superior to single-agent therapy in the treatment of advanced or metastatic breast cancer. Which combination gives the highest response rate?
    A. CAF (cyclophosphamide, doxorubicin, 5-fluorouracil)
    B. DAV (dibromodulcitol, doxorubicin, vincristine)
    C. CA (cyclophosphamide, doxorubicin)
    D. CMFP (cyclophosphamide, methotrexate, 5-fluorouracil, prednisone)
30. Pathologic features considered as risk for recurrence include the following, *except:*
    A. extensive intraductal component
    B. positive nodes
    C. vascular or lymphatic invasion
    D. tumor necrosis
31. The NSABP trial on treatment of clinical stage I breast cancer patients demonstrated which treatment is best?
    A. radical mastectomy
    B. total mastectomy plus irradiation
    C. total mastectomy
    D. no difference
32. Which adjuvant therapy should be recommended to high-risk, node-negative breast cancer patients younger than 70 years old?
    A. no adjuvant therapy
    B. tamoxifen
    C. raloxifene
    D. chemotherapy
33. Monitoring patients on tamoxifen therapy should include:
    A. routine endometrial sampling every 6 months
    B. endometrial sampling on patients who demonstrate uterine bleeding
    C. periodic transvaginal ultrasonography
    D. Pap smears every 6 months

Directions for Questions 34–52: For each numbered item, select the letter of the most appropriate answer. Each letter may be used once, more than once, or not at all.

34–37. Match the types of adjuvant therapy with types of patients.
    A. combination chemotherapy
    B. no adjuvant therapy
    C. tamoxifen
    D. chemohormonal therapy

34. Premenopausal women with positive nodes
35. Premenopausal patients with negative nodes
36. Postmenopausal women with positive nodes and positive hormone receptor levels.
37. Postmenopausal women with positive nodes and negative hormone receptor levels.

38–40. Match the stage of breast cancer with the appropriate treatments.
    A. Stages I and II
    B. Stages III and IV

38. Segmental mastectomy, axillary node dissection, radiation therapy
39. Total mastectomy, axillary node dissection
40. Aggressive preoperative radiotherapy, total mastectomy, systemic hormonal therapy, or chemotherapy

41–44. Match the relative location of malignant lesions of the breast.
    A. upper outer quadrant
    B. upper inner quadrant
    C. lower outer quadrant
    D. lower inner quadrant

41. 50%
42. 15%
43. 11%
44. 6%

45–46. Match levels of axillary nodes.
    A. level I
    B. level II
    C. level III
    D. level IV

45. Behind the pectoralis minor muscle
46. Medial to the medial border of the pectoralis minor muscle

47–52. Match carcinoma with the best entry below:
    A. ductal carcinoma in situ (DCIS)
    B. lobular carcinoma in situ (LCIS)
    C. both
    D. neither

47. Premenopausal patients
48. Multicentric lesions
49. Bilateral lesions
50. Recurrences in other breast
51. Invasive ductal carcinoma is usually the histology of recurrence
52. Diagnosis by microcalcifications on mammogram followed by needle localization biopsy

Answers

1. **D** page 385
   One of nine women will develop breast cancer. Causes of breast cancer are multifactorial: genetic predisposition, loss of host's immunologic defense mechanisms, viruses, hormones, and other factors. The increased incidence of 3% a year from 1980 to 1987 may be partly due to screening programs detecting subclinical disease. It has recently leveled off at a rate of 110 per 100,000 per year.

2. **C** page 387
Ninety-seven percent of the lymph from the breast flows to the axillary nodes, and 3% flows to the internal mammary chain.
3. **A** page 391
Because malignant lesions occur most often in the upper outer quadrant of the breast, examination of the breast should begin in that quadrant, palpating clockwise and returning to examine the upper outer quadrant a second time.
4. **B** page 393
Vitamins A and D have no role in the treatment of fibrocystic disease of the breast. Vitamin E induces a 40% complete response rate and a 46% partial response. The mechanism of action is unknown. Hormone manipulation can induce definitive improvement of the symptoms of fibrocystic disease.
5. **D** page 395
There is no greater incidence of microscopic fibrocystic disease in cancerous breasts (26%) than in noncancerous breasts (58%) studied at autopsy. Epithelial hyperplasia, often thought to be a precursor of malignant disease, is at least as common in the noncancerous breast (32%) as in the cancerous breast (23%). In a retrospective, case controlled study, the percentage of previous biopsies in patients who had cancer was quite low (8%) compared with the percentage of previous biopsies performed in patients who had benign diseases (14%).
6. **C** page 395
With a histology of atypical hyperplasia and a positive family history of breast cancer, the breast cancer risk factor is 11.0. Atypical hyperplasia, cysts with family history of breast cancer, and proliferative disease carry a risk factor of 4.5, 3.0, and 1.9, respectively.
7. **A** page 396
The most common benign tumor of the breast is fibroadenoma. It is initially seen as a firm, painless mass and may be very large, particularly in adolescents. Fibroadenomas are multiple and bilateral in about 14% to 25% of patients.
8. **C** page 396
Carcinoma infrequently occurs with adenofibroma. The prognosis of carcinoma limited to fibroadenoma is excellent. Treatment should follow the same principle used in the management of in situ or infiltrating carcinomas that occur in breast tissue in the absence of fibroadenomas. The most common carcinoma involving fibroadenomas is lobular carcinoma in situ.
9. **D** page 396
Phyllode tumors should be treated by a total excision with a wide margin of healthy tissue.
10. **A** page 398
Tubular adenomas in young women are well-defined, freely movable nodules that resemble fibroadenomas clinically. Intraductal papilloma manifests as a serous, serosanguineous, or watery type of nipple discharge. The discharge is usually spontaneous, from a single duct, and is commonly unilateral. Tranquilizers, particularly the phenothiazines, may cause bilateral nipple discharge. Ductal ectasia is manifested by a discharge that is usually multicolored and sticky, bilateral, and from multiple ducts.
11. **C** page 399
When a nipple discharge is clear and watery, a ductal carcinoma is a likely cause in 30% to 50% of cases.
12. **D** page 399
Excisional biopsy under local anesthesia remains the best diagnostic tool during pregnancy, although it may be difficult because of the edema and hypervascularity of the pregnant breast. Cytology from fine needle aspiration has a possibility of a false-positive diagnosis because of the hyperproliferative cellular state of the pregnant breast. It is not as accurate as in the nonpregnant woman.
13. **D** page 429
Multiparity is not a major risk for breast cancer. The younger a woman's age at menarche, the higher her risk of breast cancer. The later a woman's menopause occurs, the higher her risk of breast cancer. The age at first full-term pregnancy appears to be an important risk factor. Nulliparity and late maternal age at first pregnancy are major risks.
14. **D** page 402
These guidelines are recommended by the American Cancer Society, the National Cancer Institute, and the American College of Obstetricians and Gynecologists.
15. **D** page 400
An early surgically induced menopause before 50 years of age was found to have a protective effect on breast cancer.
16. **C** page 401
Cancer was less advanced clinically in patients receiving OCA. The potential risk must always be weighed against the known health benefits of OCAs and the prevention of unwanted pregnancy.
17. **D** page 400
Hereditary predisposition to breast cancer plays an important role in 5% of all breast cancers in the United States. Relative risk for patients with a first-degree relative with breast cancer is 1.8 (premenopausal) or 1.2 (postmenopausal). The relative risk with a second-degree relative is 1.5. Bilaterality of breast cancer increases the risk to 8.8 (premenopausal) and 4.0 (postmenopausal). To date, less than 10% of cancer patients have been identified as having a genetic link (*BRCA1* and *BRCA2*).
18. **D** page 411
Pathologic evaluation of the specimen should include the parameters for possible breast-conserving treatment. Not every patient with DCIS is an appropriate candidate for conservative therapy.
19. **A** page 405
Although mammography is the most accurate technique for the detection of early breast cancers, a false-negative rate of 5% to 15% occurs for clinically palpable masses. This speaks in favor of fine needle aspiration or open biopsy on a clinically suspicious mass, whether the mammogram is suspicious or not.
20. **B** page 406
Mammographic categories 4 and 5 require histologic study. Average biopsy yield of mammographic abnormalities is 21%.

21. **C** page 402
A baseline mammogram should be considered in women aged 35 to 40; for women with a family history of breast cancer, ACOG recommends annual screening .
22. **A** page 409, Table 14–12
Stage I (T_1 N_0 M_0) includes a tumor of 2 cm or less in greatest dimension with no regional lymph node metastasis and no evidence of distant metastasis. If the tumor is smaller than 0.5 cm, 0.5–1 cm, or 1–2 cm, it will be staged Ia, Ib, and Ic, respectively.
23. **B** page 409, Table 14–12
Stage IIa includes T_0 N_1 M_0 (no tumor, movable ipsilateral axillary nodes, no distant metastasis), T_1 N_1 M_0 (tumor smaller than 2 cm, movable ipsilateral axillary nodes, no distant metastasis), and T_2 N_0 M_0 (tumor 2–5 cm, no axillary node, no distant metastasis). Stage IIb includes tumor 2–5 cm and movable ipsilateral axillary nodes (T_2 N_1 M_0) or tumor 5 cm in diameter, no axillary node (T_3 N_0 M_0). If the 2-cm breast tumor has fixed axillary nodes and no distant metastasis, it will be classified as stage IIIa (T_1 N_2 M_0).
24. **B** page 405
Mammography is the most accurate technique for the detection of early stage breast cancers. However, a false negative rate of 5% to 15% has been reported for clinically palpable masses. DiSaia and Creasman encourage liberal use of biopsy or fine needle aspiration in suspicious masses, regardless of the result of mammograms.
25. **D** page 408
Large clinical series indicate a frequency of clinical stage IV disease of between 2% and 13% at the time of presentation. The 5-year survival rate for localized breast cancer is 91% today. If the cancer has spread regionally, the survival rate is 69%; with distant metastases, it is 18%. The 10-year disease-free survival rate is 38% for 1–3 positive nodes and 13% for more than 4 positive nodes.
26. **D** page 413
Similar survival figures are gathered for the three types of treatment. There is a gradual decline in use of the radical mastectomy (Halsted's operation) because of the cosmetic defect produced by loss of the pectoral muscles and the morbidity, which includes a 30% incidence of chronic arm edema. Simple mastectomy followed by radiation results in salvage rates equal to those of radical mastectomy. Modified radical mastectomy, which removes the entire breast (but not the pectoralis major muscle) and includes partial axillary dissection (levels I and II with sparing of the pectoralis minor muscle), gives similar survival figures as the Halsted operation. In Fisher's study, segmental mastectomy and axillary dissection with breast irradiation resulted in better disease-free survival than that after total mastectomy. All lesser procedures have similar end results, but none surpasses those obtained with radical surgery.
27. **D** page 417
There was a reduction of 23% in recurrence and 9% in mortality in patients with estrogen receptor–negative and progesterone receptor–positive tumors. However, objective regressions with endocrine therapy are obtained in no more than one third of patients.
28. **C** page 416
Patients 50 years of age or older showed no advantage from oophorectomy, according to a study by a collaborative group in 1996.
29. **A** page 418, Table 14–19
CAF gives the highest response rate of 82%; CA, DAV, and CMFP have a response rate of 74%, 71%, and 63%, respectively.
30. **B** page 414
Patients with positive nodes do not have an increased risk of breast recurrence when they are treated with conservative surgery and irradiation.
31. **D** page 415
A total of 1665 patients observed for 72 months found no difference among the three treatment arms in stage I. Handley was the first to suggest that some metastases were destroyed in the nodes by host defenses.
32. **D** page 418
Chemotherapy with six cycles of CMF or four cycles of AC should be given. However, tamoxifen should be given to patients older than 70 years because it is less toxic.
33. **B** page 417
Routine periodic endometrial biopsy and transvaginal ultrasonography are not recommended at this time because they are not cost effective.
34. **A** page 418
For premenopausal women with positive nodes, regardless of hormone receptor status, treatment with established combination chemotherapy should become the standard of care. The standard adjuvant therapy is a 6-month course of CMF (cyclophosphamide, methotrexate, and 5-fluorouracil) or a 3-month course of AC (cyclophosphamide, doxorubicin).
35. **B** page 418
For premenopausal patients with negative nodes, adjuvant therapy is not generally recommended. For certain high-risk patients in this group, adjuvant chemotherapy should be considered.
36. **C** page 419
For postmenopausal women with positive nodes and positive hormone-receptor levels, tamoxifen is the treatment of choice. At least 5 years of adjuvant tamoxifen may be considered the standard treatment. Tamoxifen can induce endometrial carcinoma, for a calculated risk ratio of 1.7 according to a case-controlled study by Adami in Sweden. Chemotherapy may be added for high-risk patients.
37. **A** page 419
For postmenopausal women with positive nodes and negative hormone receptor levels, chemotherapy is usually recommended.
There is no evidence that chemohormonal therapy improves long-term survival in postmenopausal women.
38. **A** page 415

39. **A** page 415
40. **B** page 415
Primary therapy for stages I and II cancer of the breast consists of total mastectomy or segmental mastectomy followed by radiation therapy. Both surgical therapies are accompanied by axillary dissection. Megavoltage radiation therapy to the entire breast to a dose of 4500 to 5000 cGy should be used. Overall patient survival is equivalent, comparing breast conservation treatment with total mastectomy with maximum follow-up of 17 years. The treatment of stages III and IV breast cancer is often palliative. Systemic endocrine therapy or chemotherapy is recommended. Several authors report good results with aggressive preoperative radiotherapy, reducing the frequency of local recurrences after mastectomy. Removal of tumor bulk by mastectomy is usually performed.
41. **A** Figure 14–5, page 391
42. **B** Figure 14–5, page 391
43. **C** Figure 14–5, page 391
44. **D** Figure 14–5, page 391
Seventeen percent of lesions are located in the areola.
45. **B** page 367
46. **C** page 367
For the purpose of determining pathologic anatomy and metastatic progression, the axillary lymph nodes are divided into three arbitrary levels: level I lymph nodes lie lateral to the lateral border of the pectoralis minor muscle; level II lymph nodes lie behind the pectoralis minor muscle; and level III lymph nodes are medial to the medial border of the pectoralis minor muscle.
47. **C** page 411
DCIS occurred in premenopausal and postmenopausal patients.
48. **B** page 412
LCIS is commonly multicentric and bilateral.
49. **B** page 412
Recurrences of DCIS are found near the original site. Recurrences of LCIS are anywhere in either breast.
50. **B** page 412
Histology of recurrences in DCIS is 50% invasive ductal carcinoma, 50% DCIS. Recurrences in LCIS are usually invasive ductal carcinoma, intraductal carcinoma, or lobular carcinoma and can occur in the other breast.
51. **C** page 412
See answer to Number 50 above.
52. **A** page 411
Diagnosis of DCIS is made on mammography on the basis of microcalcifications followed by needle localization biopsy. LCIS is usually invisible on mammography, and the diagnosis is found incidentally on biopsy of a benign disease.

chapter 15 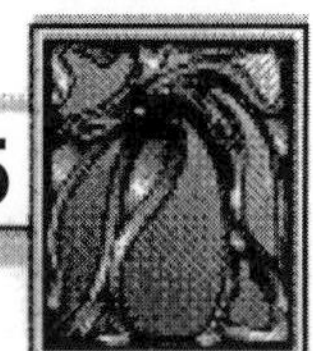

COLORECTAL and BLADDER CANCER

KEY POINTS TO REMEMBER

COLORECTAL CANCER

- Colorectal cancer (CRC) is the second leading cause of death from cancer in the United States. In 2000, 66,000 new cases of colorectal cancer were diagnosed in women, and 28,500 died from this disease. Mortality from CRC has fallen 29% for women and 7% for men over the last 30 years. Seventy percent of the incidence and 80% of deaths now involve the colon. More lesions involve the right colon.
- The majority of colorectal cancers are diagnosed in patients older than 50 years of age. Adenomatous polyps are the most common precursor lesion, estimated to occur in 93% of cases.
- Certain factors may reduce the risk of colorectal cancer: high-fiber diet, diet low in unsaturated fats, and certain micronutrients in cruciferous vegetables, calcium, and wheat bran.
- The action of bile acids appears to be related to the development of colon cancer. Patients who have undergone cholecystectomy have a higher incidence of right-sided colon cancer.
- In the sporadic type of CRC, there is an absence of family history of CRC in a first-degree relative. In the familial type, one first-degree relative has CRC. In the hereditary type, there is a family history of CRC occurring in a pattern of autosomal dominant inheritance.
- Estrogen replacement therapy decreases the risk of developing colon cancer.
- Detection of CRC at an early stage includes digital examination of the rectum, examination for occult blood in the stool, and radiographic and endoscopic procedures. Seventy percent of all CRC can be detected using fecal occult blood screening.
- Carcinoembryonic antigen (CEA) is used to monitor disease activity; its serial values can anticipate recurrence in about one third of patients by 3 to 6 months.
- Flexible fiberoptic proctosigmoidoscopy, which examines 30 cm of large bowel, should reveal nearly 65% of bowel cancers and polyps.
- Adenomatous polyps include tubular adenomas, villotubular or mixed adenomas, and villous adenomas.
- An important pathologic feature in adenomatous polyp is distinguishing between in situ carcinoma (above the muscularis mucosae) and invasive carcinoma (invasion of the submucosa).
- Two thirds of adenomas are tubular; tubular adenomas have less premalignant potential than villotubular adenomas. Five percent of patients with adenomas have high-grade dysplasia, and 2% to 3% have invasive cancer at time of presentation. Patients with an adenoma have a 40% to 50% likelihood of developing another adenoma in the future.
- Villous adenoma is the least common of neoplastic polyps but has the highest tendency toward malignant degeneration (30%). The incidence of positive nodes ranges from 16% to 39%.
- Complete polypectomy is a definitive procedure for an in situ carcinoma; polypectomy versus radical surgical resection is considered for an invasive carcinoma in a polyp depending on the degree of differentiation of the tumor and presence of lymphovascular invasion. For accurate staging of CRC, at least a dozen lymph nodes should be found in the specimen.
- The most commonly used staging classification is that of Dukes with the Astler-Coller modification, which stresses the depth of penetration as an independent variable in prognosis.
- Resection of the cancer-bearing segment of the bowel with wide excision of the lymphatic draining segment of the cancer is the only curative therapy: right colectomy or abdominoperineal resection or en bloc resection in case of extension to adjacent structures. Margin is 5 cm from the gross tumor edge.
- Five-year survival of Dukes stage A (mucosa only) is 95%; stage B (bowel wall involvement) varies from 85% to 30%; stage C (lymph node involvement) varies from 40% to 10%; and stage D (distant metastases) is 5%.
- CRC is among the most highly curable neoplasms, but almost half of the patients will relapse.
- Adjuvant chemotherapy with 5-FU and levamisole may delay recurrence without necessarily prolonging survival with Dukes stages B and C tumors.
- Preoperative radiation gives conflicting preliminary results. The incidence of local recurrence can be reduced by 50% with the use of a moderate dose of radiation, but there is no demonstrable survival benefit.
- Five-year survival in early cancer: 90% for colon cancer and 80% for rectal cancer. However, 65% of patients present with higher-staged disease, leading to an overall 5-year survival of 50%.

- Recurrences of CRC can occur locally or can metastasize to the lung or liver. Seventy-five percent of patients die from intra-abdominal causes; 25% die from lung and liver metastases. Often an elevated CEA level is the earlier sign of recurrence.
- Early detection of liver metastases and treatment with direct infusion of 5-FU into the portal system result in impressive remission.
- Thirty-five percent of patients undergoing surgery for CRC will have disease spread to regional lymph nodes, and 25% to 35% of them will survive 5 years. After surgical resection for CRC, 60% of tumor recurrences are within the first 2 years, and 90% occur within 5 years.
- Detection of recurrence at the anastomotic site by barium enema remains the most favorable pattern of recurrence in terms of secondary cure.
- Patients with localized hepatic metastasis may survive for 2 years, even without therapy. Seven percent of patients with hepatic metastases benefit from surgical resection.
- Benefits from systemic chemotherapy (5-FU, mitomycin C, nitrosoureas) are limited by low partial response rate with low duration of response.

BLADDER CANCER

- In 2000, 14,900 cancers of the bladder occurred in women (38,300 cases in men), with 4100 estimated to die. Bladder cancer is the sixth most common form of cancer in women and the seventh leading cause of cancer deaths in women.
- Hematuria with increased frequency of urination is the warning sign.
- Smoking is the greatest risk factor for bladder cancer. Workers exposed to dye, rubber, and leather are also at higher risk.
- Ninety percent of bladder tumors are transitional carcinomas and originate in the lateral and posterior bladder walls. The remainder (6% to 8%) are squamous, adenocarcinoma, or urachal carcinomas.
- Adenocarcinoma is found in the dome and trigone of the bladder.
- Urachal cancer originates from the urachus and produces CEA.
- Cystoscopy and appropriate biopsies are mandatory for diagnosis.
- Metastases involve the hypogastric, obturator nodes, and aortic chain; lung, liver, and bone are distant metastases.
- Staging is more precise with the American Joint Commission system than with the Jewett-Strong-Marshall system used in the United States (stage 0: superficial tumor; A: invasion into lamina propria; B1 and B2: tumor confined to less than or more than half of the bladder muscle; C: invasion of perivesical fat; D1: invasion of the prostate, uterus, vagina, and pelvic walls; D2: regional lymph nodes above the sacrum).
- Superficial tumors represent about 70% of new cases.
- Therapy for superficial lesions (stages 0, A) is endoscopic resection and fulguration, with cystoscopy repeated every 3 months.
- If the lesion recurs or is diffuse, intravesical instillation of thiotepa or BCG (not licensed in the United States) is performed.
- Radical cystectomy used for diffuse or recurrent superficial lesions results in a 5-year survival rate of 70% to 90%.
- Radical cystectomy with resection of local pelvic nodes is used for stages B and C with an overall 5-year survival of 30% to 50%. Preoperative and postoperative radiation therapy suggest little benefit in preventing tumor dissemination.
- Supervoltage irradiation, when surgery is contraindicated, can produce a 5-year survival rate of 20% to 30%.
- Active chemotherapeutic agents are cisplatin and methotrexate.
- Lymph node involvement (stage D2) is a poor prognostic sign, with 50% of patients who undergo surgery dying in less than 1 year and 87% in less than 2 years.
- Follow-up of patients consists of a chest film at 2- to 3-month intervals, urine cytology, and intravenous pyelogram at 6- to 12-month intervals, with baseline abdominal and pelvic CT scans at 2 months following radical cystectomy.

QUESTIONS

Directions for Questions 1–36: Select the one best answer.

1. What was the number of new cases of colorectal cancer in women and the number of deaths in the United States in 2000?
   A. 100,000/50,000
   B. 150,000/75,000
   C. 66,000/28,000
   D. 200,000/100,000
2. True statements concerning colorectal cancer in the United States are the following *except:*
   A. colorectal cancer is the second leading cause of death from cancer in the United States
   B. the majority of colorectal cancers are diagnosed after 50 years of age
   C. adenomatous polyps are the most common precursor lesion
   D. 75% of colon cancer cases occur in women
3. Choose the true statement concerning the epidemiology of colorectal cancer:
   A. high-fiber diets may decrease disease incidence
   B. diets low in unsaturated fats may be associated with a reduction in the incidence of disease
   C. certain micronutrients in cruciferous vegetables may reduce the risk of colon cancer
   D. all of the above
4. Patients with high risk for colorectal neoplasms include:
   A. patients with a personal history of breast cancer, endometrial cancer, or Crohn's disease
   B. patients who have previously had adenomas
   C. patients with a family history of colorectal polyposis or colorectal cancer
   D. all of the above

5. Common clinical manifestations of colorectal cancer are the following *except:*
   A. bleeding and anemia
   B. pain
   C. diarrhea
   D. obstructive symptoms
6. Guidelines for screening of colorectal cancer include:
   A. colorectal examination should be a part of the periodic health examination
   B. fecal occult blood testing is recommended annually at age 50 and sigmoidoscopy is recommended every 3 to 5 years
   C. special surveillance is recommended on high-risk patients
   D. all of the above
7. Advantages of the 35-cm flexible fiberoptic proctosigmoidoscope are the following *except:*
   A. it is ideally suited for office use
   B. it can detect nearly 65% of bowel cancers and polyps
   C. the cost is low and training is minimal
   D. average examination time is 30 minutes
8. Evidence that links benign polyps to an increased risk of colonic malignancy includes the following choices *except:*
   A. the risk of colonic malignancy is higher in populations with diets that are low in unsaturated fats and high in fiber
   B. benign adenomatous tissue is usually seen adjacent to a frank malignancy
   C. removal of benign lesions in large populations reduces cancer incidence
   D. the risk of malignancy is high in individuals affected by familial colonic polyposis
9. The classification of adenomatous polyps includes the following *except:*
   A. villotubular adenomas
   B. macular adenomas
   C. villous adenomas
   D. tubular adenomas
10. The microscopic tissue level beyond which malignant cells constitute an invasive malignancy is:
    A. mucosal basement membrane
    B. muscularis
    C. muscularis mucosae
    D. submucosa
11. The recommended therapy of in situ carcinoma in a polyp is:
    A. segmental resection
    B. hemicolectomy
    C. partial polypectomy
    D. complete polypectomy
12. Choose the true statement regarding villous adenoma:
    A. villous adenoma is the least common of neoplastic polyps
    B. villous adenoma has the lowest potential toward malignant degeneration
    C. cancer associated with villous adenoma has a lower risk of lymph node metastasis
    D. cancer associated with villous adenoma may be treated successfully with traditional nonradical surgery
13. The Dukes staging system relies primarily on two factors to judge the extent of a tumor. They are:
    A. depth of tumor penetration, distant metastasis
    B. depth of tumor penetration, lymph node involvement
    C. distant metastasis, lymph node involvement
    D. distant metastasis, tumor grade
14. The 5-year survival of a patient with colorectal cancer Dukes B is approximately
    A. 95%
    B. 85%
    C. 20%
    D. 15%
15. Using the Dukes classification of colon carcinoma staging, a tumor that is contained within the wall of the bowel and with mesenteric lymph node metastases would be Dukes stage:
    A. A
    B. B1
    C. C1
    D. D
16. A tumor with bowel wall involvement, negative lymph nodes, and extension to adjacent structures would be classified as what with the modified Dukes classification system?
    A. B2
    B. B3
    C. C2
    D. D
17. Using the TNM staging system for colon carcinoma, the lesion in Question 16 would be:
    A. Stage I
    B. Stage II
    C. Stage III
    D. Stage IV
18. True statements regarding surgical therapy of colon carcinoma include all *except:*
    A. surgery is the only curative primary therapy
    B. a right colectomy is standard practice for lesions in areas supplied by the superior mesenteric artery
    C. an anal-sparing procedure may be performed for rectosigmoid or high rectal cancers
    D. a surgical margin of 2 to 3 cm in the bowel wall itself is desired
19. The adenomatous polyp that has the highest incidence of malignant degeneration is:
    A. tubular adenoma
    B. villous adenoma
    C. villotubular adenoma
    D. mixed adenoma
20. What percentage of all patients with colorectal cancer can be detected using fecal occult blood screening?
    A. 30%
    B. 50%
    C. 70%
    D. 90%
21. The following are uses of the CEA test in colorectal carcinoma *except:*
    A. it is a screening and diagnostic test
    B. it is used for monitoring recurrences

C. serial values should be measured every 2 months in the first 2 years after definitive surgery and every 4 months for an additional 2 years
D. it can anticipate recurrences in one third of patients by 3 to 6 months

22. Adjuvant therapy for colorectal cancer uses the following agents *except:*
A. 5-FU or 5-FU plus methyl-CCNU
B. levamisole plus 5-FU
C. preoperative radiation
D. cisplatin

23. What percentage of patients with colorectal cancers will have a relapse?
A. 10%
B. 25%
C. 30%
D. 50%

24. The goal of preoperative radiation therapy in colorectal cancer is:
A. to decrease dissemination of cancer at surgery
B. to downstage the primary tumor
C. A and B
D. to decrease bleeding during surgery

25. Adjuvant chemotherapy in colorectal cancer uses which agent?
A. 5-FU plus methyl-CCNU
B. methotrexate
C. Adriamycin
D. cyclophosphamide

26. The most common area of recurrence in colorectal cancer is:
A. bone
B. lung
C. abdomen
D. liver

27. The tumor marker useful for monitoring recurrence of colorectal cancer is:
A. alpha-fetoprotein
B. CEA
C. CA-125
D. hCG

28. After surgical resection for colorectal carcinoma, what percentage of recurrences occurs within the first 2 years?
A. 25%
B. 30%
C. 50%
D. 60%

29. For postoperative follow-up in colorectal carcinoma, during the first year after resection of primary tumor it is recommended to perform the following *except:*
A. physical examination (and stool guaiac testing) every 3 months
B. liver function tests and CEA every 3 months
C. chest roentgenogram every 6 months
D. colonoscopy every year

30. The following statements regarding survival after therapy of recurrence of colorectal cancer are true *except:*
A. surgery for local or regional recurrences may result in secondary cure in selected patients
B. seven percent of patients who have hepatic metastases will benefit from surgical resection
C. infusion therapy with 5-FU or floxuridine in unresectable hepatic metastases has a high response rate
D. systemic chemotherapy used in widely disseminated disease results in prolongation of survival

31. The histology of most bladder cancer is:
A. transitional cell carcinoma
B. adenocarcinoma
C. squamous carcinoma
D. sarcoma

32. Which type of carcinoma often arises in lateral and posterior bladder walls?
A. transitional and squamous
B. urachal
C. adenocarcinoma
D. sarcoma

33. Metastases from bladder cancer involve the:
A. obturator and hypogastric nodes
B. para-aortic nodes
C. lung, liver, and bone
D. all of the above

34. A tumor of the bladder that does not invade beyond the lamina propria is classified, according to the Jewett-Strong-Marshall staging system, as:
A. A
B. B1
C. B2
D. C

35. Treatment of diffuse or recurrent superficial carcinoma of the bladder is:
A. endoscopic resection and fulguration
B. intravesical thiotepa
C. radical cystectomy
D. radiotherapy

36. Most active simple agents for chemotherapy of bladder cancer are:
A. cisplatin and methotrexate
B. doxorubicin
C. vinblastine
D. mitomycin C

ANSWERS

1. **C** page 423
Colorectal cancer is the Western world's most common internal malignancy and one of its leading causes of cancer deaths. In 2000, approximately 66,000 new cases of colorectal cancer were diagnosed in women in the United States alone, and approximately 28,000 people died of the disease.

2. **D** page 423
In the United States slightly more than 50% of colon cancers occur in women and slightly under 45% of rectal cancers are seen in women. The proportion involving the rectum and the colon has changed. About 70% of the incidence and 80% of deaths now involve the colon. More lesions now involve the right colon. The distribution of lesions is as follows: cecum 13%, right colon 9%, transverse colon 13%, left colon 7%, sigmoid colon 24%, rectosigmoid junction 9%, and rectum 23%.

3. **D** page 424
High-fiber diets result in high-bulk stools and rapid transit time. Theoretically, individuals with slow stool transit and low-bulk stools may be prone to higher concentrations of carcinogens adjacent to the bowel wall. The exact mechanism by which fats affect colon carcinogenesis is not clearly understood. Some micronutrients (carotenoids, terpene, and others) in vegetables may directly inhibit carcinogen formation or function by binding of carcinogens within the intestine; others may exert a more general systemic effect. The action of bile acids appears to be related to the development of colon cancer. Patients who have undergone cholecystectomy have a higher incidence of right-sided colon cancer.
4. **D** page 424
All listed groups are at high risk for colorectal neoplasms. Ulcerative colitis predisposes to malignancy but is not considered asymptomatic. Screening is not useful in patients with familial polyposis or Gardner's syndrome (Table 15–1).
5. **C** page 426
Bleeding, anemia, pain, and obstructive symptoms are the common clinical symptoms of colorectal cancer. These manifestations are most common with advanced lesions. Diarrhea is common in patients with ulcerative colitis and Crohn's disease.
6. **D** page 426
These guidelines are from the American Cancer Society, the American College of Obstetricians and Gynecologists, and the National Cancer Institute. The physician should identify high-risk patients for special surveillance, including those with a strong family history of colon cancer or with personal history of polyps, colon cancer, or inflammatory disease.
7. **D** page 427
Besides the advantages enumerated above, the average examination time is around 5 minutes and the mean insertion depth is 29 cm. The flexible 60-cm colonoscope is more expensive and requires more extensive training; the examination time requires more than 30 minutes. The rigid proctosigmoidoscope that examines the terminal 25 cm of large bowel is technically the easiest for physicians to master and is associated with a finding of unsuspected cancer in 1 of every 435 persons.
8. **A** page 427
Although the risk of colonic malignancy is lower in populations with low–unsaturated fat and high-fiber diets, diet is not linked to the presence or absence of benign colonic polyps in these populations. The remaining statements are true.
9. **B** page 427
The current classification of adenomas includes tubular adenomas, villous adenomas, and mixed (villotubular) adenomas.
10. **C** page 427
Since lymphatics are located in the submucosa, if carcinomatous foci are confined above the muscularis mucosae, the lesion is considered in situ. If it traverses the muscularis mucosae, it is considered invasive.
11. **D** page 427
Complete polypectomy is the least morbid definitive treatment for in situ carcinoma in an adenomatous polyp. It may be accomplished by proctoscope or colonoscope, or by a transperitoneal (laparotomy) approach.
12. **A** page 427
Coutsofides et al. demonstrated that malignant potential of villous adenomas was increased, as was the incidence of nodal metastasis, when invasive carcinoma was associated with villous adenomas. Most surgeons advocate radical resection of malignancy associated with villous adenoma. The therapy for malignancy associated with tubular adenoma is more individualized. It is more likely to include factors such as degree of differentiation, lymphatic or blood vessel invasion, and depth of invasion.
13. **B** page 428
The Dukes classification system uses depth of tissue penetration and degree of lymph node involvement to determine stage. The Astler-Coller modification stresses the depth of penetration as an independent variable in prognosis (Table 15–5).
14. **B** page 430
Dukes stage B denotes invasion of the bowel wall by carcinoma. If the involvement is within the intestinal wall (stage B1, according to the Astler-Coller modification), the 5-year survival is 85%; if it is grossly through the wall (stage B2), the 5-year survival drops to 50%.
15. **C** page 430
If a tumor is confined to the bowel wall but has positive lymph nodes, it is classified as Dukes C1, using the Astler-Coller modification (Table 15–5).
16. **B** page 430
A tumor with direct extension to local tissues is subclassified as B3. If regional nodes are negative, it is classified as B. If positive, it is classified as C (Table 15–5).
17. **B** page 428
This lesion is a T_4 N_0 M_0 lesion and thus is stage II. Stage II also includes T_3 N_0 M_0 lesions.
18. **D** page 430
The bowel wall margin classically desired is 5 cm from the gross tumor edge for most patients. This is most important in surgery for rectal carcinoma. A 2- to 3-cm margin may be adequate in selected patients.
19. **B** page 427
Villous adenoma is the least common of neoplastic polyps but has the highest tendency toward malignant degeneration. In a collected series reviewed by Coutsofides, the overall incidence of invasive malignancy was 30% and the incidence of positive lymph nodes ranged from 16% to 30%.
20. **C** page 426
Seventy percent of all colorectal cancers can be detected using fecal occult blood screening. However, 30% of patients do not bleed and are not detected in this manner.
21. **A** page 426
CEA is not considered as a screening or a diagnostic test for colon cancer. The other choices are true.

22. **D** page 431
Cisplatin is not used as adjuvant therapy in colorectal cancer. All those therapies have decreased the incidence of local recurrences without improving the overall survival.
23. **D** page 431
Although colorectal cancers are among the most highly curable neoplasms, almost half of the patients have a relapse.
24. **C** page 431
The goal of preoperative radiation therapy is to decrease the dissemination of cancer at surgery and to downstage the primary tumor. Postoperative radiation is used for patients at high risk for local recurrence (e.g., transmural invasion, known metastasis).
25. **A** page 431
Adjuvant chemotherapy used 5-FU or 5-FU plus methyl-CCNU. Several studies of large numbers of patients with Dukes stages B and C suggest that adjuvant therapy may delay recurrence without necessarily prolonging survival in all treated patients. Investigators have attempted to improve the therapeutic index of 5-FU by incorporating biochemical modulators such as levamisole and streptozotocin. Response rates vary from 12% to 34%.
26. **C** page 432
Autopsy studies confirm that abdominal failure is common, and almost 75% of patients die from intra-abdominal causes. Lung and liver metastases account for less than 25% of all deaths. Patients who have disease limited to a single or a few unilobular hepatic metastases may survive 18 to 24 months in many series. Treatment by direct infusion of 5-FU into the portal system or by hepatic resection has brought about impressive remissions.
27. **B** page 432
An elevated CEA is often the earliest sign of recurrence.
28. **D** page 431
After surgical resection for colorectal carcinoma, approximately 60% of recurrences are within the first 2 years, and 90% occur within 5 years.
29. **D** page 432
Colonoscopy and chest roentgenogram should be done every 6 months during the first and second year after resection of the primary tumor.
30. **D** page 433
Response rates with infusional therapy for unresectable liver metastases are high: 80%, with median survival of 26 months. Prolongation of survival with systemic chemotherapy remains an elusive goal in the treatment of recurrence of colorectal cancer.
31. **A** page 433
More than 90% of bladder cancers are transitional cell. In 1995, there were 13,200 cases of bladder cancer in women in the United States.
32. **A** page 433
Transitional and squamous cancers arise from the lateral and posterior bladder walls. Adenocarcinoma is found in the dome and the trigone of the bladder.
33. **D** page 434
Lymph nodes in the pelvis, with lung, liver, and bone, are the site of metastases of bladder cancer.
34. **A** page 434
A papillary noninvasive tumor or a carcinoma in situ is classified as stage 0. Invasion into the lamina propria is stage A (or T_1).
35. **C** page 434
Radical cystectomy for diffuse or recurrent superficial lesions of the bladder can result in a 5-year survival rate of 70% to 90%. Intravesical thiotepa has been used by certain clinicians. Endoscopic resection and fulguration with cystoscopy are used as therapy for superficial lesions (stages 0 and A).
36. **A** page 435
Cisplatin and methotrexate are the most active single agents for carcinoma of the bladder, which responds in 15% to 30% of cases.

chapter 16 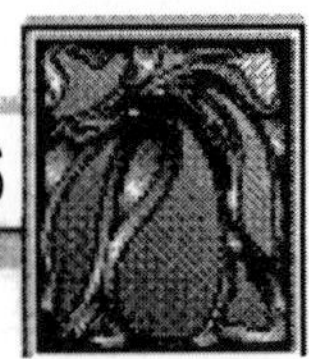

CANCER in PREGNANCY

KEY POINTS TO REMEMBER

- The most common invasive malignancy occurring in pregnancy is breast cancer, followed by gynecologic malignancies, colon cancer, and thyroid cancer.
- Despite theoretical considerations concerning the physiologic changes of pregnancy and dissemination of malignancies, there are no significant clinical data that substantiate an adverse effect of pregnancy on any malignancy.
- Vulvar cancer during pregnancy is rare (1 in 8,000–20,000 deliveries). Vulvar intraepithelial neoplasia is treated during the postpartum period. Invasive malignant disease in the first and second trimesters is treated as indicated in the nonpregnant patients. In the third trimester, many recommend wide local excision with definitive treatment postponed until the postpartum period. Some patients became pregnant after surgery and had normal deliveries.
- Primary clear cell adenocarcinoma of the vagina and cervix and primary squamous cell carcinoma of vagina during pregnancy are exceptionally uncommon.
- The evaluation of an abnormal Pap smear during pregnancy by colposcopy and directed biopsy is similar to the evaluation in a nonpregnant patient. ECC is not performed.
- In a pregnancy complicated by cervical cancer, there is no difference in fetal or maternal survival if delivery is vaginal or by cesarean section.
- A patient with microinvasive carcinoma of the cervix, diagnosed by rigid criteria on cone biopsy, may continue a pregnancy safely to term.
- Treatment decisions for pregnant patients with invasive cervical cancer should consider stage of disease and duration of pregnancy.
- For stage I and IIa lesions, patients in the first and early second trimesters can be treated with surgery or irradiation. Patients whose pregnancy is at least 20 weeks or more may have treatment delayed until fetal viability is reached. There is no appreciative difference in the 5-year survival rates of pregnant versus nonpregnant patients.
- Endometrial cancer in pregnancy is very rare, and, when it does occur, is focal and well differentiated.
- Fallopian tube cancer is extremely rare. Incidental findings of carcinoma in situ of the tube in postpartum tubal ligation are treated with total abdominal hysterectomy and bilateral salpingo-oophorectomy (TAH-BSO).
- During pregnancy a complex pelvic mass increasing in size is an indication for exploratory laparotomy on or about the 18th week of pregnancy.
- The most common ovarian neoplasms removed during pregnancy are dermoids and benign serous cystadenomas. Two adnexal conditions specifically associated with pregnancy are the luteoma and theca lutein cysts.
- Ten to fifteen percent of ovarian tumors occurring in pregnancy undergo torsion.
- Ovarian cancer in pregnancy is rare (1 in 2000 deliveries). Combination chemotherapy during pregnancy has been given without deleterious effects on the fetus. Unilateral adnexectomy and continuation of pregnancy are advised in dysgerminomas stage Ia. At laparotomy, completed surgical staging is required for tumors apparently confined to one ovary.
- Cancer of the bladder has been reported in pregnancy. Superficial and well-differentiated tumors can be managed by local fulguration, whereas others required partial or total cystectomy for cure.
- Colorectal cancer in pregnancy is managed the same way in the pregnant and the nonpregnant state.
- Cytotoxic chemotherapy administered in the first trimester of pregnancy may be associated with a significant number of fetal anomalies, especially in patients receiving antimetabolites, antifolics, or alkylators. Surprisingly few fetal anomalies are associated with exposure to chemotherapy during the second and third trimesters.
- The most critical period of embryonic development extends from the 3rd to the 8th week of development (5th to 10th week of gestational age), when susceptibility to teratogenic agents is maximal. In the human fetus, the period of organogenesis usually ends by the 13th week of gestation.
- All cancer chemotherapeutic agents should be considered teratogenic and should be avoided in the first trimester of pregnancy. When cytotoxic drugs are used in late pregnancy, the nadir should be timed to avoid the interval when delivery is expected (fetal effects).
- Women undergoing chemotherapy often experience amenorrhea and the menopausal syndrome, especially with alkylating agents. Return of menses and ovulation is the function of age. Chemotherapy also affects testicular function. The recovery of the germinal epithelium of the testes is a function of dose and may be delayed as long as 4 years.
- There is no threshold below which maternal irradiation received during pregnancy is not associated with gene mutations. Radiation doses in excess of 200 cGy during the first 20 weeks of gestation will result in congenital malformations.
- Maternal irradiation above the diaphragm with shielding to the fetus still delivers 1% to 7% of the total dose to the fetus. For the fetus, the most sensitive period is days 18 through 38. If possible, delay the initial treatment until the middle of the second trimester.

- Surgical staging of pregnant patients with Hodgkin's disease after the 18th week is feasible and important. Proper aggressive radiotherapy and chemotherapy for advanced Hodgkin's disease requires termination of pregnancy. In the second and third trimesters, or with advanced disease, the patient can be managed with chemotherapy (MOPP) until delivery.
- Hodgkin's disease does not appear to affect the outcome of pregnancy, and pregnancy does not affect the course of Hodgkin's disease. Three of four patients diagnosed with Hodgkin's disease will be cured.
- Non-Hodgkin's lymphoma adversely affects the pregnancy because patients usually have an aggressive histology and an advanced stage on presentation. Burkitt's lymphoma is usually rapidly progressive and may involve the breast and the ovary.
- In acute leukemia, premature labor is common, and postpartum hemorrhage occurs in 10% to 15% of cases. Current chemotherapy results in a 70% remission rate, but only 10% to 20% survive 5 years.
- There was no significant difference stage-for-stage in the outcome of pregnant and nonpregnant patients with melanoma. New staging system for melanoma by AJCC: Ia, localized melanoma smaller than 0.75 mm (or level II); Ib, localized melanoma larger than 0.76 to 1.5 mm (or level III); IIa, localized melanoma 1.5 to 4 mm (level IV); IIb, localized melanoma larger than 4 mm (level V); III, limited nodal metastases (one regional lymph node basin); IV, advanced regional metastases or distant metastases.
- Half of all reported malignancies metastasizing to the placenta and 90% of those metastasizing to the fetus are melanomas.
- Melanomas 1 mm in depth should be treated by wide excision with 1-cm margin; lesions larger than 1-mm thickness, excision with 2-cm margins; in advanced disease, the administration of interferon alfa–2b improved survival compared with surgery only.
- Pathologic evaluation of the sentinel node was predictive of regional lymph node metastasis in 96% to 98% of cases.
- Patients of reproductive age who have melanoma should refrain from pregnancy for 2 to 3 years.
- Patients with melanoma in pregnancy appear to have a shorter disease-free survival.
- Patients with breast cancer diagnosed early in pregnancy and with negative nodes do as well as nonpregnant patients (70% to 80% survival).
- Breast cancer diagnosed during pregnancy tends to be more advanced in stage and has a greater likelihood of nodal metastases than that in the nonpregnant patient.
- Interruption of pregnancy seems to have no effect on the survival rate of patients with breast cancer.
- Radical mastectomy is well tolerated during pregnancy. Lumpectomy or partial mastectomy is more commonly used. Local irradiation should be deferred until after delivery.
- Breast cancer in pregnant patients has the same prognosis as that in nonpregnant patients, considering similar age and stage of disease. Pregnancy after mastectomy has no influence on the disease, and future pregnancies may be protective.
- Breast feeding, in the contralateral breast, after treatment of breast cancer is traditionally discouraged to avoid vascular congestion of the breast, which may also contain a neoplasm.
- Pregnancy has no effect on the clinical behavior of bone sarcomas. Pregnancy termination is not indicated.
- Solitary thyroid nodules in pregnancy should be studied by needle aspiration.
- The most common thyroid malignancy occurring in pregnancy is papillary adenocarcinoma, which behaves in the least aggressive manner. Thyroid suppression is continued for most patients until delivery. Surgical management is indicated only if the tumor enlarges rapidly.
- Malignant melanoma is the most common tumor to spread to the fetus or placenta, followed by breast cancer. This complication is rare.

QUESTIONS

Directions for Questions 1–50: Select the one best answer.

1. What proportion of female genital tract cancer occurs in women aged 15 to 44?
   A. 35%
   B. 15%
   C. 18%
   D. 25%
2. What is the estimated incidence of invasive cancer of the cervix per 1000 pregnancies?
   A. 1
   B. 2
   C. 3
   D. 4
3. The following are true concerning cancer of the vulva in pregnancy *except:*
   A. therapy for vulvar intraepithelial neoplasia can be delayed until the postpartum period
   B. invasive cancer during the first and second trimester can be treated by radical vulvectomy with bilateral inguinal dissection
   C. invasive cancer diagnosed during the third trimester can be treated by a wide local excision, with definitive surgery postponed until the postpartum period
   D. pregnancy appears to decrease the survival of patients with carcinoma of the vulva
4. Choose the true statement(s) concerning cancer of the vagina during pregnancy:
   A. the diagnosis is exceptionally uncommon, and the prognosis appears to be unaffected by the pregnancy
   B. radical surgery appears to be appropriate only for early lesions involving the upper vagina and/or cervix
   C. when there is extensive involvement of the vagina by any primary lesion, evacuation of the uterus should be done and radiation therapy given
   D. all of the above

5. A 12-week-pregnant patient has a Pap smear suggestive of CIN III. Colposcopy visualizes the complete transformation zone and one small area of mosaicism. No atypical vessels are seen. Management consists of performing:
   A. a small biopsy of the area of mosaicism
   B. a shallow cone biopsy
   C. a repeat Pap smear
   D. a hysterectomy with pregnancy in situ
6. A 30-week pregnant patient has a Pap smear suggestive of CIN III. Colposcopic biopsy of one area of atypical vessels suggests early invasive disease. What is the next step of management?
   A. cesarean section and total hysterectomy
   B. cesarean section and radical hysterectomy
   C. repeat biopsy under colposcopy
   D. conization
7. The authors' histologic criteria of "microinvasive squamous cancer of the cervix" for conservative treatment are the following *except:*
   A. the invasive cancer does not penetrate more than 3 mm below the basement membrane of the surface epithelium
   B. there is no vascular or lymphatic invasion
   C. there are no confluent tongues of tumor
   D. margins of specimen are not free of cancer
8. Recommendations for treatment of invasive cancer of the cervix in pregnancy include the following:
   A. up to 24 weeks' gestation, patients with stages Ib–IIa could be treated by radical surgery or radiation therapy; patients with stages IIb–IIIb could be treated with irradiation
   B. with pregnancies longer than 24 weeks' gestation, patients with stages Ib–IIa should have a cesarean section at fetal viability, followed by radical hysterectomy or irradiation
   C. patients with pregnancies longer than 24 weeks' gestation in stages IIb–IIIb should have a cesarean section at fetal viability, followed by whole pelvis irradiation
   D. all of the above
9. The total 5-year survival rate of patients with pregnancy and invasive carcinoma of the cervix independent of stages of cancer and gestation is around:
   A. 40%
   B. 50%
   C. 60%
   D. 70%
10. Choose the true statement(s) concerning endometrial carcinoma in conjunction with pregnancy:
    A. it is extremely rare
    B. it is usually focal, well-differentiated, and minimally invasive
    C. the recommended primary therapy is total abdominal hysterectomy with bilateral salpingo-oophorectomy (TAH-BSO)
    D. all of the above
11. The following are true concerning fallopian tube cancer and pregnancy *except:*
    A. the possibility of fallopian tube cancer in pregnancy is extremely remote
    B. the neoplasm is usually bilateral and most often adenocarcinoma
    C. the treatment is TAH-BSO and postoperative radiation therapy or chemotherapy, depending on operative findings and residual disease after surgery
    D. carcinoma in situ of the tube can be treated by salpingectomy
12. The incidence of ovarian cancer in pregnancy is:
    A. from 1:10,000 to 1:25,000 pregnancies
    B. from 1:10,000 to 1:50,000 pregnancies
    C. from 1:5000 to 1:10,000 pregnancies
    D. from 1:5000 to 1:8000 pregnancies
13. At which gestation week should a patient undergo exploration for an ovarian cyst?
    A. 12th week
    B. 16th week
    C. 18th week
    D. 20th week
14. Of all ovarian neoplasms found in pregnancy, what proportion are carcinoma?
    A. 1%
    B. 5%
    C. 8%
    D. 10%
15. What is the most frequent ovarian neoplasm seen in pregnancy?
    A. serous cystadenoma
    B. paraovarian cyst
    C. benign cystic teratoma
    D. mucinous cystadenoma
16. Torsion of ovarian neoplasms is common in pregnancy. When does it occur?
    A. first trimester
    B. second trimester
    C. puerperium
    D. A and C
17. Philosophy for treating ovarian cancer in pregnancy consists of the following:
    A. it is necessary to properly stage the patient
    B. the management should be similar to that in the nonpregnant patient
    C. initiation of adjuvant chemotherapy should be done
    D. all of the above
18. The following statements regarding colon cancer during pregnancy are true *except:*
    A. management of the tumor is identical to that in the nonpregnant state
    B. the diagnosis is usually prompt
    C. the distribution of tumors is identical to that in the nonpregnant state
    D. the prognosis is identical to that in the nonpregnant state
19. Choose the *false* statement regarding the surgical management of colon carcinoma during pregnancy:
    A. hysterectomy may be routinely necessary if colon carcinoma is treated in the first trimester
    B. surgical management in the first trimester is identical to that in the nonpregnant state
    C. in the presence of a viable third-trimester fetus, a cesarean section and concomitant tumor resection are recommended

D. vaginal delivery followed by definitive resection several days later is allowable if the colonic lesion is above the pelvic brim

20. Choose the *true* statement relevant to the occurrence of bladder carcinoma during pregnancy:
   A. sarcoma is the usual histologic type
   B. metastasis to bone is uncommon
   C. bladder cancer is not significantly affected by pregnancy
   D. the primary tumor usually begins in the bladder apex
21. True statements relative to the use of chemotherapy agents in pregnancy include all *except:*
   A. methotrexate usually causes abortion or fetal malformations when given in the first trimester
   B. most chemotherapy drugs do not cause permanent fetal harm when given in the second or third trimester
   C. fetal pancytopenia may occur if chemotherapy agents are administered in the third trimester
   D. the time when the fetus is most susceptible to damage is the first 2 weeks after conception
22. The following are true concerning the administration of chemotherapy during pregnancy *except:*
   A. in the first trimester it is associated with morphologic abnormalities and fetal loss
   B. in the second and third trimesters it is associated with preterm delivery, fetal death in utero, and intrauterine growth retardation
   C. the effects of new drugs such as cytokines and paclitaxel are unknown
   D. for drugs used in late pregnancy, the nadir should be timed to coincide with delivery
23. Choose the *false* statement regarding chemotherapy agents and pregnancy, lactation, and fertility:
   A. cisplatin administration is a contraindication to breast feeding
   B. drugs used for gestational trophoblastic neoplasia do not increase fetal wastage or congenital anomalies in future pregnancies
   C. an increased rate of first trimester pregnancy loss is noted in women with occupational exposure to chemotherapy drugs
   D. alkylating agents reduce fertility by producing amenorrhea and oligomenorrhea
24. True statements regarding chemotherapy drugs and future fertility include all *except:*
   A. effects of chemotherapy on fertility are age- and dose-dependent
   B. prepubertal females are particularly likely to develop menstrual irregularity after alkylating agent therapy
   C. the offspring of mothers previously treated with cytotoxic drugs have no evident increase in genetic damage
   D. ovarian fibrosis is commonly seen after alkylating agent use
25. The most common abnormality attributed to irradiation of the human embryo is:
   A. CNS disorders
   B. infertility
   C. microcephaly
   D. increased risk of lymphoma and leukemia
26. If therapeutic irradiation is necessary for a pregnant patient and therapeutic abortion is refused, until when should the initiation of treatment be delayed?
   A. end of first trimester
   B. mid second trimester
   C. end of second trimester
   D. end of third trimester
27. Regarding radiation exposure, the most sensitive period of fetal development is:
   A. preimplantation
   B. days 18 to 38
   C. days 40 to 60
   D. third trimester
28. What is the radiation exposure dose that is associated with developmental abnormalities in the fetus?
   A. 5 cGy
   B. 10 cGy
   C. 15 cGy
   D. still controversial
29. True statements relative to radiation and pregnancy include all *except:*
   A. diagnostic radiographic procedures should be delayed until after second trimester and radiotherapy delayed until after delivery
   B. a chest radiograph results in exposure of the fetus to 300 mcGy
   C. a barium enema results in exposure of the fetus to 6 cGy
   D. the threshold for increased postnatal risk of tumor development in the fetus is 10 cGy
30. The following statements are true regarding Hodgkin's disease in the pregnant patient *except:*
   A. pregnancy does not adversely affect the course of the disease or survival
   B. One in 6000 pregnancies is affected
   C. nonsurgical staging is preferred over surgical staging in the pregnant patient
   D. future pregnancy in those receiving radiation plus chemotherapy is compromised
31. Young pregnant women are often affected by which subtype of Hodgkin's disease?
   A. lymphocyte predominance
   B. mixed cellularity
   C. lymphocyte depletion
   D. nodular sclerosis
32. Prognosis of Hodgkin's disease is improved in the patient who (choose the *false* statement):
   A. is younger than 40 years of age
   B. is female
   C. has substage E disease
   D. has irradiation of clinically normal lymph node groups
33. Some authors suggest that when the diagnosis of Hodgkin's disease is made before 20 weeks' gestation, therapeutic abortion should be considered as an option in the following situations *except:*
   A. infradiaphragmatic disease
   B. nodular sclerosis histology

C. visceral involvement
D. rapid progression and bulky disease in mediastinum

34. Choose the correct stage for the following patient. A pregnant 21-year-old patient at 20 weeks' gestation is found to have Hodgkin's lymphoma confined to both supraclavicular lymph node groups. All other lymph node groups are normal. Staging laparotomy reveals that all retroperitoneal lymph nodes are negative, as is the spleen.
A. I
B. II
C. III
D. IV

35. Proper therapy for Hodgkin's lymphoma includes all *except:*
A. irradiation alone is used for early stage disease
B. VAC (vincristine, dactinomycin, and cyclophosphamide) chemotherapy alone is used for advanced disease with parenchymal organ involvement
C. chemotherapy *and* radiotherapy are used for bulky disease or generalized nodal involvement
D. therapy for the pregnant patient must be individualized

36. The following statements in regard to reproduction in Hodgkin's lymphoma patients are true *except:*
A. with irradiation alone, future pregnancy outcome seems to be compromised
B. oophoropexy should be strongly considered at the time of a staging laparotomy
C. irradiation and chemotherapy together affect future reproduction to the highest degree
D. menstrual function is far less likely to be affected when therapy occurs at a younger age

37. The following are false concerning non-Hodgkin's lymphoma in pregnancy *except:*
A. it is more common than Hodgkin's lymphoma
B. it adversely affects the pregnancy
C. Burkitt's lymphoma has a good survival rate for patients treated with chemotherapy
D. lymphoma of the breast carries a good prognosis

38. Obstetric hazards noted in the pregnancies of mothers with active leukemia include all *except:*
A. premature labor
B. increase in fetal wastage and congenital anomalies
C. infection
D. postpartum hemorrhage

39. True statements relative to the therapy for leukemia in pregnancy include all *except:*
A. the asymptomatic patient with chronic myelocytic leukemia should have her pregnancy terminated
B. antimetabolite drugs should not be administered to the pregnant patient
C. pregnancy exerts no specific effect on lymphoma
D. pregnancy provides an obstacle to early therapy

40. Concerning melanoma in pregnancy, the following are true *except:*
A. spread to regional nodes appears to be more rapid in pregnant patients
B. stage for stage, there is no significant difference in the outcome for the pregnant patient
C. there is no difference in survival for women who became pregnant within 5 years of diagnosis of melanoma
D. compared with other malignancies, there is no metastasis of melanoma to products of conception

41. Which stage is a localized melanoma between 1.5 mm to 4 mm in depth?
A. Ia
B. Ib
C. IIa
D. IIb

42. According to Clark's classification, a melanoma that invades through the basement membrane to the papillary dermis is at level:
A. I
B. II
C. III
D. IV

43. Treatment of malignant melanoma in pregnancy consists of the following *except:*
A. lesions smaller than 1 mm in depth require a wide excision with a 1-cm margin
B. lesions larger than 1 mm in depth require a wide excision with a 2-cm margin
C. regional lymph node dissection should be done
D. patients in the reproductive age should refrain from pregnancy for 2–3 years

44. Concerning breast cancer in pregnancy, the following are true *except:*
A. the incidence is approximately 1 in 3000 deliveries
B. pregnant patients tend to have a higher percentage of positive nodes and an advanced stage at presentation of the disease
C. the chance of survival is the same for pregnant and nonpregnant patients if it is an early lesion
D. inflammatory carcinoma of the breast is more common in pregnancy

45. According to Haagensen, any one of the five following grave signs constitutes stage C breast cancer *except:*
A. skin edema or ulceration
B. solid fixation to chest wall
C. massive axillary nodes
D. satellite skin nodules or involved supraclavicular nodes

46. Concerning treatment of breast cancer in pregnancy, the following are true *except:*
A. the overall survival rate was 32.9% at 5 years and 19.5% at 10 years
B. physicians must treat pregnant breast cancer patients with aggressive curative intent because pregnancy does not confer a worse prognosis
C. therapeutic abortion for the treatment of localized breast cancer in the first trimester of pregnancy increases survival
D. in advanced cancer of the breast, therapeutic abortion is usually necessary to achieve palliation

47. The following are true concerning breast cancer in pregnancy *except:*
A. prophylactic surgical castration in early stage breast cancer in pregnancy has no benefit

B. there is no justification for termination of pregnancy in treated breast cancer patients without evidence of recurrence
C. most surgeons recommend artificial feeding of the infant
D. chemotherapy should not be used after the first trimester, even in very advanced disease

48. Choose the *incorrect* statement concerning bone tumors in pregnancy:
A. frequent primary tumors are Ewing's sarcoma, osteogenic sarcoma, and osteocytoma
B. they are treated by surgical excision
C. they are strong indications for termination of pregnancy
D. most recurrences occur within the first 3 years after initial diagnosis

49. The following are true concerning thyroid cancer in pregnancy *except:*
A. the most common lesion is the papillary adenocarcinoma
B. the best diagnostic tool is fine-needle aspiration with cytologic evaluation
C. thyroid suppression may be instituted in papillary adenocarcinoma during pregnancy
D. thyroid suppression is the preferred therapy for medullary thyroid carcinoma during pregnancy

50. Which is the most common malignancy metastatic to the fetus or placenta?
A. malignant melanoma
B. breast cancer
C. lymphosarcoma
D. leukemia

ANSWERS

1. **C** page 440
According to Allen and Nisker, the percentage of all genital cancers occurring in young women from 15 to 44 years old is 18%, with cancer of the cervix and cancer of the ovary representing 35% and 15%, respectively (Table 16–1).
2. **A** page 440
The estimated incidence of invasive cancer of the cervix is 1 per 1000 pregnancies; it is 1.3 for preinvasive lesions of the cervix and 0.1 for cancer of the ovary (Table 16–2).
3. **D** page 440
The pregnant state does not appear to significantly alter the course of the malignant process; survival of these patients stage for stage is similar to that of nonpregnant patients. Definitive therapy for patients diagnosed with invasive malignancies during the third trimester of pregnancy should be started within 1 week after delivery during the same hospitalization.
4. **D** page 441
Vaginal cancer during pregnancy is rare: 24 cases of clear cell adenocarcinoma of vagina have been reported by Senekjian and 12 cases by Collins and Baruah. Sarcoma botryoides of the cervix and vagina in pregnancy are recorded.
5. **A** page 442
A small biopsy could be done on the vascular pregnant cervix to confirm a histologic diagnosis. Most experienced colposcopists prefer to observe the patient each trimester with Pap smears and colposcopy and defer the entire work-up to 6 to 8 weeks after delivery, unless there is suggestion of invasive disease.
6. **D** page 442
Conization should be done to rule out invasive disease. The surgical procedure is a formidable undertaking and might be envisioned as excising a "coin" of tissue rather than a cone of tissue. Alternatively a "wedge" rather than cone, or "coin" biopsy, may be performed. If the pathology report shows microinvasion, as defined by the Society of Gynecologic Oncologists, the pregnancy may continue safely to term. In deciding on therapy for invasive cervical cancer in pregnancy, the physician must consider the stage of disease, the duration of pregnancy, and the desire of the mother.
7. **D** page 443
The margins of the cone specimen should be free of disease. DiSaia and Creasman believe that a lesion fulfilling these criteria should be treated by conization. Recommendation for postpartum hysterectomy is not essential in patients who have early stromal invasion and desire further childbearing.
8. **D** pages 449–451
Stages Ib and IIa can be treated with surgery or radiation. DiSaia and Creasman prefer a radical hysterectomy with bilateral pelvic lymphadenectomy because of the overall result, including ovarian preservation, improved sexual function, and elimination of unnecessary delays for the patient. Radiation therapy is equally efficacious in treating patients with early stage cervical cancer in pregnancy and is the treatment of choice in more advanced stages. In the first and second trimesters when the pregnancy is to be disregarded, treatment should begin with whole pelvis irradiation. Spontaneous abortion usually occurs at about 35 days in the first trimester and at 45 days in the second trimester following onset of radiotherapy (Fig. 16–5).
9. **C** page 445
The 5-year-survival rate of cervical cancer in pregnancy is 65.5% in a report by Allen and Nisker.
10. **D** page 446
The recommended primary therapy is TAH-BSO and adjuvant radiotherapy when indicated.
11. **B** page 446
The mean age of women who have fallopian tube cancer is between 50 and 55 years. Thus, the possibility of its presence in pregnancy is extremely remote. The neoplasm is usually unilateral.
12. **A** page 446
Ovarian cancer is reported to occur in from 1 in 10,000 to 25,000 pregnancies. In a survey by Kohler, about 1 in 600 pregnancies will be complicated by an adnexal mass.
13. **C** page 446
Patients operated on about the 18th week of gestation have negligible fetal wastage associated with the

exploration. Also, more than 90% of functional cysts disappear by the 14th week of gestation.

14. **B** page 447
Carcinoma of the ovary is relatively rare. The incidence is 2% to 5% of all ovarian neoplasms found in pregnancy. In nonpregnant patients about 20% of ovarian tumors are malignant, but in pregnancy this percentage drops to 5%. The size of the neoplasm is not a reliable criterion of malignancy.

15. **C** page 447
In a histological review of 69 ovarian tumors operated on during pregnancy, Struyk found dermoid cyst in 36%, serous cystadenoma in 25%, paraovarian cyst in 13%, mucinous cystadenoma in 12%, and malignancies in 4% (Table 16–4).

16. **D** page 447
The incidence of torsion of ovarian tumors in pregnancy is approximately 10% to 15%. Most torsions occur when the uterus is enlarging at a rapid rate (8 to 16 weeks) or when the uterus is involuting (in the puerperium). About 60% of the cases occur at the beginning of the pregnancy and 40% in the puerperium.

17. **D** page 448
The probability of ovarian cancer must be kept foremost in the minds of physicians caring for pregnant patients with ovarian neoplasms. Pregnancy does not appear to adversely affect the prognosis for the patient who has an ovarian malignancy.
The management of ovarian cancer in pregnancy should be similar to that in the nonpregnant patient. Malignant epithelial tumors (serous and mucinous carcinomas) should be treated appropriately for the stage of disease. Malignant germ cell neoplasms should be treated with a unilateral salpingo-oophorectomy, since they are usually stage Ia. Adjuvant chemotherapy should be given (except possibly in the case of dysgerminoma) in the postoperative period because these tumors (endodermal sinus tumors, embryonal carcinoma, immature teratoma) grow rapidly and delays can be harmful. No data concerning chemotherapy in early pregnancy are available, but all chemotherapeutic agents are theoretically teratogenic.
DiSaia and Creasman adopt conservatism for the treatment of stage Ia dysgerminomas and allow patients to continue their pregnancies because radiation and chemotherapy are successful in curing 75% of those patients with metastases or recurrences. Malignant tumors of stromal cell origin (granulosa and Sertoli-Leydig tumors) should be managed conservatively as in the young nonpregnant patient.

18. **B** page 450
The diagnosis of colon carcinoma in the pregnant patient is usually delayed for several reasons. These reasons include low level of suspicion because of young patient age or the pregnant state, procrastination in ordering appropriate diagnostic tests, and incorrectly attributing anorectal bleeding to hemorrhoids.

19. **A** page 450
During the first trimester, the size of the uterus is such that it offers little interference in the usual surgical therapies of colon carcinoma. However, as the uterus enlarges to 12- to 20-week size, experts such as Barber and Brunschwig recommend routine hysterectomy to increase surgical exposure.

20. **C** page 450
Bladder carcinoma in pregnancy is very similar to that in the nonpregnant state: it usually begins in the trigone, epithelial types predominate, bony metastases (especially to vertebrae) are common, and the usual primary treatment is surgical ablation or resection.

21. **D** page 451
The blastocyst (first 2 weeks of development) is significantly resistant to teratogenicity. Teratogenicity usually occurs when exposures to agents occur during the organogenesis stage of development (the 3rd through 8th week of life). Up to 20% of fetuses exposed during this time may exhibit fetal malformations (Table 16–7). Conversely, 80% or more do not.

22. **D** page 453
When cytotoxic drugs are used in late pregnancy, the nadir should be timed to avoid the interval when delivery is expected. Neonates should also be assessed for transient bone marrow depression; long-term neurologic and developmental follow-up is recommended.

23. **A** page 453
An investigation by Egan suggests that cisplatin is undetectable in breast milk. Doxorubicin, however, *is* detectable in breast milk, at times in concentrations exceeding that of maternal plasma. However, it is prudent to advise mothers on these antineoplastic drugs to refrain from breast feeding their children.

24. **B** page 453
Prepubertal females almost uniformly show normal menstrual development after chemotherapy; since preovulatory follicles are the most sensitive to these agents, it is the woman of menstrual age most likely to be affected by oligomenorrhea or amenorrhea. The risk of amenorrhea is proportional to the dose given and the age of the patient.

25. **C** page 454
Microcephaly is the condition most commonly attributed to irradiation of the embryo.

26. **B** page 455
Delay of initiation of treatment until at least the middle of the second trimester is recommended. Irradiation of even supradiaphragmatic structures during pregnancy will deliver fetal doses ranging from 1.2% to 7.1% of the total treatment dose. This dose to the fetus is related to interval scatter of radiation after it enters the supradiaphragmatic tissues. For the fetus, the most sensitive period is days 18 through 38. After day 40, primary organ systems have developed, and much larger doses of x-rays or gamma rays are necessary to produce serious abnormalities.

27. **B** page 455
Days 18 to 38, the phase of organ system formation, is the time at which the fetus is most susceptible to irradiation damage, which may occur with as little as **4 cGy**. Microcephaly, anencephaly, eye damage, spina bifida, growth retardation, and foot damage are

reported. During the preimplantation phase, an all-or-nothing phenomenon exists: either a blastocyst is destroyed or it is unaffected. Very high doses (250 cGy) are necessary to produce damage after organ system formation is complete.

28. **D** page 454
The exposure dose associated with developmental abnormalities in the fetus is still controversial. There is no threshold for genetic damage. A dosage of 1 cGy of radiation produces five mutations in every 1 million genes exposed. Fortunately, most mutants are recessive.

29. **D** page 455
Doses as low as 3 cGy result in increased risk of benign and malignant tumors after birth. A standard maternal chest radiograph results in 300 mcGy per plate and a maternal barium enema a 6-cGy fetal exposure. The exposure dose that is associated with developmental abnormalities is controversial. Low-dose exposure (< 100 cGy) seems acceptable only in the third trimester.

30. **C** page 457
Surgical staging in pregnancy avoids the necessity of using diagnostic techniques such as lymphangiography, intravenous pyelography, and bone and liver scans. It is feasible to perform surgical staging, including splenectomy, after the 16th week of pregnancy. The authors imply that the use of nonsurgical staging is significantly compromised without pregnancy termination.

 Although guidelines for continuing or terminating pregnancy must be individualized, most oncologists recommend terminating first-trimester pregnancies in the newly diagnosed patient and then initiating therapy. In the third trimester the pregnancy should be terminated at the time of fetal viability to reduce fetal exposure to radiotherapy and chemotherapy. Upper mantle radiotherapy, with appropriate fetal shielding, and even nonantimetabolite chemotherapy may begin before delivery of the third-trimester pregnancy.

31. **D** page 456
The nodular sclerosis subtype of Hodgkin's disease is the most common subtype encountered in pregnancy and carries a favorable prognosis.

32. **C** page 456
Substage E denotes extranodal extension of tumor. The differences in response to treatment between the non-E and E substages is most apparent in stage III disease. The younger patient and the female patient have better prognoses. Treatment (chemotherapy or irradiation) of clinically normal lymph node groups is desirable.

33. **B** page 457
Nodular sclerosis is a subtype of Hodgkin's disease with a favorable prognosis.

34. **B** page 456
The Ann Arbor classification of lymphoma states that stage I is disease in a single lymph node, stage II is disease in two or more lymph nodes on the same side of the diaphragm, stage III is disease on both sides of the diaphragm, and stage IV is disseminated extranodal involvement. Substage E includes patients with extranodal disease, and substage S signifies involvement of the spleen. This patient has stage II disease.

35. **B** page 457
MOPP (nitrogen mustard, vincristine, procarbazine, and prednisone) chemotherapy is a preferred chemotherapy for Hodgkin's lymphoma. It is added after extended-field radiotherapy in patients with extranodal parenchymal organ involvement. It is also used alone in patients with advanced disease and extensive parenchymal organ involvement.

36. **A** page 458
Future pregnancy outcome seems to be unaffected by irradiation alone and is most affected by radiation combined with chemotherapy. However, menstrual function *is* affected—least by chemotherapy, more by irradiation, and most by both.

37. **B** page 458
Non-Hodgkin's lymphoma, less common than Hodgkin's disease in pregnancy, adversely affects the pregnancy because of its aggressive histology and its advanced stage at presentation.

38. **B** page 458
Infants born of mothers having leukemia are as well as normal controls. There is no significant increase in fetal wastage and anomalies. Premature labor is common; the average period of gestation is 8 months or less. Postpartum hemorrhage, possibly associated with reduced levels of fibrinogen, occurs in 10% to 15% of cases. Infection is often the initial clinical symptom or sign in the patient with undiagnosed leukemia.

39. **A** page 459
The mother with chronic myelocytic leukemia is less likely to be harmed by deferring therapy than the (usually symptomatic) mother with acute leukemia. Conversely, Catanzarite demonstrated that the pregnancy outcome in patients treated for leukemia during pregnancy is similar to that of the untreated pregnant patient.

40. **D** page 459
Many studies demonstrate no statistically significant difference in survival between normal and pregnant patients with melanoma, stage for stage. A study by Reintgen from Duke University indicated no difference in survival for women who became pregnant within 5 years of diagnosis. Many authorities recommend avoiding pregnancy for approximately 3 years after complete surgical excision because this is the period of highest risk of relapse. Patients surviving disease-free for 5 years have a 95% chance of long-term cure.

 The incidence of metastasis of malignancies to the products of conception is low because of the unexplained resistance of the placenta to invasion by maternal cancer. Although melanoma accounts for only a small number of all cancers associated with pregnancy, almost half of all tumors metastasizing to the placenta and nearly 90% metastasizing to the fetus are melanomas.

41. **C** page 460
The new AJCC staging system for nongenital melanoma (Table 16–9) uses tumor thickness, localization, and regional metastasis as staging criteria. Stage Ia includes localized melanomas 0.75-mm thick, which are usually not associated with spread. Stage Ib includes localized melanomas between 0.76 and 1.5 mm in thickness. They are associated with 25% incidence of regional node involvement and an 8% incidence of distant metastasis. Stage IIa includes localized melanomas between 1.5 and 4 mm in thickness, having a 57% incidence of regional node involvement and a 15% incidence of distant metastasis. Stage IIb includes localized melanomas larger than 4 mm in thickness that have a high incidence of distant metastasis.

42. **B** page 460
According to Clark's classification, there are five levels of cutaneous invasion by melanoma:
Level I refers to melanoma located above the basement membrane. These lesions should be viewed as in situ lesions requiring no lymph node dissection.
Level II refers to melanoma invading through the basement membrane down to the papillary dermis. This level indicates superficial dermal penetration, with lymph node metastases seen in 1% to 5% of patients not justifying an elective lymph node dissection.
Level III refers to melanoma filling the papillary dermis at its interface with the reticular dermis.
Level IV shows melanoma penetration into reticular dermis.
Level V shows melanoma in the subcutaneous tissue.
Melanomas at the last three levels metastasize to lymph nodes in 40% to 70% of patients, necessitating lymphadenectomy after pathologic evaluation of the sentinel node. This patient has a Clark's level II melanoma.

43. **C** page 460
The value of a regional lymph node dissection is controversial and probably does not improve survival, but most authors recommend it be done with larger lesions. Reproductive-age women with melanoma should refrain from pregnancy for 2–3 years because most recurrences will occur during this period.

44. **D** page 461
Breast cancer is rare in women younger than the age of 35 and is a rare complication of pregnancy. The advanced stage at presentation of the disease in pregnancy is due to the engorgement of the breast, which can obscure the lesion, and to the increased vascularity and lymphatic drainage that assist the metastatic process to regional lymph nodes. If a lesion is detected early (present < 3 months, < 2 cm, nonanaplastic, no positive nodes) the chance of survival is the same for the pregnant and the nonpregnant patient, approximately 70% to 80%. The incidence of inflammatory carcinoma of the breast is equal before and after menopause, as well as in the pregnant and nonpregnant state.

45. **D** page 461
The Haagensen clinical staging for breast cancer is most useful in pointing out unfavorable prognostic indicators. Stage A represents no skin edema, ulceration, or solid fixation to the chest wall, axillary nodes clinically negative. Stage B is the same as stage A but with clinically palpable nodes less than 2.5 cm in diameter. Stage C includes any one of the five grave signs enumerated from A to C. Satellite skin nodules, involved supraclavicular nodes, edema of the arm, inflammatory carcinoma, and distant metastases constitute stage D.

46. **C** page 462
Therapeutic abortion is not currently believed to be an essential component of effective treatment of early disease, despite the theoretical advantage of removing the source of massive estrogen production. Reports by Peters and Rosemond and by Billroth show that termination of pregnancy has no effect on patient survival.

Although some recommend pregnancy termination to achieve palliation in the patient with extensive disease, since there have been no reports of metastasis to the fetus, a delay or termination until fetal viability may be chosen for selected patients.

47. **D** page 464
For very advanced disease, chemotherapy has been used after the first trimester. Chemotherapy should be administered when the patient is reluctant to have the pregnancy terminated and the disease appears to be progressing at an alarming rate. Peters, Cooper, and others have shown that survival is *increased* by a subsequent pregnancy, including pregnancies in the first 2 years after development of the neoplasm.

48. **C** page 465
Pregnancy does not affect the growth of bone malignancy, nor does the tumor affect the pregnancy, so strong indications for terminating the pregnancy are not present. Primary therapy for these lesions is surgical resection, disregarding the presence of the fetus. Postsurgical radiation therapy and chemotherapy are often necessary, but they are delayed until after delivery.

49. **D** page 466
Well-differentiated papillary adenocarcinoma of the thyroid behaves in the least aggressive manner (95% survival). If the lesion is medullary carcinoma of the thyroid, aggressive surgical treatment is indicated. If gestation is in the third trimester, surgery should be delayed a few weeks to ensure the viability of the fetus. Surgery results in a 50% survival at 5 years. In a poorly differentiated carcinoma of the thyroid, the main concern is to keep the mother alive until delivery, since these tumors are almost uniformly lethal lesions: 90% to 95% of patients are dead within 1 year of diagnosis.

50. **A** page 467
Metastatic lesions to the fetus and placenta are rare: fewer than 50 cases have been reported. Malignant melanoma was by far the most common tumor metastatic to the placenta and fetus.

chapter 17 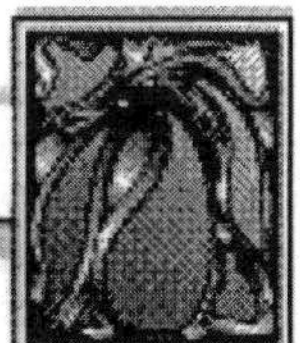

COMPLICATIONS of DISEASE and THERAPY

KEY POINTS TO REMEMBER

- Hemorrhage from large tumors can be stopped with sclerosing agents (Monsel solution) or large packs soaked in acetone. More aggressive management consists of hypogastric embolization or hypogastric ligation.
- Ureteral obstruction, most often caused by lateral parametrial extension of carcinoma of the cervix, can be relieved by percutaneous nephrostomy. The advisability of diversion must be individualized.
- Genitourinary fistulae, which sometimes can be multiple and complex, should be treated only after knowledge of the exact abnormalities. In most instances, diversion procedures should be considered.
- Gastrointestinal obstruction, most commonly seen in patients with ovarian cancer, is first managed conservatively (NPO, IV hydration, nasogastric suction) and then, if the first method is not successful, with bypass surgery. Survival of many of these patients is brief (median survival, 149 days). Percutaneous gastrostomy is used in patients with upper tract obstruction from malignancy. Octreotide (0.1 to 0.2 mg tid) may decrease the nausea and vomiting in inoperable patients.
- Gastrointestinal fistulae, most often encountered in radiation-treated patients with cervical and vaginal cancers, should be treated with a primary colostomy for diversion before a second repair procedure. Colostomy is also recommended in patients with fistulae and vulvar cancer.
- Thromboembolic disease is one of the leading causes of significant morbidity and mortality after pelvic surgery for malignancy. Forty percent of patients with deep venous thrombosis (DVT) who do not have pulmonary symptoms have diagnostic evidence of a pulmonary embolus (PE). Conversely, patients with PE have an 80% documented evidence of DVT (longer half-life in plasma treatment as outpatient with subcutaneous injections without laboratory monitoring).
- Low-dose heparin prophylaxis does not appear to be of benefit in preventing thromboembolic (TE) complications in the gynecologic oncology patient. External pneumatic calf compression appears to decrease TE complications.
- A high index of suspicion and constant monitoring with impedance plethysmography or ^{125}I fibrinogen scanning appear to be the best means of early diagnosis and treatment.
- Anticoagulation should be started immediately if DVT or PE is diagnosed. There is an increased interest in the use of low-molecular-weight heparin for the treatment of DVT.
- Superior vena cava syndrome due to metastatic gynecologic cancer is treated with radiation.
- Jaundice is due to direct involvement of liver parenchyma by tumor or to obstruction of the common bile duct, which can be relieved by stenting the duct endoscopically.
- Venous oozing during surgery can be stopped with the use of Avitene when packing has not succeeded. Large-vessel injuries need to be closed by arterial suture.
- Intraoperative ureteral injuries (1.3%) can be avoided by identification of the ureter and immediate surgical correction. Both ureterovaginal and vesicovaginal fistulae manifest within a week to 10 days after surgery. Genitourinary injuries are similar whether radical or simple hysterectomy is done. Repair surgery is contraindicated in the presence of chronic infection or calculi. Combined use of radical surgery and radiation therapy increases the rate of genitourinary complications.
- Bladder dysfunction after radical surgery is due to disruption of sympathetic fibers that travel through the paracervical web. Suprapubic continuous drainage for 1 week followed by attempts at voiding and training of spontaneous voiding "by the clock" for several weeks should be performed to correct the dysfunction. The most important determinant for poor bladder function after radical hysterectomy is the extent of parametrial and ureterovesical ligament dissections.
- Mechanical bowel preparation should be done on all patients undergoing abdominal surgery. Antibiotic bowel preparation is necessary in case of bowel surgery.
- The use of somatostatin in conjunction with total parenteral nutrition has been successful in the spontaneous closure of enteric fistulae, both large and small bowel.
- Large bowel fistula should be repaired using three-stage procedure: diverting colostomy, repair of rectovaginal fistula, and closure of colostomy.
- Diarrhea due to *Clostridium difficile* infection is treated with vancomycin and fluids and electrolyte replacement. Metronidazole is also effective.
- Lymphocysts are decreasing in incidence when the pelvic peritoneum is left open after lymph node sampling. They are treated expectantly in most instances, rarely with surgical drainage.
- Prophylactic antibiotics in gynecologic cancer patients have decreased the febrile morbidity.

- Wide excision should be done in life-threatening necrotizing fasciitis, which is due to polymicrobial infection. Fluid and electrolyte replacement with broad-spectrum antibiotics should be started before surgery.
- Management of septic shock includes adequate oxygenation, fluid replacement, cardiac output monitoring, and administration of broad-spectrum antibiotics. The infected tissue should be removed.
- Empiric antibiotic coverage is given to neutropenic patients when they become febrile. The most common combination is that of an aminoglycoside with an antipseudomonal beta-lactam. The neutrophil count should be 500 cells/mL before the antibiotics are stopped.
- Alkylating agents and epipodophyllotoxins (etoposide and teniposide) have been related to the development of subsequent leukemias. Acute myeloid leukemia occurring after use of epipodophyllotoxins has a relatively short latency period (mean 35 months) and a good response to chemotherapy (60% CR). The contrary exists for AML occurring with alkylating agents. A new report in 1999 by Travis concluded that women who are treated for ovarian cancer with platinum-based chemotherapy have a two- to eight-times greater chance for development of leukemia.
- Hypercalcemia is treated with hydration and biphosphonates (pamidronate).
- Chemotherapy-produced nausea and vomiting can be controlled with granisetron (Kytril) and dexamethasone given before chemotherapy.
- Older patients (older than 65 years) can withstand radical surgery as well as younger patients. Complications from radiation therapy are increased.
- The greatest use for invasive monitoring in gynecologic oncology is to determine the cause of hypotension and low urinary output, particularly during the postoperative period.
- Radiation complications are related to the dose, field size, and type of equipment used.
- Radiation proctitis and enteritis (diarrhea, tenesmus) resolve within 1 week after therapy is completed.
- The most common offending agent in proctitis is vaginal radium.
- One half of small bowel injuries occurred within 1 year after radiation and three fourths occurred within 2 years. Any anastomosis for bypass or resection should be done with nonradiated bowel. Anemia resulting from significant small bowel irradiation can be treated with vitamin B_{12}.
- Radiation-induced rectovaginal fistulae occurred at a median of 13 months post-treatment and rectal strictures at 24 months. All patients with rectovaginal fistulae should have diverting colostomy performed with subsequent fistula repair postponed for several months.
- Acute radiation cystitis with hemorrhage is controlled with continuous bladder irrigation using 0.5% or 1% acetic acid or 1/1000 potassium permanganate solution.
- Vesicovaginal fistulae are more frequent in patients treated with radiation and surgery (4.1%) than in those treated with radiation only (1.4%).
- Serious morbidity of pelvic irradiation is less than 5% if the external irradiation is less than 5000 cGy (10% to 20% if more than 5000 cGy).

QUESTIONS

Directions for Questions 1–31: Select the one best answer.

1. Management of bleeding in a female with cancer of the lower genital tract after failure of conservative management includes the following *except:*
   A. ligation of the posterior branch of the hypogastric artery
   B. vasopressin infusion
   C. transcatheter embolization techniques
   D. balloon catheter technique
2. The most frequent complication of percutaneous nephrostomy in the cancer patient is:
   A. hemorrhage
   B. obstruction of catheter
   C. urinary infection
   D. expulsion of catheter
3. The most effective management of gastrointestinal obstruction by a malignant pelvic neoplasm is:
   A. conservative management
   B. bowel resection
   C. bypass surgery
   D. adhesiolysis
4. The most significant preoperative risk factor associated with thromboembolic complications is:
   A. weight in excess of 190 lb
   B. advanced age
   C. advanced clinical stage of malignancy
   D. radiation therapy within 6 weeks of operative procedure
5. The best means of early diagnosis and treatment of thromboembolic disease is:
   A. a high index of suspicion
   B. constant monitoring with impedance plethysmography
   C. ^{125}I fibrinogen scanning
   D. a combination of the above
6. Which of the following is true concerning the prevention of thromboembolic disease in the gynecologic oncology patient?
   A. use of low-dose heparin
   B. use of antiembolism stockings
   C. use of external pneumatic compression
   D. nothing
7. Successful treatment of superior vena cava syndrome caused by metastatic gynecologic cancer is offered by:
   A. ligation of the superior vena cava
   B. drainage of the superior vena cava
   C. drainage of pleural and pericardial effusions
   D. radiation to the mediastinum
8. If the ureter cannot be located on the medial leaf of the broad ligament, one should search for:
   A. the round ligament
   B. the origin of the external and internal iliac arteries
   C. the hypogastric artery
   D. the external iliac artery
9. Best treatment for an operative ureteral fistula within 5 cm of the bladder is:
   A. percutaneous nephrostomy
   B. reimplantation into the bladder (ureteroneocystostomy)

C. ureteroureteral anastomosis (ureteroureterostomy)
D. ureteroileoneocystostomy

10. Incidence of genitourinary fistulae after radical hysterectomy is:
A. 1%–2%
B. 2%–3%
C. 3%–4%
D. 4%–5%

11. Ureterovaginal and vesicovaginal fistulae manifest how many days after surgery?
A. 3–5 days
B. 7–10 days
C. 12–15 days
D. 20–30 days

12. Reduction in genitourinary fistulae after radical surgery has been credited to the following changes in surgical procedure *except:*
A. suspension of the ureter to the obliterate hypogastric and encasing the ureter in peritoneum
B. prolonged bladder drainage
C. suction drainage to the retroperitoneal space
D. peritonealization of the retroperitoneal space

13. Bladder dysfunction after radical surgery is due to:
A. postoperative edema and hematoma
B. urethral drainage of the bladder
C. suprapubic drainage of the bladder
D. radicality of the surgery

14. In the patient with postoperative large rectovaginal fistula, the following procedure is recommended:
A. three-stage procedure
B. expectant management—the fistula will heal spontaneously
C. vaginal repair of the fistula
D. abdominal repair of the fistula

15. The following are true concerning lymphocysts *except:*
A. they occur anteriorly in the pelvis and are more easily appreciated on abdominal examination
B. they often become infected
C. surgical drainage is imperative when lymphocysts are large
D. preventive measures include ligating multiple lymphatic branches during a lymphadenectomy and leaving the pelvic peritoneum open

16. In case of neutropenia with fever, DiSaia and Creasman recommend the use of which antibiotics for empiric coverage?
A. aminoglycosides only
B. aminoglycoside with an antipseudomonal beta-lactam
C. monotherapy with third-generation cephalosporins
D. vancomycin with aminoglycoside and an antipseudomonal penicillin

17. The following statements are true concerning infection in the neutropenic cancer patient *except:*
A. if the neutrophil count is less than 100 cells/mL, almost one fourth of the febrile episodes will have an associated bacteremia
B. primary sites for infection are the alimentary tract and the skin
C. it is necessary to perform multiple site cultures, including blood cultures
D. *Staphylococcus aureus* and coagulase-negative staphylococci are the most frequent causes of catheter-induced infection

18. There is correlation between deep venous thrombosis (DVT) and pulmonary embolism (PE), which clinically represent two separate entities. In patients with DVT who are pulmonary asymptomatic, how many will have diagnostic evidence of a PE?
A. 10%
B. 20%
C. 30%
D. 40%

19. Concerning the older cancer patient, the following are *not* true *except:*
A. older patients cannot withstand radical surgery
B. postoperative small bowel obstruction, bladder dysfunction, and pulmonary emboli are less frequent in the individual 65 years of age or older
C. complications from radiation therapy are more frequent
D. fistula rate after radiation therapy reaches 50%

20. Normal pressure values in the wedged pulmonary artery are:
A. 4–12 mm Hg
B. 0–8 mm Hg
C. 15–25 mm Hg
D. 4–25 mm Hg

21. Causes of hypotension and low urinary output in the postoperative period of cancer patients may be due to:
A. hypovolemia
B. congestive heart failure or myocardial infarction
C. sepsis
D. all of the above

22. Radiation complications are related to:
A. the dose
B. field size
C. type of equipment used
D. all of the above

23. The majority of small bowel injuries occur how many years after irradiation?
A. 1–2 years
B. 2–3 years
C. 3–4 years
D. 4–5 years

24. Initial treatment for postradiation rectovaginal fistula is:
A. vaginal closure of fistula
B. abdominal closure of fistula
C. diverting colostomy
D. low-residue diet

25. The following are true concerning radiation complications *except:*
A. radiation proctitis manifests many months to years after treatment
B. acute radiation cystitis is occasionally encountered during or in the immediate post-therapy period
C. fistulae of GU and GI tracts usually occur in extensive disease of the cervix and upper vagina
D. there is no difference in the rate of vesicovaginal fistulae if surgery is added to radiation

26. Appropriate management of the rectovaginal fistula in pelvic malignancy is:
    A. primary repair
    B. diverting colostomy
    C. low resection and anastomosis
    D. low-residue diet
27. After radical hysterectomy, suprapubic catheter for continuous drainage is maintained for 1 week. Then attempted voiding is begun. Two weeks after the operation, how many patients have residual urine?
    A. 50%
    B. 60%
    C. 70%
    D. 80%
28. Patients who have an enterovaginal fistula can be cured successfully with:
    A. repeat laparotomy and suture of the fistula
    B. total parenteral nutrition (TPN) and somatostatin
    C. gastrointestinal tubing
    D. continuous suction and cleaning of the fistula
29. The hallmark of therapy of necrotizing fasciitis is:
    A. extensive surgical débridement
    B. fluid and electrolyte replacement
    C. broad-spectrum antibiotic therapy
    D. oxygen therapy
30. Which is the drug of choice to be used in septic shock for improving cardiac function:
    A. isoproterenol
    B. ephedrine
    C. digitoxin
    D. dopamine
31. Chemotherapeutic agents that may be related to the development of acute myeloid leukemia are:
    A. alkylating agents
    B. methotrexate
    C. epipodophyllotoxins
    D. A and C

Answers

1. **A** page 474
   Because of the availability of less invasive and successful methods of hemorrhage control, hypogastric artery ligation is usually limited to the control of intraoperative bleeding. The anterior branch should be isolated for ligation.
2. **C** page 475
   Urinary infection was the most frequent complication of percutaneous nephrostomy (70%). Hemorrhage was seen in 28% and blockage of catheter in 65% of patients.
3. **C** page 476
   Bypass surgery is usually the quickest and easiest method of alleviating the obstruction and has proved to be more prudent than attempts at lysis of adhesions or bowel resection. Conservative management in the form of nothing by mouth, intravenous hydration, and nasogastric suction is initially prudent. The survival of many of these patients is brief (50% are dead within 3 months).
4. **A** page 478
   According to a review at Duke University Medical Center, preoperative risk factors found to be associated with thromboembolic (TE) disease are, in order of significance, weight in excess of 190 lb, advanced clinical stage of malignancy, and radiation therapy within 6 weeks of the operative procedure.
5. **D** page 479
   A high index of suspicion and constant monitoring with impedance plethysmography or ^{125}I fibrinogen scanning appear to be the best means of early diagnosis and treatment of thromboembolic complications after surgery.
6. **C** page 479
   According to a study from Duke University Medical Center, low-dose heparin and the use of antiembolism stockings as preventive measures did not appear to reduce the incidence of TE complications. Also, from another Duke study comparing three groups of patients receiving, respectively, no heparin, low-dose heparin 2 hours preoperatively and 7 days postoperatively, and heparin 1 day preoperatively and 7 days postoperatively, there was a statistically significant difference in the scan-detected calf thromboses between the control group (16%) versus the two low-dose groups (8% and 2%). There was no difference among any of the three groups for proximal deep venous thromboses or pulmonary emboli. A prospective, controlled trial of external pneumatic compression (EPC) compared with a control group showed 13% of thromboembolic complication in the EPC groups versus 35% in the control group ($P < 0.005$).
7. **D** page 480
   The use of accelerated radiation therapy to the mediastinum to a total dose of 3000 to 5000 cGy has been successful in relieving the vascular compromise with its resultant physical characteristics (edema and plethora of the head, neck, and upper extremities and trunk, pleural, and pericardial effusions).
8. **B** page 482
   The bifurcation of the common iliac artery should be sought because the ureter usually crosses the vessels near this point.
9. **B** page 482
   If the ureteral fistula is within 4 to 5 cm of the bladder, reimplantation of the ureter can usually be done. If the fistula is higher, a ureteroureteral anastomosis is recommended.
10. **A** page 483
    Previous studies suggest that as many as 10% of patients treated with radical hysterectomy and pelvic lymphadenectomy develop a vesicovaginal or ureterovaginal fistula. Current studies suggest that this incidence has dropped to approximately 1% to 2%.
11. **B** page 483
    Ureterovaginal and vesicovaginal fistulae manifest within a week to 10 days after surgery. After a vesicovaginal fistula has been identified, an attempt is made to keep the patient dry by inserting a Foley

catheter. Repair is attempted after 3 to 6 months. If the fistula is small and high, an immediate repair with the Latzko technique may be successful. Surgery is contraindicated in the presence of infection and calculi formation. Combined use of radiation and surgery increases the complication rate of genitourinary fistulae.

12. **D** page 483
The routine of *not* reperitonealizing the retroperitoneal space may also contribute to the reduction of fistulae.
13. **D** page 484
It is the degree of radicality of the surgery and not the method of drainage that appears to be important relative to bladder function after radical hysterectomy. Kader found that incomplete division of the cardinal ligament resulted in decreased postoperative detrusor hypertonia compared with complete division. Photopulos suggested that a less radical operation (type II vs. type III) would decrease the morbidity, including bladder dysfunction.
14. **A** page 483
In a patient with large bowel fistula, it is usually necessary to perform a three-stage procedure. This usually means a diverting colostomy with a subsequent repair of the rectovaginal fistula a few months later and reanastomosis of the large bowel with closure of the colostomy site after healing of the fistula.
15. **B** page 486
Unmanipulated lymphocysts rarely become infected. In most instances they are small and can be treated expectantly. Most will slowly resolve. If the lymphocyst is large or critically placed (obstruction of ureter or pelvic veins), surgical drainage through a retroperitoneal incision is imperative.
16. **B** page 487
Although some authors suggest prophylactic antibiotics in afebrile patients with neutropenia less than 1000 cells/mL, DiSaia and Creasman use antibiotics only when fever is associated with neutropenia. The most common combination is an aminoglycoside with an antipseudomonal beta-lactam. If a patient is known to have coagulase-negative staphylococci, methicillin-resistant *Staphylococcus aureus*, *Corynebacterium*, or an alpha-hemolytic streptococci, vancomycin is added. The authors recommend that antibiotics be continued for a minimum of 7 days.
17. **C** page 489
The role of multiple-site cultures, including blood cultures, appears to have limited clinical usefulness. The reason for this is because no single site is a predictable source of infection. Many investigators do not recommend routine cultures in the neutropenic patient. An exception to this might be the individual who has an indwelling intravenous device.
18. **D** page 478
Several studies have found that in patients with DVT who are pulmonary asymptomatic, 40% will have diagnostic evidence of a PE. Conversely, patients with a PE will have an 80% documented evidence of DVT. Chemotherapy, particularly in combination with tamoxifen and progestins, seems to increase the incidence of PE.
19. **C** page 491
Complications from radiation therapy in the older patient are increased. The rate of fistula is 10% according to Kennedy's study. Older patients can withstand radical surgery. Febrile morbidity is less frequent in the older patient, but postoperative small bowel obstruction, bladder dysfunction, and pulmonary emboli are more frequent. It is thought that functional age is a more important criterion than chronologic age in determining whether a patient is a tolerable surgical risk.
20. **A** page 492
Normal pressure ranges in millimeters of mercury measured by Swan-Ganz catheter are as follows: right atrium, mean 5 to 12; right ventricle, systolic 15 to 25, diastolic 0 to 8; pulmonary artery, systolic 15 to 25, diastolic 8 to 15, mean 10 to 17; pulmonary artery wedged, mean 5 to 12.
21. **D** page 492
The greatest utility of invasive monitoring in gynecologic oncology is to determine the cause of hypotension and low urinary output, particularly during the postoperative period. These may be caused by hypovolemia, congestive heart failure, myocardial infarction, and sepsis, all of which require different treatments. In the postoperative patient, hypovolemia could result from dehydration, hemorrhage, or third-space fluid loss (ovarian cancer with ascites).
22. **D** page 492
The larger the field, the greater the risk of problems if the dose remains constant. With the newer megavoltage equipment, the 100% absorption isodose level may be several centimeters beneath the skin. This has nearly completely eliminated skin complications that occurred with orthovoltage equipment.
23. **A** page 493
In a study from MD Anderson Hospital, about one half of small bowel injuries occurred within 1 year after radiation and three fourths occurred within 2 years. Patients usually are seen initially with partial or complete obstruction with or without perforation or intestinal fistulae. Many surgeons prefer an intestinal bypass procedure to relieve the obstruction. Resection with reanastomosis is an option. Any anastomosis should be done with nonradiated bowel if at all possible.
24. **C** page 493
Rectovaginal fistula is the most common significant radiation injury to the large bowel. All patients should have diverting colostomies performed and a postponed fistula repair. Radiation-induced rectovaginal fistulae occur at a median of 13 months after treatment, and rectal strictures occur at 24 months.
25. **D** page 493
The addition of hysterectomy to irradiation will increase the fistula rate. In an MD Anderson series, Boronow and Rutledge noted 4.1% vesicovaginal

fistula rate if radiation and surgery both were used, in comparison with 1.4% if radiation alone was used.

26. **B** page 493
Colostomy is the most efficient and effective way to manage rectovaginal fistulae. Likewise, vesicovaginal fistulae are usually best managed with urinary diversion if the patient would have significant remaining functional life or symptom relief.

27. **C** page 484
According to a study by Ralph, 2 weeks after operation, all patients had small spastic bladders and 68% had residual urine. Bladder sensation was impaired in all patients at 2 weeks and in 63% at 1 year.

28. **B** page 485
An enterovaginal fistula not complicated by active tumor or high-dose irradiation can be cured medically with TPN and somatostatin. There is a synergistic effect of TPN and somatostatin. Up to 75% of fistulae will heal with this medical management.

29. **A** page 487
Extensive surgical débridement, which may be frequent, is the hallmark of therapy of necrotizing fasciitis. All necrotic tissue should be removed and wide excision to bleeding edges should be done. Nonviable muscle should be removed. The wound is packed. Secondary closure or skin grafting may be performed, after infection has resolved.

30. **D** page 488
If cardiovascular function is suboptimal, dopamine is usually the drug of choice for improving cardiac function. Before dopamine is administered to patients in shock, hypovolemia should be corrected.

31. **D** page 489
Alkylating agents and epipodophyllotoxins (etoposide and teniposide) are related to the development of subsequent leukemias.

chapter 18 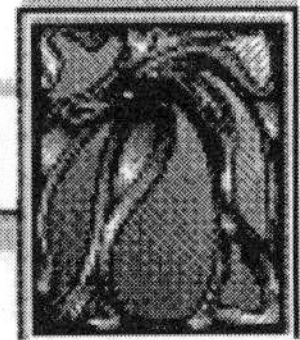

BASIC PRINCIPLES of CHEMOTHERAPY

KEY POINTS TO REMEMBER

- Chemotherapy is used to treat disseminated neoplasia. The use of adjuvant chemotherapy soon after eradicating surgery is increasing, especially in the treatment of uterine and ovarian cancer.
- The rationale for the use of drugs in the treatment of cancer is to achieve the selective killing of tumor cells. A given dose of a drug kills a constant fraction of cells, not a constant number, regardless of the cell numbers present ("cell kill" hypothesis by Skipper et al.).
- As tumor mass increases in size, its mass-doubling time becomes progressively longer. The Gompertzian aspect of tumor growth is recognizable only when a tumor is measured in its clinical palpable range. In the subclinical period the growth is assumed to be exponential.
- As a mass responds to treatment (i.e., gets smaller) the doubling time is assumed to decrease as a consequence of a greater number of cells moving into cycle. Cell cycle–nonspecific agents (e.g., cyclophosphamide) reduce the size of the mass; cell cycle–specific agents (e.g., methotrexate) kill the larger percentage of metabolically active cells.
- Metastases can be expected to be more sensitive to chemotherapy in general, and to cell cycle–specific agents in particular, than the primary tumor from which they arise.
- The larger the total malignant mass, the higher the proportion of the permanently drug-resistant variance to any compound or regimen.
- Metastases will generally have a shorter doubling time than the primary lesion.
- A 1-cm mass has undergone 30 doublings.
- The growth fraction and cell death regulate the growth speed of tumors. In humans, the growth fraction ranges from 25% to 95%. In a tumor mass, there is only a small fraction of rapidly proliferative cells—the majority of cells are often out of the cell cycle and resting.
- High-dose intermittent drug treatment is substantially more effective treatment than low-dose daily treatment. Adjuvant chemotherapy assumes subclinical cell masses (10^1 to 10^4 cells) that can produce failure but undetectable after the initial surgery therapy. This small burden is vulnerable to effective chemotherapy.
- Chemotherapeutic agents appear to work by first-order kinetics; that is, they kill a constant fraction of cells rather than a constant number.
- Alkylating agents appear to act in all phases of the cell generation time from G_0 to mitosis; they are termed *cycle-nonspecific agents*.
- Hydroxyurea, doxorubicin, and methotrexate appear to act in the S phase; bleomycin appears to act in the G_2 phase; and vincristine appears to act in the M phase—they are termed *cycle-specific agents*.
- Steroids, 5-FU, and cisplatin have rather uniform activity around the cell generation cycle.
- Extent of disease is the most important factor when considering curative radiation or surgery, but in using chemotherapy, the total mass is most important. In a reduced tumor volume, tumor cells are propelled from the G_0 phase into the more vulnerable cell generation cycle, susceptible to chemotherapy.
- Chemotherapy of cancer requires the differential killing of cancer cells and the sparing of normal cells as much as possible. At any given time, a large number of cancer cells are in the DNA synthesis (S phase) of the cell cycle and are susceptible to cycle-dependent agents. Unfortunately, a small portion of bone marrow cells, epithelial cells of gastrointestinal tract, and hair follicles have generation times comparable to those of tumors and are also vulnerable to compounds that inhibit DNA synthesis.
- The effectiveness of any cancer treatment is limited by the development of acquired drug resistance (due to limited drug accumulation of structurally unrelated agents by cells, cross resistance between agents, spontaneous mutation, P glycoprotein on cell membrane, and gene amplification).
- Alkylating agents prevent cell division primarily by crosslinking strands of DNA: cyclophosphamide, chlorambucil, melphalan, thiotepa, and ifosfamide (only cyclophosphamide inhibits DNA synthesis).
- Antimetabolites act by inhibiting essential metabolic processes that are required for DNA and/or RNA synthesis: 5-FU, methotrexate, and cytarabin.
- Cytotoxic antibiotics are dactinomycin, bleomycin, and doxorubicin.
- Plant alkaloids arrest cells in metaphase and comprise vinblastine, vincristine, etoposide, paclitaxel (Taxol), and vinorelbine (Navelbine).
- Other antineoplastic agents include cisplatin, carboplatin, hexamethylmelamine, hydroxyurea, dacarbazine, and nitrosoureas.
- Hematologic toxicity is the most frequently seen side effect; most clinicians consider patients with absolute

granulocyte counts lower than 500/mm^3 for 5 days or longer to be at high risk for sepsis. Thrombocytopenic patients with platelet counts lower than 20,000/mm^3 are at increased risk for spontaneous hemorrhage.

- Other toxicities include gastrointestinal toxicity (mucositis, necrotizing enterocolitis), skin reactions (alopecia, skin necrosis: doxorubicin [Adriamycin], actinomycin D, methotrexate, paclitaxel), hepatic toxicity, interstitial pneumonitis (doxorubicin, alkylating agents), cardiac toxicity (doxorubicin), genitourinary toxicity (chronic hemorrhagic cystitis, renal tubular toxicity: cyclophosphamide), neurologic toxicity (neuropathies, ototoxicity, cerebellum toxicity: vinca alkaloids, cisplatin), and gonadal dysfunction (azoospermia, amenorrhea: alkylating agents).
- Trials for new therapeutic agents are defined: phase I for evaluation of toxicity and tolerance of various doses; phase II for therapeutic effectiveness and extent of toxicity; phase III for comparison with the treatment currently in use.
- Assays for chemosensitivity testing do not provide useful clinical correlations.
- Performance status (Karnofsky score) should be watched carefully in patients undergoing combination chemotherapy. Supportive care should always be available in case of complications.
- Hematopoietic growth factors of granulocyte and macrophage lineage (G-CSF, GM-CSF) stimulate hematopoiesis and enhance host defense to infection.
- Erythropoietin may stimulate erythropoiesis.
- Other growth factors, G-CSF (filgrastim) and IL-11 (oprelvekin), may be used to increase neutrophils and platelets, respectively.
- Treatment of the most common side effects: nausea and vomiting with high-dose steroids, metoclopramide, ondansetron; alopecia with scalp tourniquet, use of wigs; renal toxicity with adequate hydration and mannitol-induced diuresis; and peripheral neuropathy with vitamin B_6 (doubtful effect).
- Calculation of chemotherapy dosages should be discussed as milligrams per square meter of total body surface area, or milligrams per kilogram of body weight. Dose adjustments should be made in compromised patients. In adults, milligrams per kilogram can be converted with reasonable accuracy to milligrams per square meter by multiplying by 40.
- Many antineoplastic agents are mutagenic and teratogenic. The second malignancy commonly occurs 4 to 7 years after successful therapy. The incidence of acute leukemia is increased in patients who have been treated with high-dose alkylating agents (cyclophosphamide, melphalan, chlorambucil).

QUESTIONS

Directions for Questions 1–20: Select the one best answer.

1. The Gompertzian growth process expresses the following *except:*
   A. as tumor mass increases in size, its mass-doubling time becomes progressively longer
   B. the doubling time is also applicable for tumors < 1 mm
   C. as a mass responds to treatment by getting smaller, the doubling time decreases as a consequence of a greater number of cells moving into cycle
   D. metastases can be expected to be more sensitive to cell cycle–specific chemotherapy agents than the primary tumor
2. An "early" lesion detected by the clinician is approximately a 1-cm mass. How many doublings has the tumor undergone, considering that the malignancy begins from a single cell?
   A. 10 doublings
   B. 20 doublings
   C. 30 doublings
   D. 40 doublings
3. Chemotherapeutic agents appear to work by first-order kinetics. That means:
   A. they kill a constant fraction of cells
   B. they kill a constant number of cells
   C. they kill only cells in the premitotic phase
   D. they kill only cells in the resting phase
4. Significance of the S phase in the cell generation time:
   A. resting phase
   B. DNA synthesis
   C. mitosis
   D. premitotic phase
5. Alkylating agents include the following drugs *except:*
   A. cyclophosphamide
   B. chlorambucil
   C. melphalan
   D. methotrexate
6. The following drugs are antimetabolites *except:*
   A. paclitaxel (Taxol)
   B. 5-FU
   C. methotrexate
   D. cytarabine
7. Cytotoxic antibiotics include the following *except:*
   A. dactinomycin
   B. bleomycin
   C. cisplatin
   D. doxorubicin
8. Plant alkaloids are the following *except:*
   A. paclitaxel (Taxol)
   B. vincristine
   C. etoposide
   D. hexamethylmelamine
9. A patient with ovarian cancer who is ambulatory, capable of self-care, unable to work, and out of bed greater than 50% of working hours has a Karnofsky score of:
   A. 90–100
   B. 70–80
   C. 50–60
   D. 30–40
10. Which is the most leukemogenic alkylating drug used in ovarian cancer?
    A. cyclophosphamide
    B. thiotepa

C. busulfan
D. chlorambucil and melphalan

11. Dosages of chemotherapeutic agents are usually discussed as milligrams per kilogram of body weight or milligrams per square meter of total body surface area. In adults, milligrams per kilogram can be converted with reasonable accuracy to milligram per square meter by multiplying by:
A. 10
B. 20
C. 30
D. 40

12. Chemotherapy agents used in gynecologic oncology that frequently cause bone marrow depression include all *except:*
A. doxorubicin
B. bleomycin
C. methotrexate
D. carboplatin

13. Chemotherapy agents known to cause severe inflammatory or ulcerative reactions after extravasation include all *except:*
A. cisplatin
B. doxorubicin
C. mitomycin C
D. actinomycin D

14. The chemotherapy agent *least* likely to cause severe alopecia is:
A. ifosfamide
B. doxorubicin
C. 5-fluorouracil
D. melphalan

15. Drugs groups demonstrating substantial activity against epithelial carcinoma of the ovary include all *except:*
A. antibiotic drugs such as actinomycin D and bleomycin
B. alkylating agents such as cyclophosphamide and melphalan
C. the platinum drugs: cisplatin and carboplatin
D. hexamethylmelamine, paclitaxel (Taxol)

16. Drugs known to cause neurotoxicity include the following *except:*
A. hexamethylmelamine
B. cyclophosphamide
C. cisplatin
D. vincristine, vinblastine

17. Which drug listed below is *least* likely to cause bone marrow depression?
A. cisplatin
B. carboplatin
C. cyclophosphamide
D. doxorubicin

18. The following statements comparing cisplatin and carboplatin toxicity and activity are true *except:*
A. both drugs exhibit substantial antitumor activity in epithelial ovarian carcinoma
B. carboplatin is more myelotoxic than cisplatin
C. cisplatin is more nephrotoxic than carboplatin
D. carboplatin is more neurotoxic than cisplatin

19. Drugs found to be effective antiemetic agents include all *except:*
A. metoclopramide
B. high-dose steroids
C. ondansetron
D. nonsteroidal anti-inflammatory drugs

20. Some unusual but potentially fatal toxicities of cytotoxic antitumor drugs include all *except:*
A. hypertension with etoposide
B. cardiotoxicity with paclitaxel (Taxol)
C. hepatic fibrosis with methotrexate
D. myocardial toxicity with doxorubicin

Directions for Questions 21–27: For each numbered item, select the letter of the most appropriate answer. Each letter may be used once, more than once, or not at all.

21–24. Match the following toxicities with the drugs:
A. hemorrhagic cystitis
B. pulmonary fibrosis
C. cardiac toxicity
D. ototoxicity and peripheral neuropathy

21. Cisplatin
22. Adriamycin
23. Cyclophosphamide
24. Bleomycin

25–27. Match the trial phases for the regular use of a newly developed agent:
A. phase I
B. phase II
C. phase III

25. Therapeutic effectiveness of new drug and extent of toxicity against specific tumor types.
26. Comparison of new drug to the drug currently in use.
27. Toxicity and tolerance to new drug at various doses.

ANSWERS

1. **B** page 502
The Gompertzian aspect of tumor growth is recognizable only when a tumor is measured in its clinically palpable range. In the subclinical period (e.g., 1-mm diameter), the growth is considered to be exponential.

2. **C** page 503
If it is assumed that exponential growth occurs early in the malignancy's history and the malignancy begins from a single cell, a 1-mm mass will have undergone approximately 20 tumor doublings, a 5-mm mass (size first recognizable on a radiograph) 27 doublings, and a 1-cm mass 30 doublings. This "early lesion" has already undergone 30 doublings, with significant DNA change being possible. Once a tumor becomes palpable (1 cm in diameter), only three more doublings will produce a very large tumor mass (8 cm in diameter).

3. **A** page 503
Chemotherapeutic agents kill a constant fraction of cells rather than a constant number. This concept of "log kill hypothesis" provides a rationale for multiple-drug or combination chemotherapy, as well as for the philosophy of adjuvant chemotherapy.

4. **B** page 503
S phase is the phase of DNA synthesis and usually lasts between 10 and 20 hours. Drugs such as hydroxyurea, doxorubicin, and methotrexate appear to act primarily in the S phase.
5. **D** page 510
Methotrexate is an antimetabolite.
6. **A** page 510
Paclitaxel (Taxol) is a plant alkaloid.
7. **C** page 511
Cisplatin does not fit into any category of antineoplastic drugs used against cancer in women.
8. **D** page 511
Hexamethylmelamine does not fit into any category.
9. **C** page 514
A Karnofsky score of 90–100 is assigned to a fully active patient with unrestricted activities of daily living; a score of 70–80 describes a patient who is ambulatory but restricted in strenuous activity.
10. **D** page 519
The risk of leukemia is greatest 4 to 5 years after chemotherapy begins, and the risk is elevated for at least 8 years after cessation of chemotherapy. Chlorambucil and melphalan were the most leukemogenic drugs.
11. **D** page 517
Dosage based on surface area is preferable to that based on weight because surface area and the variation in total dose between very obese and very thin people is minimized.
12. **B** page 510
Bleomycin rarely affects the bone marrow.
13. **A** page 510
Cisplatin is the only drug listed that is not a vesicant—a drug that, if extravasated, may cause severe inflammatory or ulcerative soft tissue change. Other vesicants include nitrogen mustard (mechlorethamine), 5-fluorouracil, vinblastine, and vincristine.
14. **D** page 509
Severe alopecia is not commonly seen with melphalan (Table 18–5).
15. **A** page 509
Antibiotic drugs commonly used for sarcomas, germ cell tumors, choriocarcinoma, and squamous cell cancer are rarely used for epithelial ovarian carcinoma (Table 18–5).
16. **B** page 509
Peripheral neuropathy is regularly seen in patients receiving cisplatin, vincristine, hexamethylmelamine, and occasionally vinblastine (Table 18–5).
17. **A** page 509
Other drugs less frequently affecting the bone marrow are bleomycin and vincristine (Table 18–5).
18. **D** page 511
Carboplatin is markedly less neurotoxic and nephrotoxic than cisplatin. It is somewhat less emetogenic but significantly more myelotoxic (Table 18–5).
19. **D** page 516
Drugs found to be most effective for the intense vomiting associated with cisplatin are metoclopramide and ondansetron. Phenothiazines, droperidol, and cannabinoids are also effective in some patients.
20. **A** page 510
Severe hypotension is occasionally seen with the rapid infusion of etoposide (Table 18–5). Pulmonary fibrosis can occur with bleomycin.
21. **D** page 510
22. **C** page 510
23. **A** page 509
24. **B** page 510
25. **B** page 513
26. **C** page 513
27. **A** page 513

chapter 19 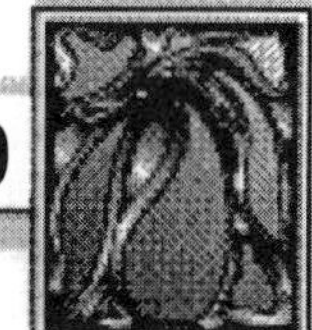

TUMOR IMMUNOLOGY, HOST DEFENSE MECHANISMS, and BIOLOGIC THERAPY

KEY POINTS TO REMEMBER

- Tumor cells express most of the same cell surface antigens (e.g., transplantation or HLA antigens) as normal cells. In addition many tumor cells express specific tumor-associated antigens (TAAs).
- Oncofetal antigens (CEA, AFP) are found in fetal and malignant tissue and occur more commonly than TAA. CEA and AFP are not disease specific.
- Each human tumor may express many TAAs. There is considerable heterogenicity in the expression of many TAAs between different tumors of the same type and between different cells of the same tumor. Heterogeneity is reflected even in a different expression of a TAA in a primary tumor and its metastases.
- For the detection of malignant disease, serum markers (like CA-125) should have a high sensitivity (to detect early disease) and a sufficient specificity (to discriminate from benign conditions). Tumor markers have been used also to monitor response to therapy.
- CA-125, which is used to monitor patients with epithelial ovarian cancer, has a day-to-day 12% to 15% variation for the assay and requires a doubling or halving of antigen levels to be considered significant.
- Antibodies are secreted by plasma cells, which are responsible for humoral immunity.
- The unique variable region of an antibody can act as an antigen, called *idiotype*. An idiotype can trigger complementary antibody called *anti-idiotype*.
- There are five classes of antibodies: IgG, IgM, IgA, IgE, and IgD. An antibody directed toward a particular antigen does not confer protection against other antigens. Interaction between the tumor cell and some of the antibodies activates the complement system, leading to lesions in the cell membrane and eventually to lysis. Antibodies specifically bound to membranes of tumor cells may result in loss of adhesive properties important to the establishment of blood-borne metastatic foci.
- Thymus-dependent (T) lymphocytes recognize and destroy foreign cells and regulate immune reactions. T lymphocytes carry out these functions directly by cell-to-cell contact or indirectly by using factors they produce and secrete (cytokines). T lymphocytes, after leaving the thymus, are found in the blood and thymic-dependent areas of the lymphoid tissues (spleen, lymph nodes, Peyer's patches). They are divided into three functional subgroups: helper, suppressor, and cytotoxic lymphocytes. T cells simultaneously recognize cell-associated antigens and a portion of one of the self-class I or II major histocompatibility complex (MHC) gene products. Activated lymphocytes can produce cytokines. T cells are distinguished by their stages of differentiation (T1 through T11) and their surface markers (CD1 to CD86).
- B lymphocytes derived from the hematopoietic stem cells produce immunoglobulins on activation. There are seven different cell types in the B-lymphocyte differentiation pathway. Plasma cells, the final stage in B-cell differentiation, secrete large amounts of immunoglobulin. An individual plasma cell initially secretes antibodies of the IgM class but can switch to producing antibodies of other subclasses with the same antigen specificity.
- Natural killer (NK) cells, a subpopulation of lymphoid cells, do not result from a classic immune response. They have spontaneous cytolytic activity against a variety of tumor cells and some normal cells, and their reactivity can be rapidly augmented by interferon. They are closely associated with large granular lymphocytes and share several features with macrophages and polymorphonuclear leukocytes. NK cells can recognize several widely distributed antigenic specificities.
- Lymphokine-activated killer (LAK) cells result from culturing lymphocytes with high doses of IL-2. They are activated cells derived from NK cells and T cells. They selectively lyse a broad spectrum of fresh autologous, syngeneic, and allogeneic cells in an independent fashion.
- Macrophages, dendritic cells, and B cells that have class II MHC expressed on cell surfaces can present antigens to CD4-bearing T cells. The macrophage can be activated by lymphocytes and exert a killing effect on tumor cells. Macrophage cells form a critical part of the immune defense system by serving three distinct functions: secretion of active molecules, antigen clearance, and antigen presentation to lymphocytes. Dendritic cells can be isolated from peripheral blood by use of cytokines (CSF, IL-4, TNF-α). Dendritic cell–based cancer vaccines offer the potential of an effective, nontoxic, and outpatient approach to cancer therapy.
- There are two categories of immune responses: cell-mediated immunity (CMI) and humoral immunity. The key to both responses is the small lymphocyte. Formed in the bone marrow, the small lymphocytes pass through

the thymus and participate in CMI (T cells) or bypass the thymus and differentiate into B cells (humoral immunity). In addition to B and T cells, a central role in the inductive phase of the immune response is played by "accessory cells" of the monocyte-macrophage series.

- Activation of CD4 T cells begins with the engagement of T1-CD3 receptors that recognize the specific antigen in association with the class II molecule on an "accessory cell," followed by the further stabilization of this molecular interaction through CD4 class II association and through the cellular interaction of adhesion molecules. T-cell activation results in the secretion of lymphokines that belong to the general category of cytokines. T cells act as potentiators (helper cells) or inhibitors (suppressor cells) of the B-cell transition into immunoglobulin-secreting plasma cells. Suppressor cells may terminate excessive immune responses after antigenic exposure, and they probably provide a safeguard against autoimmune reactions.
- Humoral immunity is mediated by antibody globulins produced by the B cell. B cells originate from the bone marrow and are distributed in areas of lymphatic tissue (spleen, lymph nodes, tonsils, appendix). With suitable stimulation, B cells become metabolically active and begin to synthesize antibodies.
- There is T-B cooperation in the immune response. The presence of healthy T cells is necessary for production of many antibodies by B cells.
- Suppression of immunologic responses is a natural result of certain biologic processes such as pregnancy and aging. It also occurs in several systemic diseases, as a result of radiation or drug therapy, and following severe injuries. In most instances CMI is suppressed more rapidly or profoundly than humoral immunity.
- In tumor surveillance the assumption is made that the mutant cell will express one or more antigen(s) than can be recognized as non-self. The role of immunity in immunosurveillance against newly arising tumors remains controversial. NK cells may be the effectors of immune surveillance.
- Mechanisms by which mutant cells might avoid interaction with the immune system are lowered tumor antigenicity (antigenic modulation) privileged sites, immunoresistance, vascularization, immunosuppression, and blocking factors.
- Immunoprophylaxis is the induction of resistance to a tumor before its origination. It may theoretically be achieved by immunization against the etiologic agents of cancer. It may also lead to induction of immune complexes (e.g., blocking antibodies) that enhance rather than impede tumor growth and metastasis.
- Before the institution of immunotherapy it is crucial to reduce the tumor mass to a minimum (preferably 10^8 cells). Immunotherapy, still in an embryonic state, includes two categories: active and passive.
- Nonspecific active immunotherapy uses adjuvants, which are substances that increase response to an antigen: BCG, MER, *Corynebacterium parvum*, levamisole, cyclophosphamide, cytokines (interferons, IL-2).
- Specific immunotherapy can be active or passive (adoptive).
  1. Active specific immunotherapy calls for administration to the cancer patient of tumor cells (tumor vaccines). To date, trials in humans have been disappointing.
  2. Passive adoptive immunotherapy can be (1) nonspecific, using LAK cells generated by IL-2, or (2) specific, using heterologous antiserum from an immunized human or monoclonal antibodies (murine or human). Limited success has been found to date.
- Monoclonal antibodies (MABs) directed to tumor antigens or markers help to stage disease by identifying sites of tumor involvement that might go unrecognized (photoscanning after injection of radiolabeled MABs). Detection of circulating tumor antigen is helpful in initial diagnosis and serial monitoring of the results of therapy.
- Biologic response modifiers are molecules produced by the body to regulate modulation of the individual's own biologic responses: cytokines, interferons, interleukins, and tumor necrosis factor. Lymphokines and other cytokines may regulate certain components of the immune response that can alter the growth of cancer. They may also enhance immune response by lessening the effects of suppressive factors. Interferons have antiviral activity and profound effects on the immune system. Interleukins may stimulate an immune reaction (IL-2, IL-4). Tumor necrosis factor, cytokines produced by activated monocytes and lymphocytes, can destroy tumor cells in the absence of the cells of the immune system. Retinoid acid, a derivative of vitamin A, is thought to act by inducing cell differentiation and thus cell death. It has been tried on cervical intraepithelial neoplasia.
- Antiangiogenesis agents (thalidomide, angiostatin) are planned for testing.

QUESTIONS

Directions for Questions 1–23: Select the one best answer.

1. The following are true concerning tumor-associated antigens (TAA) *except:*
   A. they have a low degree of tumor specificity
   B. each human tumor may express many TAAs
   C. there is considerable homogeneity in the expression of TAAs
   D. most TAAs are shared by neoplasms of many different types
2. CA-125, used to monitor patients with epithelial ovarian cancer, is found in the following *except:*
   A. normal ovary
   B. nonmucinous epithelial ovarian cancers
   C. carcinomas of endometrium, fallopian tube, and endocervix
   D. carcinomas of pancreas, colon, breast, and lung
3. What percentage of increase or decrease in CA-125 levels is considered significant?
   A. 10%
   B. 20%
   C. 30%
   D. 50%

4. The following are true concerning natural killer (NK) cells *except:*
   A. they are a subpopulation of lymphoid cells present in most normal individuals
   B. they depend on the thymus for maturation
   C. they have cytolytic activity against various tumor cells
   D. they may be important in the first line of defense against tumor growth and against infection by some microbial agents
5. Choose the *false* statement relevant to lymphokine-activated killer (LAK) cells:
   A. they result from culturing lymphocytes with high doses of IL-2
   B. they are derived from B cells
   C. they are cytotoxic for tumor cells
   D. they lyse a broad spectrum of fresh autologous, syngeneic, or allogeneic cells
6. True statements concerning the macrophage are the following *except:*
   A. it is derived from the bone marrow
   B. it secretes a wide range of biologically active molecules
   C. it processes and presents antigens to T cells to generate an immune response
   D. it is distributed in the connective tissue only
7. The key element in cell-mediated immunity and humoral immunity is the:
   A. small lymphocyte
   B. polynuclear neutrophil
   C. eosinophil
   D. monocyte
8. Activation of T cells requires the following steps *except:*
   A. direct engagement of T cells by free antigen
   B. processing by accessory cells of the polypeptide antigens into smaller peptides
   C. association of these peptides with major histocompatibility complex (MHC) molecules and recognition by T-cell receptor
   D. enhancement of the above interaction by CD4
9. The activated T cell secretes several antigen-nonspecific soluble factors known as:
   A. immunoglobulins
   B. interleukins
   C. lymphokines
   D. monokines
10. The following statements are true regarding T cell function *except:*
    A. suppressor T cells potentiate excessive immune response to a given antigen stimulus
    B. suppressor T cells are capable of "switching off" antibody production by B cells
    C. helper T cells stimulate B-cell conversion to immunoglobulin-secreting plasma cells
    D. suppressor T-cell impairment can lead to autoimmune disease
11. The following statements regarding principles of immunotherapy are true *except:*
    A. the most highly antigenic tumors are the least responsive
    B. surgery, radiotherapy, or chemotherapy *must* first be used
    C. active immunotherapy attempts to stimulate the host to induce an immune response to tumor
    D. passive immunotherapy transfers to the host immunologically active substances that mediate an antitumor response themselves
12. Mechanisms whereby tumor cells are theorized to decrease their interaction with the host immune system include all *except:*
    A. lowered antigenicity of tumor cells
    B. protection of tumor cell by oncogene expression
    C. immunoresistance by secretion of blocking factors (excess-free antigen)
    D. protection by vascularization against influx of host immune cells
13. The following are true concerning monoclonal antibodies (MABs) that recognize tumor-associated antigens *except:*
    A. MABs directed against tumor cell determinants can inhibit tumor cell proliferation in cultures and in animals
    B. MABs administered directly to patients can eradicate all small tumors
    C. MABs can diminish the amount of circulating tumor antigens that could have a blocking effect on subsequent immunotherapy
    D. MABs can be attached to antitumor drugs, which can destroy tumor cells and spare normal cells
14. Concerning interleukins (ILs):
    A. IL-1 activates resting T cells, stimulates synthesis of other cytokines
    B. IL-2 augments lymphocyte killer activity
    C. IL-3 stimulates early growth of monocyte, granulocyte, erythrocyte, and megakaryocyte progenitor cells
    D. all of the above
15. Vitamin A:
    A. is essential for the integrity of mesenchymal cells
    B. plays a major role in the induction of control in differentiation in mucus-secreting and keratinizing tissues
    C. when in excess, will be associated with epithelial atrophy
    D. when in excess, will be associated with proliferation of basal cells
16. Retinoids:
    A. are the immediate precursors of most human vitamin A
    B. have been associated with epithelial tumor regression when applied topically
    C. have shown no activity against intraepithelial neoplasia of the cervix when applied topically
    D. have shown no effects when used to protect against chemically induced tumors in animals
17. Which is *not* true regarding tumor necrosis factor (TNF)?
    A. TNF is primarily produced by fibroblasts
    B. TNF can induce hemorrhagic necrosis of tumors in a laboratory setting
    C. clinical toxicity of TNF is similar to the toxicity of recombinant interferon (i.e., chills, fever, and malaise)
    D. TNF may modulate cell-mediated immunity

18. Regarding clinical trials with nonspecific immunotherapy such as BCG or *Corynebacterium parvum:*
    A. most trials involving gynecologic neoplasms have been negative trials, indicating little, if any, anticancer activity
    B. intravenous *C. parvum* has been associated with an improved response rate to radiation therapy in patients with advanced carcinoma of the cervix
    C. BCG administration to patients with advanced ovarian cancer has never been reported to have an effect on the response rate to doxorubicin and cyclophosphamide
    D. intravenous *C. parvum* seems to potentiate the effect of melphalan when used to treat patients with advanced carcinoma of the ovary
19. When applied to the cervix of patients with carcinoma in situ, interferon:
    A. can normalize cytologic findings
    B. has little effect on long-term rates of CIN in treated patients when compared with patients treated with placebo
    C. may have some activity, but it should be avoided in women of reproductive age
    D. most responding patients relapse by 6 months
20. Alpha-interferon has been used to treat patients with advanced carcinoma of the ovary. All of the following are true *except:*
    A. when administered with cytotoxic chemotherapy, myelosuppression is cumulative and significant
    B. use of intraperitoneally administered interferon is associated with increased NK cell activity in peripheral blood
    C. when administered intraperitoneally to patients with persistent disease at second-look laparotomy, more than 30% of patients were reported to have complete responses
    D. when given intraperitoneally, there is a significant reduction in systemic side effects such as fever and malaise
21. When monoclonal antibodies are used to treat patients with malignancy, radionuclides as the lethality-inducing moiety have many attractive features. All of the following are true regarding radionuclide-labeled monoclonal antibodies *except:*
    A. there is the possibility of diagnosis through imaging
    B. the use of radionuclides reduces the problem of tumor cell antigen heterogeneity because the isotope can have a killing distance of several centimeters
    C. the ideal isotope has a short half-life and high energy at short distance
    D. cell damage is highly specific to the tumor
22. The following are true concerning interferons *except:*
    A. they have an antibacterial and antiviral activity
    B. they have profound effects on the immune system
    C. they prolong and inhibit cell division
    D. they have antitumor activity
23. Concerning immunoprophylaxis, the following are true *except:*
    A. immunoprophylaxis is the induction of resistance to a tumor before its origination
    B. it may be achieved by immunization against the etiologic agent of cancer or the specific antigens of the tumor
    C. it can induce immune complexes
    D. it has the same goal as immunotherapy

Directions for Questions 24–75: For each numbered item, select the letter of the most appropriate answer. Each letter may be used once, more than once, or not at all.

24–27. Match the genetic relationship with the type of antibodies.
    A. autologous
    B. isologous
    C. heterologous

24. Identical twin
25. Different species
26. Different individual, same species
27. Identical, same individual

28–31. Match the type of transplant with the genetic relationship.
    A. autologous
    B. syngeneic
    C. allogeneic
    D. xenogeneic

28. Different species
29. Same species, different individual
30. Identical twin
31. Identical, same individual

32–35. Match the definition of sensitivity and specificity.
    A. sensitivity
    B. specificity

32. $$\frac{\text{true positives}}{\text{true positives + false negatives}}$$

33. $$\frac{\text{true negatives}}{\text{true negatives + false positives}}$$

34. Needed to detect disease at an early stage
35. Must be sufficient to discriminate malignant disease from a broad spectrum of intercurrent, benign conditions

36–46. Match the attributes of T and B cells.
    A. T cells
    B. B cells
    C. both
    D. neither

36. Mature in the thymus
37. Make up 80% to 90% of the total lymphocytes
38. Produce immunoglobulins on activation
39. Are divided into three functional groups: helper, suppressor, and cytotoxic
40. Plasma cells
41. Produce cytokines
42. Surface markers used to identify phenotypes

43. Lymphoid series
44. Polymorphonuclear neutrophils
45. Seven different cell types
46. Bone marrow stem cells

47–53. Match the location and role of the following cells.
   A. B cell
   B. helper T cell
   C. suppressor T cell
   D. plasma cell
   E. all

47. An activated B cell
48. Originates from bone marrow precursors
49. Actual production of antibodies
50. Stimulates transformation of B cell
51. Present in peripheral lymph node
52. Germinal center of lymph node
53. Peripheral blood lymphocytes

54–61. Match the attributes of T and B cells.
   A. T cells
   B. B cells
   C. both
   D. neither

54. Bone marrow origin
55. "Hairy" electron microscopic appearance
56. Lymphokines
57. Immunoglobulins
58. Long lived
59. Delayed hypersensitivity
60. Easily suppressed by illness
61. Independent of other cell types

62–66. Match the agents with the type of immunotherapy.
   A. nonspecific immunotherapy
   B. specific immunotherapy
   C. neither
   D. both

62. Cyclophosphamide
63. Antitumor monoclonal antibodies
64. Interferons
65. Activated lymphocytes
66. BCG

67–72. Match the agents with the type of immunotherapy.
   A. active immunotherapy
   B. passive immunotherapy
   C. neither
   D. both

67. Activated macrophages
68. Interferons
69. Monoclonal antibodies
70. BCG
71. Cultured T lymphocytes
72. Inactivated tumor vaccines

73–75. Match the letters with the numbers.
   A. immunoprophylaxis
   B. immunotherapy
   C. immunodiagnosis

73. Radiolabeled monoclonal antibodies
74. Tumor necrosis factor
75. Low prevalence of leukemias in BCG-vaccinated children

Answers

1. **C** page 525
   There is considerable heterogeneity in the expression of many tumor-associated antigens, both between different tumors of the same type and between different cells of the same tumor. This heterogeneity is even reflected by the different expression of a TAA in a primary tumor versus its metastases.
2. **A** page 525
   CA-125 has not been found in sections of normal ovary in the fetus or the adult. The antigen is present at the cell surface in more than 80% of nonmucinous epithelial ovarian cancers, as well as in a smaller fraction of carcinomas of endometrium, fallopian tube, endocervix, pancreas, colon, breast, and lung.
3. **D** page 525
   Antigen activity of CA-125 is expressed on an arbitrary scale from 1 to 20,000 units/mL. The day-to-day coefficient of variation for the assay is 12% to 15%. A doubling or halving of antigen levels is considered significant.
4. **B** page 528
   Natural killer (NK) cells do not depend on the thymus for maturation. They have spontaneous cytolytic activity against various tumor cells and some normal cells. Their reactivity can be augmented by interferon. NK cells are closely associated with large granular lymphocytes, and they share several features with macrophages and polymorphonuclear leukocytes. NK cells can recognize widely distributed antigenic specificities; such recognition is clonally distributed. Additional research is needed to determine the lineage of NK cells and their role in immunosurveillance.
5. **B** page 530
   Lymphokine-activated killer (LAK) cells are activated cells derived from NK cells and T cells exposed to high doses of IL-2. The cytotoxic mechanisms of LAK cells appear to be similar to those of NK cells and cytotoxic T lymphocytes.
6. **D** page 530
   Macrophages are widely distributed throughout the body (blood, bone marrow, lymphoid tissue, liver, connective tissue). Their secretory products include enzymes, complement products, growth and differentiation factors, cytotoxins, and prostaglandins. Macrophages can be activated directly by endotoxin or other stimulants, and they can be activated indirectly by lymphokines released by lymphocytes. Macrophages can independently exert a killing effect on tumor cells.
7. **A** page 533
   The small lymphocyte is the key element in cell-mediated immunity and humoral immunity. It is formed in the bone marrow from precursor stem cells and then is released into the circulation, coming to rest in the lymphoid organs. The small lymphocyte differentiates into T and B cells. In addition to T and B cells, a central role in the inductive phase of the immune response is played by "accessory cells" of the monocyte-macrophage series.

8. **A** page 533
The way in which T cells bind antigen is a useful mechanism for avoiding engagement of T cells by free antigen. The interaction with free antigen is a role that is left to antibodies. The sequence of events leading to the activation of CD4 T cells begins with the engagement of the T1-CD3 receptors that recognize the specific antigen, in association with the class II molecule on an accessory cell, followed by the further stabilization of this molecular interaction through CD4 class II association, as well as by the cellular interaction of adhesion molecules.
9. **C** page 534
Lymphokines are soluble products released by lymphocytes; they belong to the general category of substances known as cytokines. Cytokines are soluble substances produced by cells that have various effects on other cells. Other cytokines include monokines, soluble products of monocytes, and interleukins, produced by leukocytes. Immunoglobulins are produced by plasma cells.
10. **A** page 535
Suppressor T cells seem to terminate excessive immune response to antigens.
11. **A** page 540
The most highly antigenic tumors (melanoma, Burkitt's lymphoma, neuroblastoma) are the *most* responsive to immunotherapy.
12. **B** page 538
Oncogene expression is thought to induce malignant transformation, not to decrease ability of the host to defend against the transformed cell.
13. **B** page 550
The potential use of monoclonal antibodies that recognize tumor-associated antigens may be far reaching. Unfortunately, their administration directly to patients has found limited success to date.
14. **D** page 546
The interleukins belong to a family of polypeptide growth and differentiation factors called lymphokines. These are factors produced by lymphocytes or macrophages that stimulate the proliferation, differentiation, and function of T and B lymphocytes and other cells involved in the immune response.
15. **B** page 547
Vitamin A plays a major role in the induction and control of differentiation in mucus-secreting and keratinizing tissues, with little effect on mesenchymal tissues. Surface epithelial atrophy and basal cell proliferation are associated with vitamin A deficiency. Excessive retinol will lead to the production of a thick layer of mucin with a predominance of goblet cells and inhibition of keratinization.
16. **B** page 547
Retinoids are derivatives of dietary vitamin A. Although clinical trials in humans are just under way, preliminary data suggest protective effects orally and topically against chemically induced tumors in animals and some epithelial neoplasms in humans. Topical retinoic acid has reversed carcinoma in situ in early trials. Unfortunately, retinoids and high doses of vitamin A may be teratogenic in humans; clinical use of these preparations should be avoided in patients who may be pregnant.
17. **A** page 546
Tumor necrosis factor (TNF) is produced by properly stimulated monocytes and lymphocytes. It is now produced by recombinant DNA technology. In laboratory settings such as the xenogenic nude mouse model using transplanted tumors, hemorrhagic necrosis and tumor regression have been observed in a wide spectrum of tumor implants, including ovarian cancer, cervical cancer, breast cancer, and others. The main toxicity in humans is a flulike syndrome characterized by fever and malaise. Additional side effects include neurologic symptoms, reversible hypotension, and a dose-related myelosuppression.
18. **A** page 548
Most trials involving gynecologic neoplasms using nonspecific immunotherapy such as BCG or *Corynebacterium parvum* have been negative, indicating little, if any, anticancer activity. Patients receiving intravenously administered *C. parvum* demonstrate an enhanced ability to respond to mitogenic stimuli, but there have been no positive clinical trials using *C. parvum* in gynecologic neoplasms. Alberts et al. reported a positive BCG phase III clinical trial performed by the Southwest Oncology Group comparing patients with Stage III ovarian cancer treated with doxorubicin-cyclophosphamide (AC) and BCG vs. patients treated with AC alone. There was a significant improvement in response and survival. A Gynecologic Oncology Group trial using similar treatment arms did not corroborate these results.
19. **A** page 548
Clinical trials of topically administered alpha-interferon are encouraging. When administered topically for 14 to 21 days, most patients demonstrate return to normal cytologic findings. These regressions have high durability (Ikic et al. reported no recurrences during 6 months of observation). A major role of topically applied interferon may be in women of reproductive age to obviate the need for surgery.
20. **D** page 549
Use of alpha-interferon in patients with metastatic ovarian cancer is encouraging when used in certain settings. Berek reported a 36% complete response rate, and an additional 9% partial response rate, in patients after intraperitoneally administered alpha-interferon. In these patients NK activity in the peripheral blood was significantly increased. The side effects of IP interferon are essentially the same as systemically administered interferon (i.e., fever and malaise). In addition, the myelosuppressive effects of cytotoxic chemotherapy seem to be enhanced by simultaneous administration of interferon. In a Gynecologic Oncology Group pilot trial of CAP and interferon, the study was terminated due to unacceptable myelotoxicity.
21. **D** page 551
Radionuclide-tagged monoclonal antibodies (MABs) can theoretically be used for treatment and diagnosis

by imaging. Another theoretical advantage of the use of radionuclide tagged MABs is their circumvention of the problem of tumor heterogeneity, since the isotope can have a killing distance of several centimeters. There is no need for the malignant cell to integrate the MAB, just to be relatively near its final site of deposition. The ideal radioisotope has a short half-life and high energy and is safe when excreted. These advantages decrease the specificity of the treatment, since high energy can damage adjacent normal cells, e.g., liver.

22. **A** page 545
Interferons do not have antibacterial activity. Antitumor effects of interferon were demonstrated in tumors considered to be induced by oncogenic viruses. The greatest therapeutic usefulness of interferon is in the treatment of hairy cell leukemia.
23. **D** page 539
Immunoprophylaxis should be clearly separated from immunotherapy, which is the treatment of established neoplasms. Immunotherapy is a more difficult problem.
24. **B** page 522
25. **C** page 522
26. **B** page 522
27. **A** page 522
The term *autologous antibody* applies to identical, same individual; *isologous antibody* to identical twins or different individuals from the same species, and *heterologous antibody* to different species (Table 19–1).
28. **D** page 522
29. **C** page 522
30. **B** page 522
31. **A** page 522
The term *autologous transplant* applies to the same individual, *syngeneic transplant* to identical twins; *allogeneic transplant* to different individuals of the same species; and *xenogeneic transplant* to different species (Table 19–1).
32. **A** page 525
33. **B** page 525
34. **A** page 525
35. **B** page 525
Sensitivity is defined as the proportion of assay positives to true positives. Sensitivity notes the number of those with the disease who are correctly identified by the test. *Specificity* is defined as the proportion of assay negatives to true negatives. Specificity measures the number of those without disease who are correctly identified as disease free by the test. High sensitivity is needed to detect disease at an early stage. Specificity must be sufficient to discriminate malignant disease from a broad spectrum of intercurrent benign conditions. For effective monitoring the degree of specificity is somewhat less critical than that of sensitivity. Assays for persistent and recurrent disease are of greatest value in settings in which there is an effective salvage therapy.
36. **A** page 527
37. **A** page 527
38. **B** page 528
39. **A** page 527
40. **B** page 528
41. **A** page 527
42. **A** page 527
43. **C** page 527
44. **D** page 527
45. **B** page 528
46. **C** page 532
Polymorphonuclear neutrophils do not arise from T or B cells. T and B cells are lymphocytes derived from primordial marrow stem cells. T cells differentiate in the thymus and regulate the activity of other T cells, macrophages, B cells, neutrophils, eosinophils, and basophils. They have been characterized by monoclonal antibody and are divided into three functional subgroups: helper, suppressor, and cytotoxic lymphocytes. They can produce substances called *cytokines* (interferons, interleukins, tumor necrosis factor, and others). Various surface markers are useful to identify their differentiation and function: CD1, CD3, CD4, and so on. T lymphocytes are found in the deep cortex and in areas between germinal centers of lymph nodes.
The production of immunoglobulins on activation to plasma cells is characteristic of the B lymphocyte. There are seven different cell types in the B lymphocyte differentiation pathway: pro-B cells, pre-B cells, late pre-B cells, immature B cells, mature B cells, memory cells, and effector cells. There are also five classes of immunoglobulins: IgM, IgG, IgA, IgE, and IgD. Plasma cells, the final stage in B cell differentiation, secrete large amounts of immunoglobulins. An individual plasma cell initially secretes antibodies of the IgM class, but it can switch to produce antibodies of other subclasses having the same antigen specificity. B lymphocytes are found in germinal centers of lymph nodes and in the spleen.
47. **D** page 527
B cells are stimulated by helper T cells to become plasma cells.
48. **E** page 527
All of these cells are thought to originate from a primordial bone marrow stem cell, although they are distributed later to all loci of lymphoid tissue.
49. **D** page 527
It is the plasma cell that is thought to actually produce antibodies; B cells do not.
50. **B** page 527
Helper T cells stimulate transformation of B cells to antibody-producing plasma cells.
51. **E** page 527
In a typical lymph node, the germinal centers are occupied by B cells and plasma cells, and the cortical areas harbor T cells.
52. **A** page 527
See answer to Question 51.
53. **A** page 527
Resting B cells are the typical small peripheral blood lymphocytes.
54. **C** page 527
Both cells originate in the bone marrow. T cells then mature in the thymus; B cells mature in peripheral lymphatic tissue.

55. **B** page 527
B cells have multiple, small, hairlike projections; T cells are smoother.
56. **A** page 527
The majority of lymphokines (bioactive proteins) are produced by T cells, although some B cells may produce lymphokines as well.
57. **B** page 528
B cells, when transformed into plasma cells in the presence of an antigen, produce immunoglobulins.
58. **A** page 527
T cells remain viable for months to years; B cells remain viable for only days to weeks.
59. **A** page 527
T cells and derivatives are responsible for delayed hypersensitivity reactions.
60. **A** page 527
In systemic illness, with radiation or cytotoxic drug therapy, cell-mediated immunity (a function of T-cell derivatives) is suppressed to a greater degree than is humoral immunity.
61. **D** page 527
B- and T-cell function, cell-mediated immunity, and humoral immunity are interdependent.
62. **A** page 540
63. **B** page 540
64. **A** page 540
65. **B** page 540
66. **A** page 540
Nonspecific immunotherapy is the use of substances such as cytokines, immune-stimulating chemicals, immune-stimulating microbial products, and some chemotherapy drugs that directly or indirectly cause a general, nonspecific host immune response. Specific immunotherapy is the use of substances, such as antitumor antibodies, activated lymphocytes, inactivated tumor vaccines, and serum from immune individuals that have (or cause) a specific and direct immune response.
67. **B** page 542
68. **D** page 542
69. **B** page 542
70. **A** page 542
71. **B** page 542
72. **A** page 541
Active immunotherapy is the use of a substance that causes the host to mount an immune response. Passive immunotherapy is the use of substances that act directly against the target cells. There is some overlap: some cytokines, such as interferon, have direct (passive) and indirect (active) actions.
73. **C** page 543
Immunodiagnosis uses the host, animal, or hybridoma immune mechanism to conjugate a diagnostic substance to a tumor antigen, structure, or product.
74. **B** page 546
The use of cytokines, such as TNF, is one type of immunotherapy.
75. **A** page 539
Immunoprophylaxis is the induction of resistance to a tumor in a host *before* the tumor originates.

chapter 20 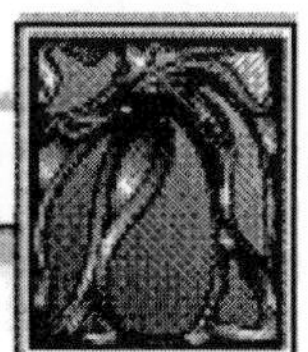

GENES and CANCER

KEY POINTS TO REMEMBER

- Cancer requires several different mutations in many different genes to allow irreversible and uncontrolled growth.
- Three broad classes of genes are involved in the development of cancer: tumor suppressor genes (inhibit cell growth), oncogenes (promote cell growth), and mismatch repair genes (repair DNA damage).
- The human genome contains 3 billion base pairs and between 50,000 and 100,000 genes and 3000 centimorgans. The average chromosome contains about 5000 genes in 130 million base pairs and 130 centimorgans (functional length).
- Genes consist of coding sequences of DNA called *exons* ("expressed DNA") interrupted by noncoding sequences called *introns* ("filler DNA"). DNA is transcribed into RNA that is translated into protein.
- Various mutations identified in cancers are single base pairs substitutions and point mutations, larger deletions, insertions, duplications, inversions, and translocations.
- Examples of genomic imprinting and cancer are hydatidiform mole (only paternal chromosomes) and teratoma (only maternal chromosomes).
- In a normal mammalian genome, there is at least one gene in the normal cellular DNA that possesses potent transforming ability when appropriately activated by viruses or chemical or physical conditions (proto-oncogenes) by changing the sequence of the gene. Such agents activate the proto-oncogene and convert it to a powerful oncogene. A cell carrying such a mutant gene might respond to this damage with a program of deregulated growth and become a cancer cell. Oncogenes cannot explain most cancers by themselves, because only 20% of tumors turn out to carry expected alterations. Oncogene mutations do not appear to be inherited through the germline.
- Tumor suppressor genes are equally important in the development of cancer. The first tumor suppressor gene cloned was the *RB* gene; it is the defective gene in retinoblastoma. The tumor suppressor gene *TP53* is a gene associated with many cancers. Tumor suppressor gene inactivations are loss of function events usually requiring a mutational event in one allele followed by a loss or inactivation of the other allele. This loss of gene function leads to loss of cellular control and unchecked growth.
- Apoptosis means programmed death and is important in the growth and development of an organism. If a cell does not die and becomes immortal, a cancer will result. Apoptosis is controlled at the molecular level by genes associated with malignant changes. Apoptosis is important in the development of the normal organism, and it is important in the development and growth of cancers. In cancer, apoptosis appears to be a mechanism for deleting cells from the population that have sustained carcinogenic DNA damage; however, when apoptosis of such cells is blocked or inhibited by mutations in genes that help control that process, such as *BCL2* or *TP53*, these cells are suddenly free to continue replicating and propagating their mutations.
- If a cell cannot repair DNA damage that occurs during the course of normal cell division, mutations can continue to accumulate; eventually enough mutations occur in genes critical for cell control, and cancer results. This is how the absence of DNA repair can lead to cancer. Germline mutations in mismatch repair genes are present in many families with hereditary cancers (colon cancers, endometrial cancers).
- Normal cells lack telomerase activity. Telomerase, enzyme complex, add back telomere sequences (structures at the end of chromosomes) lost during replication. Telomerase becomes reactivated in most cancer cells or germ cells.
- Gene therapy for cancer involves the abrogation of oncogene activity or the restoration of tumor suppressor gene function. The tumor suppressor gene *TP53* seems a likely target for gene therapy. Transforming the effects of oncogene function can be done by either removing the oncogene product, blocking its function, or using exogenous or intracellular antisense nucleotides to block the production of oncogenes. Research also revolves around cytokine gene transfer to tumor cells to enhance the development of immunity.
- Molecular technologies include restriction enzymes, Southern blot analysis (DNA probes), Northern blot (RNA sequences), Western blot (proteins), and polymerase chain reaction that simplifies DNA analysis, shortens laboratory time, and requires minute quantities of DNA (0.1 to 1 μg).
- Genes associated with the development of colon cancer are *ras* genes, adenomatous polyposis coli (*APC*) tumor suppressor gene (loss on the long arm of chromosome 5), and *TP53* tumor suppressor gene (17P). The development of colorectal cancers requires the sequential acquisition of a series of mutations.
- Familial breast cancer is associated with *BRCA1* (chromosome 17), which is a nuclear phosphoprotein responsible for some aspect of cell cycle control. Carriers of a second breast susceptibility gene *BRCA2* (chromosome

13q) have a lifetime risk for development of breast cancer of 80% to 90% and a risk for development of ovarian cancer.

- Overexpression of *ERB-B2 (Her-2/neu)*, amplification of c-*myc*, and inactivation of *TP53* play a role in the development or progression of ovarian cancer. Six percent of 145 families with multiple cases of ovarian and breast cancer demonstrate the presence of *BRCA1* gene. *BRCA2* confers a lifetime ovarian cancer risk of 10% to 20%.
- HPV infection alone is insufficient to bring about cervical carcinoma. *TP53* may function as an "emergency brake" in cells that have sustained DNA damage. Oncogenic HPV-16 expression may disrupt the *TP53*-mediated cellular response to DNA damage. When HPV-16 E_6 is transfected into cells exhibiting normal DNA damage response, TP53 protein levels are undetectable and cell cycle arrest after DNA damage is abolished. Genomic instability is achieved, leading to further genetic alterations and tumorigenesis.
- HPV infection (HPV-16–18) may play a role in the occurrence of molecular alterations that lead to tumor development and progression of vulvar cancer.
- It is estimated that 6% of endometrial cancers have a heritable component. Between 5% and 50% of endometrial cancers express the p53 protein, which may be associated with a poorer prognosis. Oncogenes associated with endometrial cancers included the K-*ras* gene and *Her-2/neu* gene.

Questions

Directions for Questions 1–6: Select the one best answer.

1. The following are true for the development of cancer, *except:*
   A. cancer is the result of a single mutation
   B. cancer is due to the accumulation of somatic mutations that result from the process of normal living.
   C. three broad classes of genes are involved in the development of cancer: oncogenes, tumor suppressor genes, and mismatch repair genes.
   D. tumor suppressor genes are expressed in a recessive manner.
2. The *TP53* suppressor gene is contained in the region of which chromosome?
   A. 13
   B. 15
   C. 16
   D. 17
3. The following are true of apoptosis *except:*
   A. it means programmed cell death
   B. it is controlled at the molecular level by genes associated with malignant changes
   C. it occurs spontaneously in malignant tumors
   D. histologically, it is associated with inflammation
4. The following are true of telomerase activity *except*:
   A. normal cells have plenty of telomerase activity
   B. telomerase adds back telomere sequences lost during replication
   C. telomerase becomes reactivated in most cancer cells
   D. it is the most prevalent cancer maker known
5. The polymerase chain reaction allows the exponential amplification of the targeted gene. Which is the typical number of cycles of denaturation often used?
   A. 10
   B. 20
   C. 30
   D. 40
6. Carriers of *BRCA2* gene have a lifetime ovarian cancer risk of:
   A. 5%–10%
   B. 10%–15%
   C. 10%–20%
   D. 10%–25%

Directions for Questions 7–10: For each numbered item, select the letter of the most appropriate answer.

7–10. Match the gene type with its characteristics
   A. Oncogene
   B. Tumor suppressor gene

7. Two mutational events in cancer
8. Germline mutation
9. Activates cell proliferation
10. Suppresses malignant phenotype

Answers

1. **A** page 564
   Cancer requires several different mutations in many different genes to allow this irreversible, uncontrolled growth. One does not inherit cancer as one would inherit cystic fibrosis or sickle cell disease. Progression from a normal to a malignant cell is the result of a series of mutations.
2. **D** page 568
   The *TP53* tumor suppressor gene–containing region of chromosome 17p is deleted or mutated in a wide variety of human cancers.
3. **D** page 572
   Apoptosis is a distinct mode of cell death in normal tissues. It occurs also spontaneously in malignant tumors, markedly retarding their growth. It is increased in tumors responding to radiation, chemotherapy, heat, and hormone damage. Apoptotic bodies are formed during apoptosis; there is no associated inflammatory response.
4. **A** page 575
   Normal cells lack telomerase activity. Telomerase may be used as a generic cancer marker and as a possible treatment.
5. **C** page 578
   After one cycle of denaturation, annealing, and primer extension, the DNA content is doubled. Amplification increases exponentially with each cycle so that the final amount of amplified DNA is 2^n, in which n equals the number of cycles. After 30 cycles, which is the typical number of cycles used, the gene of interest may be amplified over 2^{30} times, to well above 1 million times.

6. **C** page 582
   Characterization of *BRCA2* gene is currently under way.
7. **B**
8. **B**
9. **A**
10. **B** Table 20–6, page 572

chapter 21 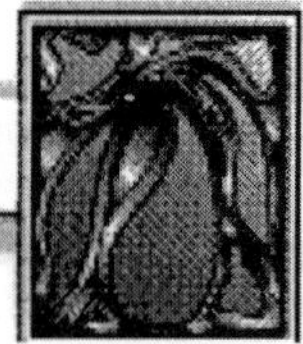

PALLIATIVE CARE and QUALITY of LIFE

KEY POINTS TO REMEMBER

- *Palliative care* is defined as interdisciplinary care that seeks to prevent, relieve, or reduce the symptoms of a disease or disorder without effecting a cure.
- The gynecologic oncologist is in a unique position to function collectively as a primary care provider, surgeon, radiation oncologist, and chemotherapist, allowing comprehensive transfer of treatment with an emphasis on the patient's quality of life.
- Palliative care is collaboratively provided by an interdisciplinary team prompted by issues and concerns of the patient and family.
- Fatigue is the most prevalent (60% to 90%) and one of the least understood symptoms that affect cancer patients. It is characterized by diminished energy, mental capacity, and psychological condition. Efforts should be made to correct potential etiologies (sleep disorders, depression, anemia). Several drug classes such as psychostimulants (methylphenidate, pemoline) and low-dose corticosteroids (dexamethasone, prednisone) may yield favorable results.
- Cancer pain can be managed effectively in up to 90% of patients. Drug therapy is the cornerstone of cancer pain management. For mild to moderate pain, nonsteroidal anti-inflammatory drugs are often effective. Moderate to severe pain requires opioids of higher potency and dose. Dosing should be on a regular schedule to maintain a certain level of drugs that helps prevent the recurrence of pain. Oral administration is preferred. Adjuvant drugs are valuable: corticosteroids, anticonvulsants, and antidepressants.
- Nausea and vomiting are controlled with 5-HT3 serotonin antagonists (ondansetron), phenothiazines, and dexamethasone.
- Diarrhea and constipation are managed with anticholinergic drugs (Lomotil) or laxatives.
- Breaking bad news is a difficult and emotionally laden task for the physician. It is critical to project reasonable hope and confidence. Most patients (70%) express their resolve to continue fighting against their disease.
- Psychosocial and spiritual care requires the assistance of social workers and chaplains.
- In advanced and recurrent ovarian cancer, small bowel obstruction can be dealt with by intestinal bypass, ileostomy, or gastrostomy; ascites can be relieved with therapeutic paracentesis.
- In advanced and recurrent uterine and cervical cancer, bilateral ureteral obstruction can be considered for urinary diversion, followed by appropriate radiation therapy; diversion of the urinary or the fecal stream (colostomy) is an option in dealing with urinary and intestinal fistulae. The use of regular vaginal dilation, hormone replacement therapy, and lubricants can improve vaginal length and elasticity.
- Physicians should respect the patient's decision for her own medical care and her right to formulate an advance directive.
- In futility cases, a process-based approach has been proposed that includes four distinguishable steps aimed at deliberation and resolution, two steps aimed at securing alternatives in case of irresolvable differences, and a final step aimed at closure when all alternatives have been exhausted (AMA).
- Patients entering hospice care have a life expectancy of 6 months or less, a focus on comfort measures, and a preference for care at home.

QUESTIONS

Directions for Questions 1–6: Select the one best answer.

1. Some barriers to optimal end-of-life care identified by ASCO include the following *except*:
   A. reluctance to discuss death and dying by health care professionals and patients
   B. unrealistic expectations and treatment options by patients
   C. universal access to care
   D. lack of systematic education for physicians about clinical and psychosocial aspects of care
2. Fatigue in cancer patients may be due to:
   A. underlying disease
   B. treatment for the disease (chemotherapy, radiotherapy, surgery, etc.)
   C. intercurrent systemic disorders (anemia, infection, pulmonary disorders, etc.)
   D. all of the above
3. Epoetin alfa, the recombinant form of erythropoietin, is used to treat anemia in cancer patients and reduce the need for transfusion. Which is the level of increased hematocrit that shows improvement in energy levels and daily activities?

A. >2%
B. >4%
C. >6%
D. >10%

4. When fatigue is nonresponsive to symptomatic therapies, the physician should empirically try:
   A. antidepressants
   B. vitamins
   C. herbs
   D. no other therapy
5. For the reversal of opioid-induced respiratory depression, the physician should use judiciously:
   A. ketorolac (Toradol)
   B. naproxen
   C. naloxone
   D. ibuprofen
6. A study on end-of-life preferences of gynecologic cancer patients reported what percentage of patients will continue fighting against their disease when the prognosis is poor?
   A. 40%
   B. 50%
   C. 60%
   D. 70%

Directions for Questions 7–10: For each numbered item, select the letter of the most appropriate answer. Each letter may be used once, more than once, or not at all.

Match the symptoms with the use of the drugs.

A. fatigue
B. pain
C. nausea and vomiting
D. dyspareunia

7. Hormone replacement therapy
8. Methylphenidate
9. Ondansetron (Zofran)
10. MS Contin

Answers

1. **C** page 590
   One of the important barriers to optimal end-of-life care is economic, including lack of universal access to care and underfunding of end-of-life care.
2. **D** page 592
   Fatigue in cancer patients has multiple etiologies. In addition to the physiologic factors already mentioned, there are also psychological factors (anxiety, depression), financial concerns, and spiritual distress. Efforts should be directed to correct potential etiologies.
3. **C** page 592
   Many controlled studies have shown that epoetin alpha increases hematocrit. Of patients with an increase in hematocrit, more than 6% demonstrated significant improvement in energy level and daily activities and in overall quality of life.
4. **A** page 593
   The physician should empirically try antidepressants such as selective serotonin reuptake inhibitors, secondary amine tricyclics (nortriptyline and desipramine) or bupropion, which are sometimes associated with increased energy.
5. **C** page 596
   Administration of naloxone is indicated for the reversal of opioid-induced respiratory depression. It should be used with titration in small increments to improve respiratory function without reversing analgesia. Ketorolac (Toradol), ibuprofen, and naproxen are NSAIDs used for pain control.
6. **D** page 603
   Seventy percent of gynecologic cancer patients expressed their resolve to continue fighting against their disease, even under the poorest prognostic circumstances.
7. **D** page 607
   Dyspareunia resulting from gynecologic cancer therapy can lead to loss of desire and can cause women to avoid sex. Regular vaginal dilation with appropriate use of hormone replacement therapy and lubricants may improve coital function.
8. **A** page 592
   Methylphenidate, pemoline, and dextroamphetamine are psychostimulants. Their empiric administration may yield favorable results in some patients.
9. **C** page 601
   Ondansetron (Zofran) is a 5-HT3 antagonist that blocks serotonin receptors of the chemoreceptor trigger zone to prevent vomiting.
10. **B** page 599
    MS Contin is controlled-release morphine.

appendix 1

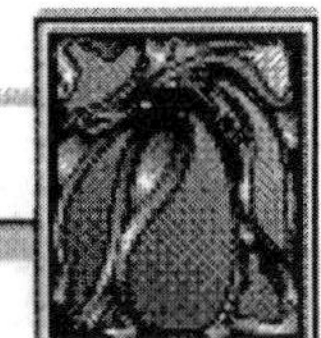

APPENDICES

The following Questions and Answers pertain to Appendices C (Blood Component Therapy), D (Commonly Used Statistical Terms), E (Suggested Recommendations for Routine Cancer Screening), F (Nutritional Therapy), and G (Radiotherapy).*

QUESTIONS

APPENDIX C

Directions for Questions 1–7: Select the one best answer.

1. Concerning packed red blood cells (RBCs), the following are true *except:*
   A. they are prepared from whole blood by centrifugation and subsequent removal of plasma
   B. they contain the white blood cells from the original whole blood unit
   C. the risk of hepatitis after the transfusion of one unit of packed erythrocytes is the same as for whole blood
   D. they are contraindicated for use in anemic patients with heart failure
2. How much of an increase in the platelet count usually occurs after a transfusion of one unit of platelet concentrate?
   A. 5000/mm^3
   B. 10,000/mm^3
   C. 20,000/mm^3
   D. 30,000/mm^3
3. Choose the *incorrect* statement concerning cryoprecipitate:
   A. it contains fibrinogen, factor VIII, factor XIII, and von Willebrand factor
   B. the shelf-life after thawing is 4 hours
   C. viral hepatitis transmission and allergic and febrile reactions can occur
   D. compatibility testing is necessary
4. True statements concerning the origin and use of albumin are the following *except:*
   A. albumin is obtained from heat-treated pooled plasma
   B. 5% albumin is used for rapid expansion of vascular volume
   C. 25% albumin is used for treatment of hypoalbuminemia
   D. albumin transfusion can increase hepatitis transmission risk
5. Each unit of packed RBCs (180–200 mL) should increase the hematocrit in a 70-kg adult by:
   A. 2%–3%
   B. 3%–4%
   C. 4%–5%
   D. 5%–6%
6. The following are true concerning transfusion of concentrates *except:*
   A. a patient should have a platelet count of 100,000/mm^3 before going to surgery
   B. repeated platelet transfusion can lead to immunization to HLA antigen
   C. one unit of platelet concentrate will increase the platelet count by 7,000–10,000/mm^3
   D. thrombocytopenia to 50,000/mm^3 produces serious bleeding
7. Concerning autologous blood, the following are true *except:*
   A. donor should maintain a hemoglobin level of 10 g/dL
   B. the blood should be taken at least 2 weeks before surgery
   C. if a large amount of blood is required, frozen cells are an option
   D. intraoperative blood salvage requires sterile collection and reinfusion of shed blood that is free of infecting agents

APPENDIX D

Directions for Questions 1–4: Select the one best answer.

1. The null hypothesis states:
   A. that there is an association between two variables and it is not due to chance
   B. that there is no association between two variables
   C. that the likelihood of any association occurring by chance is less than .05
   D. that the likelihood of any association occurring by chance is greater than .95
2. The erroneous rejection of the null hypothesis is:
   A. a type I (alpha) error
   B. a type II (beta) error

*__Note__: Appendices A and B are not included in this chapter for these reasons:
a. Appendix A concerns staging of female genital cancer. The questions are included in various chapters of the book.
b. Appendix B concerns GOG toxicity criteria and is used for reference only.

C. a measure of sensitivity
D. a measure of specificity

3. The predictive value of a negative test:
A. is a proportion of those with a condition to those who test positive for the condition (i.e., the sum of the true positive and the false positives)
B. is a proportion of those with a condition to those who have false test results (i.e., the sum of the false positives and false negatives)
C. is a proportion of those free of a condition to those who test negative for the condition (i.e., the sum of the true negatives and the false negatives)
D. is a proportion of those free of a condition to the total tested

4. The best evidence on which medical decisions are made in evidence-based medicine is:
A. a nonrandomized, controlled trial
B. case-control studies
C. opinions of respected authorities or extensive clinical experience
D. a well-designed randomized, prospective, controlled trial

Directions for Questions 5–12: For each numbered item, select the letter of the most appropriate answer. Each letter may be used once, more than once, or not at all.

5–8. Match the definition of:
A. mean
B. median
C. one-tailed test
D. two-tailed test

5. Middle value when they are arranged in the order of the smallest to the largest
6. Average of a sample of observations
7. A test to determine a difference in only one direction
8. A test to determine any difference between the variable

9–12. Match the definition of:
A. incidence
B. prevalence

9. Measures the proportion of a population affected by disease at a given point in time
10. Measures the probability of having the disease at a specific time
11. Measures the probability of developing a disease
12. Measures the new cases of a specific disease that develop over a defined period

APPENDIX E

Directions for Questions 1–3: For each numbered item, select the letter of the most appropriate answer. Each letter may be used once, more than once, or not at all.

1. Choose the *incorrect* statement concerning screening guidelines for cervical cancer:
A. an annual Pap test and pelvic examination for all women who have been sexually active
B. an annual Pap test and pelvic examination for all women who have reached the age of 18
C. after three normal annual examinations and findings, a Pap test may be performed less frequently at the discretion of the physician
D. after one normal annual examination and finding, a Pap test should be performed every 3 years

2. A baseline mammogram should be obtained between the ages of:
A. 25 and 30
B. 30 and 35
C. 35 and 40
D. 40 and 45

3. The following are American College of Obstetricians and Gynecologists recommendations for cancer screening:
A. for endometrial cancer, high-risk patients may require endometrial sampling
B. for ovarian cancer and lung cancer, there is no available technique for routine screening
C. for colorectal cancer, women aged 40 to 49 should undergo a digital rectal examination and fecal occult test every year and sigmoidoscopy every 5 years or colonoscopy every 10 years
D. all of the above

APPENDIX F

Directions for Questions 1–3: Select the one best answer.

1. Candidates for nutritional assessment should have the following requirements *except:*
A. 5% decrease in body weight 2 months before assessment
B. serum albumin 3.4 g/dL
C. anergy to four or five standard skin text antigens
D. low total lymphocyte count (1200)

2. Which is the most important test for determining protein calorie undernutrition?
A. serum globulin
B. serum albumin
C. serum transferrin
D. serum folate

3. The following are true for total parenteral nutrition (TPN) *except:*
A. it can increase body weight
B. it can reverse the serum marker of malnutrition
C. it can correct nutritional deficits
D. it can eliminate toxicity due to cancer therapy

APPENDIX G

Directions for Questions 1–32: Select the one best answer.

1. The correct order, in terms of least to most radiosensitive areas of an individual cell, is:
A. enzymes, membranes, chromosomes
B. membranes, enzymes, chromosomes
C. membranes, chromosomes, enzymes
D. enzymes, chromosomes, membranes

2. True statements relative to biologic effects of radiation include all *except:*
   A. neoplastic cells are more sensitive to radiation than normal cells
   B. radioresistant tumors are potentially curable with irradiation
   C. cell nuclei are the major sites of radiation damage leading to cell destruction
   D. radiosensitivity and radiocurability are equivalent concepts
3. Choose the *false* statement regarding genetic effects of radiation:
   A. the dose that doubles the human mutation rate is estimated to be 10 to 100 cGy
   B. radiation exposure is known to increase the mutation rate in humans
   C. detectable mutations were not increased in survivors of the Hiroshima and Nagasaki nuclear explosions
   D. U.S. government recommendations state that no individual younger than 30 years should be exposed to 10 cGy of manmade irradiation to the gonads
4. True statements relative to fetal effects of radiation include all *except:*
   A. the peak incidence of gross malformations occurs during the early organogenesis period (10 to 40 days of gestation)
   B. acute in utero exposure to 25 cGy results in no detectable effect
   C. all embryos will be affected in some way by a 100-cGy dose
   D. when exposure occurs after 30 weeks of gestation, fetal structural abnormalities usually result
5. Characteristics of supervoltage, when compared with orthovoltage radiation, include all *except:*
   A. reduced absorption in bone
   B. higher proportional skin doses
   C. better vascular tolerance
   D. increased "forward scattering"
6. Choose the isotope commonly used in gynecologic brachytherapy with the *longest* half-life:
   A. ^{137}Cs
   B. ^{192}Ir
   C. ^{198}Au
   D. ^{226}Ra
7. Choose the isotope commonly used in gynecologic brachytherapy with the *shortest* half-life:
   A. ^{137}Cs
   B. ^{192}Ir
   C. ^{198}Au
   D. ^{226}Ra
8. Relative disadvantages of the clinical use of radium for brachytherapy when compared with cesium include all *except:*
   A. long half-life of radium
   B. production of radon gas
   C. radium is enclosed in tubes and needles
   D. as a powder, it is difficult to incorporate into solid materials (e.g., ceramics)
9. The dose of radiotherapy at point R from source X is 900 units. Choose the correct dose at point T.
   A. 30 units
   B. 100 units
   C. 300 units
   D. 450 units

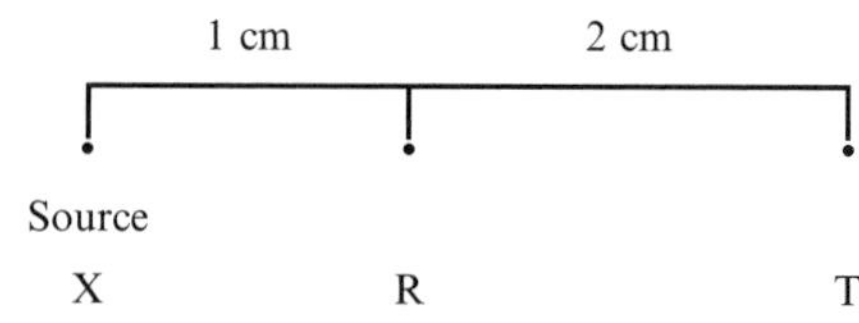

10. The dose delivered to point *A* (2 cm lateral to the point source) by the tandem is 2500 cGy. What is the dose delivered to point *B* (pelvic sidewall lymph nodes)?
    A. 100 cGy
    B. 400 cGy
    C. 1000 cGy
    D. 1111 cGy

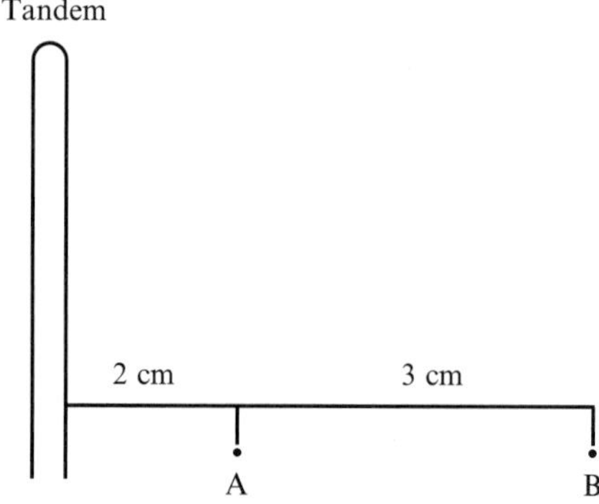

11. Choose the *false* statement relative to cellular radiosensitivity:
    A. cellular radiosensitivity is directly dependent on tissue oxygen tension
    B. cellular radiosensitivity is directly dependent on cell cycle
    C. cellular radiosensitivity is directly dependent on tumor size
    D. cellular radiosensitivity is dependent on ability to repair damaged DNA
12. The following statements regarding tolerance of tissues to radiotherapy are true *except:*
    A. increased tolerance occurs with increased volumes of irradiated tissue
    B. increased tolerance occurs with lower dose rates
    C. increased tolerance occurs with increased fractionation
    D. increased tolerance occurs with lower total dose
13. Choose the *false* statement regarding tissue tolerance of radiation:
    A. the cervix and corpus can withstand radiotherapy doses better than any other tissue
    B. the bladder tolerates more radiotherapy than the rectum
    C. the large intestine is the least radiosensitive pelvic tissue

D. the sum of external beam dose in centigray plus milligram-hours of radium (or equivalent) should not exceed 10,000

14. Choose the *false* statement relative to irradiation-associated tissue damage:
   A. 90% of radiation damage to normal tissue is reversible
   B. essentially all radiated normal tissue is damaged
   C. pelvic radiation usually spares the small intestine because of normal peristaltic motion
   D. radiated tissues should generally *not* undergo a second course of radiation
15. New radiation modalities are generally geared toward increasing irradiation damage to the hypoxic cell. Choose the *false* statement in regard to a specific modality and its activity:
   A. hyperbaric oxygen delivery increases radiotherapy efficacy in clinical studies
   B. hyperthermia is a significant radiosensitizer
   C. metronidazole and related compounds increase the efficacy of radiotherapy
   D. neutrons and pions are more effective against hypoxic cells
16. Choose the *false* statement in regard to absorbed irradiation dose:
   A. 100 cGy = 1 Gy
   B. 1 Gy = 1 J/kg
   C. 1 cGy = 100 rad
   D. 1 rad = 100 erg/g
17. Radiosensitivity of a tumor depends on:
   A. degree of hypoxia of its cells
   B. proportion of clonogenic and radiosensitive cells in the radiation therapy fields
   C. proportion of tumor cell lines having potential lethal damage incapable of repair
   D. all of the above
18. The radiation sensitizer that has been found to increase survival in advanced cervical cancer is:
   A. hydroxyurea
   B. misonidazole
   C. 5-FU
   D. cisplatin

Directions for Questions 19–32: For each numbered item, select the letter of the most appropriate answer. Each letter may be used once, more than once, or not at all.

19–22. Match the description/treatment with the most appropriate voltage.
   A. low voltage
   B. orthovoltage
   C. supervoltage
   D. megavoltage

19. Linear accelerator, used for most external beam gynecologic radiotherapy
20. ^{137}Cs
21. ^{226}Ra
22. Transvaginal radiotherapy, as for cervical stump carcinoma

23–27. Match the following definitions with the appropriate letter.
   A. x-rays
   B. gamma rays
   C. photons
   D. electrons
   E. all of the above

23. Originate from decay of atomic nucleus
24. Used to stimulate electromagnetic radiation emission
25. Emitted from a target bombarded by high-energy particles
26. Charged particles
27. Interact with tissue to ionize molecules and/or form free radicals

28–32. Match the average radiation dose to fetus and maternal gonads from various diagnostic examinations:
   A. 8 mcGy
   B. 185 mcGy/film
   C. 585 mcGy
   D. 330 mcGy
   E. 465 mcGy

28. Chest roentgenography
29. Abdominal roentgenography
30. Intravenous or retrograde pyelography
31. Upper gastrointestinal roentgenography
32. Lower gastrointestinal roentgenography

Answers

APPENDIX C

1. **D** page 625
   Since packed erythrocytes, or packed red blood cells (PRBCs), have the same red blood cell mass as whole blood, they provide the same oxygen-carrying capacity but in a smaller volume. If not diluted before administration, the decrease in volume reduces the possibility of circulatory overload and cardiovascular failure. The removal of plasma also reduces the amount of citrate, sodium, potassium, and ammonia, rendering PRBCs superior to whole blood transfusion to patients with cardiac, renal, or hepatic disease.
2. **B** page 625
   One unit of platelet concentrate increases the platelet count by 7000 to 10,000/mm^3, if the patient does not have any condition causing platelet destruction. The shelf life of platelet concentrates is 72 hours at room temperature.
3. **D** page 626
   Compatibility testing is not necessary when one uses cryoprecipitate. Approximately 10 units of cryoprecipitate are needed to increase the patient's serum fibrinogen by 100 mg/dL.
4. **D** page 626
   There is no risk of hepatitis transmission since the albumin is filtered and pasteurized by heating for 10 hours at 60°C.
5. **B** page 626
   Adequate oxygenation can be maintained with a hemoglobin content of 70 g/L in the normovolemic patient without cardiac disease. Each unit of packed RBCs increases Hb 10 g/L and Hct 3%. In most patients requiring transfusion, levels of Hb of 100 g/L are sufficient to keep oxygen supply from being critically low.
6. **D** page 625

Thrombocytopenia does not usually produce serious bleeding, unless the platelet count is less than 20,000, except when there is a platelet function defect, a coagulation defect, or a local cause of hemorrhage (e.g., trauma, surgery).

7. **A** page 626
   The patient must maintain a hemoglobin level of at least 11 g/dL.

APPENDIX D

1. **B** page 631
   The null hypothesis states there is no relationship between two variables. Testing for statistical significance allows one to accept or reject the null hypothesis but does not prove the null hypothesis. *P* value is the main tool used to test the null hypothesis. The point of significance is traditionally 5% ($P = .05$). If P is less than .05, the null hypothesis is rejected (i.e., there is a relationship between the two variables).
2. **A** page 631
   The erroneous rejection of the null hypothesis is the same as stating that there is an association between two variables, even though this association may have occurred by chance alone. *P* levels are set to state the level of confidence that no type I error occurred. If the *P* level is .05, there is a 5% chance that a type I error may have occurred, even though significance was demonstrated.
   The erroneous acceptance of the null hypothesis is the same as stating that there is no association, even though there may, in fact, be a true relationship. The ability to detect a type II error is called *statistical power*. The most common cause of a type II error is too small a sample size.
   Sensitivity denotes the number of those with a condition who are correctly identified by a test. *Specificity* denotes the number without the disease who are correctly identified as being disease free.
3. **C** page 631
   Where:
   a = number of individuals with disease who test positive (true positive)
   b = number of individuals disease free who test positive (false positive)
   c = number of individuals with disease who test negative (false negative)
   d = number of individuals disease free who test negative (true negative)

$$\text{sensitivity} = \frac{a}{a + c}$$

Sensitivity notes the number of patients with the disease who are correctly identified by the test.

$$\text{Specificity} = \frac{d}{b + d}$$

Specificity measures the number of patients without disease who are correctly identified disease free by the test.

$$\text{Positive predictive value} = \frac{a}{a + b}$$

The *predictive value of a positive test result* refers to the proportion of patients with a positive test result who are diseased.

$$\text{Negative predictive value} = \frac{d}{c + d}$$

The *predictive value of a negative test result* refers to the proportion of patients with a negative test result who are disease free.

4. **D** page 631
   The best evidence is a properly designed, randomized, controlled trial. Medical decisions should be based on quality evidence.
5. **B** page 631
6. **A** page 631
7. **C** page 631
8. **D** page 631
9. **B** page 632
10. **B** page 632
11. **A** page 631
12. **A** page 631

APPENDIX E

1. **D** page 633
   In view of the appreciable false-negative rate of the Pap test, the American College of Obstetricians and Gynecologists propose that guidelines of annual cervical cytology are warranted for most women.
2. **D** page 633
   A baseline mammogram should be obtained at the age of 40. Thereafter, mammography is suggested every 1 to 2 years for women aged 40 to 50 years and annually for women older than 50 years of age.
3. **D** page 634
   The cost-effectiveness of screening asymptomatic women for endometrial cancer and its precursors is very low and therefore is unwarranted. However, abnormal bleeding in perimenopausal or postmenopausal women should be investigated without delay. Concerning ovarian cancer, peritoneal fluid profiles, tumor-associated antigens, and ultrasonography are being investigated as a possible screening tool, but to date none has proved practical or effective. Because colorectal cancer is a significant risk to women and because available data do not substantiate the cost-effectiveness of various screening recommendations, the ACOG task force has suggested that the recommendations of the American Cancer Society and the National Cancer Institute be used as a guide. Concerning lung cancer, the only effective way

to reduce mortality is to promote a "stop smoking" message to the public.

APPENDIX F

1. **A** page 636
   Dundrick suggests that patients who have a 10-lb weight loss or a 10% decrease in body weight 2 months before assessment should undergo a nutritional assessment.
2. **B** page 635
   Serum albumin is the single most important test for determining protein calorie undernutrition. Albumin is the main plasma protein necessary to maintain plasma osmotic pressure, as well as other functions. Serum transferrin is also a good indicator of protein nutritional status.
3. **D** page 636
   Results of TPN as an adjuvant to cancer therapy are not encouraging. TPN has not decreased the complications of cancer therapy, nor has it increased the survival rate.

APPENDIX G

1. **A** page 642
   Enzymes are the least radiosensitive of the listed cellular structures, requiring up to 1 million cGy to be significantly affected. Membranes are more sensitive, requiring 1000 cGy or more. Only a few hundred centigrays are necessary to produce lethal chromosomal aberrations.
2. **D** page 642
   Localized radioresistant tumors may be cured when treated with high-dose radiotherapy, whereas a metastatic radiosensitive tumor may not be curable with local irradiation.
3. **B** page 645
   Direct evidence of radiation-induced mutations in humans is lacking, even in descendants of those exposed to radiation in the Hiroshima or Nagasaki atomic explosions. Estimates of human mutational rates are extrapolated from studies conducted in mice.
4. **D** page 647
   Studies of pregnant survivors of Hiroshima and Nagasaki reveal that at more than 30 weeks' gestation, there is little chance of structural damage, but functional/learning disabilities may result. Exposure at 2 to 3 weeks leads to an all-or-nothing phenomenon—abortion or a normal embryo; at 4 to 11 weeks—severe abnormalities of many organs in most children; at 11 to 16 weeks—few structural abnormalities, but stunted growth or mental disorders; at 16 to 30 weeks—mild growth or mental retardation.
5. **B** page 647
   As voltage used to accelerate particles increases, a higher proportion of its energy is absorbed more deeply, thus sparing skin and superficial structures (Fig. G–7). Bone absorption of radiation approaches water or tissue doses at supervoltage energies, whereas with megavoltage, a significantly higher proportion of energy is absorbed by bone. There is less damage to vasculoconnective tissue. Forward scattering (as opposed to lateral particle scatter) in tissue increases as voltage increases.
6. **D** page 649
   Radium has the longest half-life of 1620 years. Cesium is next with a half-life of 30 years, then iridium with 74 days (Table G–5).
7. **C** page 649
   Gold has the shortest half-life of 2.7 days (Table G–5).
8. **A** page 648
   The longer half-life of radium, when compared with that of cesium, is a clinical advantage. Measurement or calibration of emitted dose does not need to occur as often as with cesium.
9. **B** page 648
   The inverse square law states that energy from a source is proportional to the inverse square of the distance from the source. Therefore, the dose at point T is:

$$900 \times \frac{(1)^2}{(1+2)^2} = 100 \text{ units}$$

10. **B** page 648
    Again, using the inverse square law, the dose at point B is:

$$2500 \times \frac{(2)^2}{(2+3)^2} = 400 \text{ cGy}$$

    The inverse square law is exploited to deliver high doses of irradiation to areas near the isotopes but to spare surrounding tissues (Figs. G–7 and G–8).
11. **C** page 645
    Cellular radiosensitivity is most dependent on DNA repair mechanisms, tissue oxygenation, and position in the cell cycle. Tumor size does not *directly* affect cellular radiosensitivity, although increasing tumor size increases cellular hypoxia and *indirectly* affects radiosensitivity. Hypoxic cells are three times more resistant to radiation than "oxic" cells. Mitotic cells (M and G_2 phases) are more radiosensitive than late S phase or G_0 cells (Fig. G–6).
12. **A** page 650
    The volume of tissue irradiated is an integral factor in tolerance; tolerance is inversely proportional to the volume of tissue affected. The authors use as an example a 1-cm circular field of skin, which easily tolerates a single 1000 cGy fraction weekly for 5 weeks. The patient would not tolerate identical dosing and fractionation if given via standard whole pelvic fields.
13. **C** page 650
    Of all pelvic tissues, the sigmoid and rectum are thought to be the *most* sensitive to radiation.

14. **A** page 651
Injury occurs to all radiated tissue to some extent. Radiobiologists estimate that only 5% to 20% of this damage is repaired, however.
15. **A** page 653
Clinical studies with hyperbaric oxygen and pelvic tumors show mixed results. A British Medical Research Council study shows significant impact in stage III cervical cancer and advanced head and neck cancer. Further studies of pelvic tumors by other investigators fail to validate these original observations.
All of the other modalities are considered to be hypoxic cell sensitizers. Each continues to be investigated. Another promising area of research is the use of other radiopotentiators (substances *not* thought to work by increasing oxygen sensitivity, or with an unknown mechanism) such as cytotoxic chemotherapy drugs and cytokines, concurrent with radiotherapy.
16. **C** page 641
1 Gy = 100 cGy = 100 rad = 1 J/kg. 1 cGy = 100 erg/g
17. **D** page 642
Radiosensitivity, which is defined as the response of the tumor to irradiation, depends on the enumerated factors. Hypoxic cells are less responsive to radiation. Proliferating cells are very sensitive to it. Cellular repair of sublethal irradiation damage varies from one tumor to another.
18. **A** page 653
The addition of hydroxyurea to radiation has been shown to improve local control and increased survival in comparison to radiation alone, or radiation and misonidazole.
19. **D** page 640
Most external radiotherapy units in use in North America today are megavoltage units (>8 mV). In general, the higher the energy used to accelerate photons, the more deeply the majority of the energy is absorbed, thus reducing superficial tissue complications compared with those occurring from giving the same tumor dose with a supervoltage (500 kV–8 mV) machine (Table G–2, Fig. G–7).
20. **C** page 640
^{137}Cs and ^{226}Ra are supervoltage (500 kV–8 mV) emitters of photons and gamma rays.
21. **C** page 640
See Answer 20.
22. **B** page 640
Transvaginal radiotherapy is designed for low penetration, with maximum deposition of its energy and maximum effect in the superficial-most tissues. Orthovoltage or medium-voltage (180–400 kV) machines are commonly used for this purpose, as are some low-voltage (85–150 kV) machines. (**A** is a correct response, also.)
23. **B** page 640
Gamma rays are electromagnetic radiation that originates from the decay of an "excited" atomic nucleus.
24. **D** page 640
Electrons, high-energy charged particles, are used to bombard a target. As they approach the fields around a nucleus of the target substance, they are deflected from their path and emit particulate energy in the form of x-rays. X-rays can also be generated by the electron colliding with, and "exciting," the orbital target electron to an outer higher-energy orbit. As the target electron then falls back to its inner, original orbit, it emits electromagnetic energy in the form of x-rays.
25. **A** page 640
X-rays are particulate forms of electromagnetic radiation that result from electron bombardment of a target such as tungsten. The energy of the x-ray is determined by the energy with which the electrons are accelerated. Gamma rays and x-rays are collectively called *photons*; therefore, **C** is a correct response, also.
26. **D** page 640
Electrons are negatively charged particles. X-rays and gamma rays are composed of uncharged photons.
27. **E** page 640
Photons interact directly with target tissues by ionizing molecules within the tissue or indirectly by free radical formation. Electrons may also ionize molecules in tissue but to a much more superficial depth.
28. **A** page 646, Table G–4
29. **B** page 646, Table G–4
30. **C** page 646, Table G–4
31. **D** page 646, Table G–4
32. **E** page 646, Table G–4